HANDBOOK OF
HIV MEDICINE

THIRD EDITION

Disclaimer
While every effort has been made to check drug dosages in this handbook, it is still possible that errors have been overlooked. Dosages continue to be revised and new side-effects recognised. Oxford University Press makes no representation, express or implied, that the drug dosages in this book are correct. For these reasons the reader is strongly urged to consult the *South African Medicines Formulary* or the drug manufacturer's printed instructions before administering any of the drugs recommended in this clinical handbook. The authors and the publishers do not accept responsibility or legal liability for any errors in the text or for the misuse or misapplication of material in this work.

Dosages
Unless otherwise stated, drug dosages are for oral administration and recommendations are for the non-pregnant adult who is not breastfeeding.

HIV Type 1 and Type 2
Unless otherwise stated, throughout the text HIV refers to HIV-1.

HANDBOOK OF
HIV MEDICINE

THIRD EDITION

Editors
Gary Maartens
Mark Cotton
Douglas Wilson
Francois Venter
Linda-Gail Bekker
Tammy Meyers

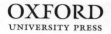

OXFORD

UNIVERSITY PRESS
Southern Africa

Oxford University Press Southern Africa (Pty) Ltd

Vasco Boulevard, Goodwood, Cape Town, Republic of South Africa
P O Box 12119, N1 City, 7463, Cape Town, Republic of South Africa

Oxford University Press Southern Africa (Pty) Ltd is a wholly-owned subsidiary of
Oxford University Press, Great Clarendon Street, Oxford OX2 6DP.

The Press, a department of the University of Oxford, furthers the University's objective of
excellence in research, scholarship, and education by publishing worldwide in

Oxford New York

Auckland Dar es Salaam Hong Kong Karachi
Kuala Lumpur Madrid Melbourne Mexico City Nairobi
New Delhi Shanghai Taipei Toronto

With offices in

Argentina Austria Brazil Chile Czech Republic France Greece
Guatemala Hungary Italy Japan Poland Portugal Singapore South Korea
Switzerland Turkey Ukraine Vietnam

Oxford is a registered trade mark of Oxford University Press
in the UK and in certain other countries

Published in South Africa
by Oxford University Press Southern Africa (Pty) Ltd, Cape Town

Handbook of HIV Medicine third edition
ISBN 978 0 19 905366 7

© Oxford University Press Southern Africa (Pty) Ltd 2012

The moral rights of the author have been asserted
Database right Oxford University Press Southern Africa (Pty) Ltd (maker)

First edition published 2002

Second edition published 2008

Third edition published 2012

Publishing manager: Alida Terblanche
Publisher: Marisa Montemarano
Project manager: Sarah Floor
Editor: Dr Bridget Farham
Designer: Judith Cross
Illustrator: Bronwen Lusted
Indexer: Michel Cozien

Set in 8.5 pt on 10.5 pt Utopia Std by Raimund Theiner, Aurora 7325
Printed and bound by ABC Press, Cape Town
118572

Contents

Contributors   viii
Preface   xv
Acknowledgements   xvi
Abbreviations   xvii

Part 1   General introduction to HIV medicine   1
1   Epidemiology   3
2   Virology   16
3   The immune system and HIV infection   23
4   Interactions between HIV and tuberculosis   36
5   Laboratory investigations   41
6   HIV transmission and natural history   53
7   Counselling   69
8   Sex and sexuality   79
9   Preventing HIV infection: individuals and populations   84

Part 2   Approach to HIV infection in children   93
10   Clinical assessment (paediatric)   95
11   Childhood vaccination   109
12   HIV and infant feeding   121
13   Expressed breastfeeding in hospital   130
14   Nutrition   145
15   Diarrhoea   152
16   Paediatric tuberculosis   160
17   Sexual abuse   174
18   Setting up an HIV/AIDS clinic for children   178

Part 3   Approach to HIV infection in adults   187
19   Clinical assessment   189
20   Common emergencies   198
21   Evaluation of fever   213
22   Primary prophylaxis and immunization   219
23   Diet and nutrition   224
24   Adult tuberculosis   232

25 Sexually transmitted infections   262
26 Gynaecology   273
27 Contraception   280
28 Sexual assault   285

Part 4   Systemic approach to HIV infection   291
29 Cardiology   293
30 Haematology   303
31 Nephrology   311
32 Pulmonology   322
33 Intensive care management   342
34 Endocrinology and metabolic
    abnormalities   346
35 Neurology   354
36 Psychiatry   381
37 Ophthalmology   389
38 Gastroenterology and hepatology   400
39 Oral medicine   413
40 Dermatology   426
41 Oncology   443
42 Rheumatology   448

Part 5   Antiretroviral drug management   457
43 Antiretroviral drug classes   459
44 Adult antiretroviral therapy   465
45 Paediatric antiretroviral therapy   474
46 Prevention of mother-to-child
    transmission of HIV   498
47 Antiretroviral drug resistance   508
48 Adherence to antiretroviral therapy   512
49 Drug-drug interactions   520
50 Immune reconstitution inflammatory
    syndrome   526
51 Principles of managing adverse drug
    reactions   531
52 Occupational post-exposure prophylaxis 543

Part 6   **Patient-centred care**   **551**

53   Primary care approach   553

54   Integrating HIV and TB services   569

55   Palliative care   576

56   Women's health   596

57   Gay sex and sexuality   602

58   Ethical issues   608

59   Health care worker burnout   624

60   Micronutrient and complementary therapies   629

Contributors

Contributors to the 1st Edition

Dr Aziz Aboo, Department of Medicine, Groote Schuur Hospital and University of Cape Town

Dr Steve Andrews, Brooklyn Medical Centre, Cape Town

Dr Pieter Barnardt, Department Radiation Oncology, Tygerberg Hospital and University of Stellenbosch

Prof Solomon Benatar, Department of Medicine, Groote Schuur Hospital and University of Cape Town

Dr Linda-Gail Bekker, Infectious Diseases Clinical Research Unit, UCT Lung Institute

Prof Raziya Bobat, Department of Paediatrics and Child Health, Nelson R Mandela School of Medicine, University of Natal

Prof Patrick JD Bouic, Immunology Section, Department of Medical Microbiology, University of Stellenbosch

Dr Abdul Cariem, GIT Clinic, Groote Schuur Hospital

Dr Nicole Cockburn, Department of Ophthalmology, Groote Schuur Hospital

Dr Karen Cohen, Division of Pharmacology, University of Cape Town

Dr Myles Connor, Division of Neurology, Department of Neurosciences, University of the Witwatersrand

Dr Ruth Cornick, UCT Lung Institute

Prof Mark Cotton, Paediatric Infectious Diseases Clinical and Research Unit, Faculty of Health Sciences, Tygerburg Children's Hospital and University of Stellenbosch

Prof Anna Coutsoudis, Department of Paediatrics and Child Health, Nelson R Mandela School of Medicine, University of Natal

Dr Carol Cragg, City Of Cape Town Health Services

Dr Sinead Delaney-Moretlwe, Department of Obstetrics and Gynaecology, Reproductive Health Research Unit, Chris Hani Baragwanath Hospital

Prof Lynette Denny, Department of Obstetrics and Gynaecology, Groote Schuur Hospital and University of Cape Town

Prof Brian Eley, School of Child and Adolescent Health, Red Cross War Memorial Children's Hospital, University of Cape Town

Prof Arderne Forder, Emeritus Professor, Department

of Medical Microbiology, University of Cape Town

Colleen Gibbon, Division of Pharmacology, University of Cape Town

Dr Clive M Gray, AIDS Research Unit, National Institute for Communicable Diseases, Johannesburg

Dr Elizabeth Gwyther, St Luke's Hospice

Dr Beth Harley, South Peninsula Administration, City of Cape Town

Dr Prudence Ive, Clinical HIV Research Unit, University of the Witwatersrand

Carroll Jacobs, Western Cape AIDS Training, Information and Counselling Centre Metropole Region, Provincial Administration of the Western Cape

Prof Prakash Jeena, Department of Paediatrics and Child Health, Nelson R Mandela School of Medicine, University of Natal

Dr Sue Jessop, Department of Dermatology, Groote Schuur Hospital and University of Cape Town

Dr Henry Jordan, Department of Dermatology, Tygerberg Hospital and University of Stellenbosch

Roy Kennedy, Department of Human Nutrition, Medunsa

Prof Gert Kirsten, Head of Neonatal Intensive Care Unit, Department of Paediatrics and Child Health, Tygerberg

Children's Hospital and University of Stellenbosch

Stephen Kramer, AIDS Research Unit, Metropolitan Group

Dr Johan H Lamprecht, Department of Pharmacology, University of Stellenbosch

Prof Gary Maartens, Division of Infectious Diseases, Groote Schuur Hospital and University of Cape Town

Prof Shabir Madhi, MRC/Wits/NHLS Respiratory and Meningeal Pathogen Research Unit, and Paediatric Infectious Diseases Research Unit, University of the Witwatersrand

Prof James McIntyre, Perinatal HIV Research Unit, University of the Witwatersrand

Prof Mervyn Mer, Department of Medicine, Division of Pulmonology, Johannesburg Hospital and University of the Witwatersrand

Prof Girish Modi, Division Of Neurology, Department of Neurosciences, University of the Witwatersrand

Dr Mala Modi, Division of Radiology, Department of Radiation Sciences, University of the Witwatersrand

Dr Andre Mochan, Division of Neurology, Department of Neurosciences, University of the Witwatersrand

Prof Lynn Morris, National Institute for Communicable Diseases and University of the Witwatersrand

Prof Sudeshni Naidoo, School for Oral Health Sciences, Faculty of Health Sciences, University of Stellenbosch

Dr Ettiene Nel, Faculty of Health Sciences, Tygerberg Children's Hospital and University of Stellenbosch

Dr Catherine Orrell, Diana Princess of Wales HIV/AIDS Clinical Research Unit, Somerset Hospital

Dr Robert Pawinski, HIV/AIDS Public Health Unit, Department of Medicine, Nelson R Mandela School of Medicine, University of Natal

Dr Frank Post, Infectious Diseases Research Unit, University of Cape Town

Dr Kevin Rebe, Department of Medicine, University of Cape Town

Prof Helen Rees, Department of Obstetrics and Gynaecology, Reproductive Health Research Unit, Chris Hani Baragwanath Hospital, University of the Witwatersrand

Dr Paul Roux, Department of Paediatrics, Groote Schuur Hospital and University of Cape Town

Dr Ian Sanne, Clinical HIV Research Unit, University of the Witwatersrand

Dr Jane Saunders, Department of Psychiatry, University of Cape Town

Dr Hendrik Simon Schaaf, Department of Paediatrics and Child Health, Tygerberg Children's Hospital and University of Stellenbosch

Dr Helgo Schomer, Department of Psychology, University of Cape Town

Claudia Schubel, Department Human Nutrition, Faculty of Health Sciences, University of Stellenbosch

Dr Piers Stead, Renal Unit, Groote Schuur Hospital and University of Cape Town

Dr Wendy Stevens, Molecular Diagnostic Unit, Department of Haematology and Molecular Medicine, University of the Witwatersrand

Dr Katrin Stuve, Victoria Hospital, GIT Clinic Groote Schuur Hospital, and HIV Clinic, Somerset Hospital

Dr François Venter, HIV Clinic, Johannesburg General Hospital and Clinical HIV Research Unit, University of the Witwatersrand

Marianne Visser, Nutrition and Dietetics Unit, Department of Medicine, University of Cape Town

Dr Andrew Whitelaw, Department of Medical Microbiology, University of Cape Town

Prof Carolyn Williamson, Division of Medical Virology, Institute of Infectious Diseases and Molecular Medicine, University of Cape Town

Dr Douglas Wilson, HIV Clinic, Somerset Hospital and

Dr Trevor Gernholtz, Dumisani Mzamane African Institute of Kidney Disease, Chris Hani Baragwanath Hospital

Dr Elizabeth Gwyther, St Luke's Hospice

Prof Hilard Goodman, Department of Radiology, University of Cape Town

Dr Anneke Hesseling, Desmond Tutu TB Centre, University of Stellenbosch

Dr Steve Innes, KID-CRU, Stellenbosch University

Dr Heather Jaspan, Fellow in Infectious Diseases, Seattle Children's Hospital

Prof Prakash Jeena, Department Paediatrics and Child Health, University of KwaZulu-Natal

Prof Gert Kirsten, Department of Paediatrics, Tygerberg Hospital, University of Stellenbosch

Tamara Kredo, Division of Clinical Pharmacology, University of Cape Town

Dr Barbara Laughton, Department of Paediatrics and Child Health, Tygerberg Children's Hospital, University of Stellenbosch

Dr Steven Lawn, Desmond Tutu HIV Foundation, Cape Town

Dr John Lawrenson, Cardiology Service, Red Cross Children's Hospital and Tygerberg Children's Hospital, Western Cape

Dr Angela Loyse, Centre for Infection, Department of Cellular and Molecular Medicine, St George's Hospital, University of London

Prof Gary Maartens, Division of Clinical Pharmacology, University of Cape Town

Dr Mignon McCulloch, Nephrology Service, Red Cross Children's Hospital, University of Cape Town

Prof Shabir Madhi, Department of Science and Technology/ National Research Foundation: Vaccine Preventable Diseases, University of Witwatersrand

Prof Ben Marais, Desmond Tutu TB Centre, University of Stellenbosch

Prof James McIntyre, Perinatal HIV Research Unit, University of the Witwatersrand

Dr Tammy Meyers, Harriet Shezi Clinic, Chris Hani Baragwanath Hospital, University of Witwatersrand

Dr Graeme Meintjes, Institute of Infectious Diseases & Molecular Medicine, University of Cape Town

Michelle Meiring, Chris Hani Baragwanath Hospital, University of Witwatersrand

Dr Fazile Mohammed, Department of Medicine, Grey's Hospital

Dr Anand Moodley, Department of Neurology, Grey's Hospital, University of KwaZulu-Natal

Fritse Muller, Lifeline Rape Crisis Centre, Pietermaritzburg

Dr Landon Myer, Department of Medicine, University of Cape

Infectious Diseases Research Unit, University of Cape Town

Prof Robin Wood, Department of Medicine, Somerset Hospital and Diana Princess of Wales HIV/AIDS Clinical Research Unit, University of Cape Town

Dr Jane Yeats, Diagnostic Virology Laboratory, University of Cape Town and National Health Laboratory Service

Dr Heather Zar, Department of Paediatric Pulmonology, School of Child and Adolescent Health, Red Cross Children's Hospital, University of Cape Town

Editors 1st Edition
Douglas Wilson
Sudeshni Naidoo
Linda-Gail Bekker
Mark Cotton
Gary Maartens

Contributors to the 2nd Edition
Dr Gonzalo Alvarez, Ottawa Health Research Institute of the University of Ottawa and Respirology Division, Ottawa Hospital

Dr Steve Andrews, Private Practitioner, Claremont and Honorary Senior Lecturer, Division of Infectious Disease, University of Cape Town

Dr Linda-Gail Bekker, Desmond Tutu HIV Foundation, Cape Town

Prof Marc Blockman, Division of Clinical Pharmacology, University of Cape Town

Prof Raziya Bobat, Department of Paediatrics and Child Health, University of KwaZulu-Natal

Dr Roy Breeds, Milnerton Mediclinic, Cape Town

Dr Jonathan Burns, Department of Psychiatry, University of KwaZulu-Natal

Dr Karen Cohen, Division of Clinical Pharmacology, University of Cape Town

Prof Anna Coutsoudis, Department of Paediatrics and Child Health, University of KwaZulu-Natal

Prof Mark Cotton, Department of Paediatrics and Child Health, University of Stellenbosch

Clair Craig, Department of Dietetics, Edendale Hospital

Prof Lynette Denny, Gynaecology Oncology Unit-Institute of Infectious Disease & Molecular Medicine, University of Cape Town

Dr Hlubi Dlwati, Antiretroviral Clinic, Edendale Hospital

Dr Krista Dong, Division of Infectious Diseases, Massachusetts General Hospital, Harvard University

Dr Robin Draper, Department of Medicine, Edendale Hospital

Prof Brian Eley, Infectious Diseases Service, Red Cross Children's Hospital, University of Cape Town

Prof Aderne Forder, Discipline of Medical Microbiology, Tygerberg Hospital

Town

Prof Sudeshni Naidoo, Faculty of Dentistry, University of the Western Cape

Dr Ettiene Nel, Department of Paediatrics and Child Health, Tygerberg Children's Hospital, University of Stellenbosch

Dr Peter Nourse, Division of Nephrology, Tygerburg Children's Hospital, University of Stellenbosch

Dr James Nuttall, Red Cross Children's Hospital, University of Cape Town

Dr Catherine Orrell, Desmond Tutu HIV Foundation, Cape Town

Paddy Paisley, The Coaching Centre & The Learning Centre, Cape Town

Dr Prinitha Pillay, Médecins Sans Frontières

Dr Helena Rabie, Clinical Infectious Diseases Service

Dr Kevin Rebe, Department of Medicine, GF Jooste Hospital, University of Cape Town

Prof Helen Rees, Reproductive Health and HIV Research Unit, University of the Witswatersrand

Dr Paul Roux, Paediatric HIV/AIDS Service, Groote Schuur Hospital, University of Cape Town

Dr Faieza Sahid, Division of Infectious Diseases, University of KwaZulu-Natal

Prof Simon Schaaf, Department of Paediatrics and Child Health, University of Stellenbosch

Dr Chris Sutton, Dept Paediatrics and Child Health, Pietersburg/Mankweng Hospital Complex, University of Limpopo

Dr Gilles Van Cutsem, Médecins Sans Frontières

Dr Ronald Van Toorn, Department of Paediatrics and Child Health, Tygerberg Children's Hospital, University of Stellenbosch

Dr Francois Venter, Reproductive Health and HIV Research Unit, University of the Witswatersrand

Dr Heinrich Weber, Private practice, Bellville, Cape Town

Prof Carolyn Williamson, Department of Medical Virology, University of Cape Town

Dr Douglas Wilson, Department of Medicine, Edendale Hospital, University of KwaZulu-Natal

Prof Robin Wood, Desmond Tutu HIV Foundation, Cape Town

Dr Colleen Wright, Anatomical Pathology, University of Stellenbosch

Prof Heather Zar, Chair of Paediatrics and Child Health, Head of Paediatric Pulmonology, Red Cross Children's Hospital, University of Cape Town

Dr Ekkehard Werner Arthur Zöllne, Tygerberg Children's Hospital, University of Stellenbosch

Editors for the 2nd Edition
Douglas Wilson
Mark Cotton
Linda-Gail Bekker
Tammy Meyers
Francois Venter
Gary Maartens

Assistant Editor
Angela Loyse

Contributors for the 3rd edition
Dr Linda-Gail Bekker, Desmond
  Tutu HIV Foundation, Cape
  Town
Dr Vivian Black, Wits
  Reproductive Health and
  HIV Institute, South African
  National AIDS Council
Prof Raziya Bobat, Department of
  Paediatrics and Child Health,
  University of KwaZulu-Natal
Prof Mark Cotton, Division of
  Paediatric Infectious Diseases,
  Department of Paediatrics
  and Child Health, Tygerberg
  Children's Hospital
Prof Anna Coutsoudis,
  Department of Paediatrics and
  Child Health, University of
  KwaZulu-Natal
Louise Goosen, Milk Matters,
  Mowbray Hospital
Cheryl Kirsten, Department of
  Paediatrics and Child Health,
  Tygerberg Children's Hospital,
  University of Stellenbosch
Prof Gert Kirsten, Department of
  Paediatrics and Child Health,
  Tygerberg Children's Hospital,

University of Stellenbosch
Dr Max Kroon, Mowbray
  Maternity Hospital, Neonatal
  Medicine, Department of
  Paediatrics, University of Cape
  Town
Prof Gary Maartens, Division
  of Clinical Pharmacology,
  University of Cape Town
Dr Elke Maritz, South to
  South Treatment and Care
  Programme, Stellenbosch
  University
Prof Graeme Meintjies, Institute
  of Infectious Diseases and
  Molecular Medicine, University
  of Cape Town
Dr Tammy Meyers, Harriet Shezi
  Clinic, Chris Hani Baragwanath
  Hospital, University of the
  Witwatersrand
Dr Helena Rabie, Clinical
  Infectious Diseases Service,
  Department of Paediatrics and
  Child Health, Stellenbosch
  University
Dr François Venter, Reproductive
  Health and HIV Research Unit,
  University of the Witwatersrand
Dr Douglas Wilson, Department
  of Medicine, Edendale Hospital,
  University of KwaZulu-Natal

Editors for the 3rd edition
Gary Maartens
Mark Cotton
Douglas Wilson
François Venter
Tammy Meyers
Linda-Gail Bekker

Preface

Since the publication of the 1st Edition of the *Handbook of HIV Medicine* in 2002 the practice of HIV medicine has been transformed by the increasing availability of antiretroviral therapy in southern Africa. Clinicians have had to learn new skills including how to set up robust systems to cope with large numbers of patients on antiretroviral therapy and working with international donor agencies, and how to recognize and manage mitochondrial toxicity and the immune reconstitution syndrome. Ethical issues have become more complex, including equitable access to antiretroviral therapy and management of non-adherence. Multidrug resistant tuberculosis has become a clinical reality in HIV care.

The updated 3rd edition features a revised section on the approach to HIV infection in children, including breastfeeding and paediatric tuberculosis. Content on managing antiretroviral toxicity has also been considerably expanded. HIV drug management principles have been thoroughly updated to keep abreast of the latest advancements in HIV medicine.

Acknowledgements

Prof Sudeshni Naidoo obtained funding from BMS Secure the Future to coordinate the 1st edition of the Handbook, on which this edition is based. The editors are grateful to the expert contributors who willingly gave their time and expertise. Dr Bridget Farham edited and proof-read the final version of the text. Marisa Montemarano from Oxford University Press Southern Africa consistently supported this edition to publication. Proceeds from the sale of the Handbook are donated to the HIV Clinicians Society.

Abbreviations

3TC	lamivudine
ABC	abacavir
ACEI	angiotensin-converting enzyme inhibitor
ACTG	AIDS Clinical Trial Group
ADA	adenosine deaminase
ADEM	acute disseminated encephalomyelitis
ADH	anti-diuretic hormone
ADR	adverse drug reaction
AFB	acid-fast bacilli
AGN	acute glomerulonephritis
AIDP	acute inflammatory demyelinating polyneuropathy
AIDS	acquired immune deficiency syndrome
AIN	acute interstitial nephritis
ALP	alkaline phosphatase
ALT	alanine aminotransferase
ANCA	anti-neutrophil cytoplasmic antibody
APC	antigen-presenting cell
ARDS	adult respiratory distress syndrome
ARF	acute renal failure
ARN	acute retinal necrosis
ART	antiretroviral therapy
ASOT	antistreptolysin titre
AST	aspartate amino transferase
ATN	acute tubular necrosis
ATNR	asymmetrical tonic neck reflex
AZT	zidovudine
BAL	bronchoalveolar lavage
BCG	bacille Calmette-Guérin
BMI	body mass index

BOOP	bronchiolitis obliterans organizing pneumonia
BRVO	branch retinal vein occlusion
BSA	body surface area
CAM	complementary and/or alternative medicines
CAP	community-acquired pneumonia
CBO	community-based organization
CDC	Centers for Disease Control and Prevention
CI	confidence interval
CK	creatine kinase
CKD	chronic kidney disease
CMO	cardiomyopathy
CMV	cytomegalovirus
CMVR	cytomegalovirus retinitis
CNS	central nervous system
CPAP	continuous positive airways pressure
CRF	circulating recombinant forms
CRP	C-reactive protein
CSF	cerebrospinal fluid
CT	computerized tomography
CTL	cytotoxic T-lymphocyte
CXR	chest radiograph
d4T	stavudine
ddC	zalcitabine
ddI	didanosine
DIC	disseminated intravascular coagulation
DILS	diffuse infiltrative lymphocytosis syndrome
DOTS	directly observed treatment short-course
DTwP	Diptheria-Tetanus-Pertussis
DWI	diffusion-weighted imaging
EBV	Epstein-Barr virus
ECG	electrocardiogram
EEG	electroencephalogram
EF	eosinophilic folliculitis

EFV	efavirenz
EIA	enzyme immunoassay
ELISA	enzyme-linked immunosorbent assay
EMB	ethambutol
EMG	electromyography
EPI	expanded programme of immunization
EPSE	extra-pyramidal side effects
ERCP	endoscopic retrograde cholangiopancreatography
ESR	erythrocyte sedimentation rate
FACS	fluorescent-activated cell sorter
FBC	full blood count
FDA	Food and Drug Administration
FDC	follicular dendritic cell
FMS	fibromyalgia syndrome
FSGS	focal segmental glomerular sclerosis
FTA	fluorescent treponema antibody
FTC	emtricitabine
FUO	fever of unknown origin
γ-GT	gamma-glutamyl transpeptidase
GFR	glomerular filtration rate
GIT	gastrointestinal tract
HAD	HIV-associated dementia
HBC	home-based care
HBeAg	hepatitis B e antigen
HBIG	hepatitis B-specific immunoglobulin
HBsAg	hepatitis B surface antigen
HBV	hepatitis B virus
HCV	hepatitis C virus
HCW	health care worker
HHV-8	human herpesvirus 8
Hib	*Haemophilus influenzae* type b
HIV	human immunodeficiency virus
HIVAN	HIV-associated nephropathy

HIVICK	HIV immune complex kidney disease
HLA	human leukocyte antigen
HPCSA	The Health Professions Council of South Africa
HPV	human papillomavirus
HSV	herpes simplex virus
HTLV	human T-cell leukaemia/lymphoma virus
HUS	haemolytic uraemic syndrome
HZO	herpes zoster ophthalmicus
HZV	herpes zoster virus
ICP	intracranial pressure
IDV	indinavir
Ig	immunoglobin
IL	interleukin
IFN	interferon
IFN-α	interferon-alpha
IFN-γ	interferon-gamma
IMCI	integrated management of childhood illnesses
INH	isoniazid
IDA	iron deficiency anaemia
IRIS	immune reconstitution inflammatory syndrome
IVIg	intravenous immunoglobulin
KCS	keratoconjunctivitis sicca
KS	Kaposi's sarcoma
LAM	lactational amenorrhoea
LBM	lean body mass
LDH	lactate dehydrogenase
LFT	liver function tests
LGE	linear gingival erythema
LIP	lymphocytic interstitial pneumonitis
LP	lumbar puncture
LPVr	lopinavir/ritonavir
LRTI	lower respiratory tract infections
LTS	long-term survivors

MAC	*Mycobacterium avium* complex
MC	molluscum contagiosum
MCV	mean cellular volume
MDR	multi drug-resistant
MHC	mean haemoglobin concentration
MHC-1 and MHC-2	major histocompatibility complex
MMSE	mini-mental state examination
MRI	magnetic resonance imaging
MRS	magnetic resonance spectroscopy
MRSA	methicillin resistant *S. aureus*
MSM	men who have sex with men
MTCT	mother-to-child transmission
NASBA	nucleic acid sequence based amplification
NFV	nelfinavir
NGO	non-governmental organization
NHL	non-Hodgkin's lymphoma
NNRTI	non-nucleoside reverse transcriptase inhibitor
NRTI	nucleoside reverse transcriptase inhibitor
NSAID	non-steroidal anti-inflammatory drug
NSI	non-syncitium inducing
NTP	national tuberculosis programme
NUG	necrotizing ulcerative gingivitis
NUP	necrotizing ulcerative periodontitis
NVP	nevirapine
OCD	obsessive compulsive disorder
OHL	oral hairy leukoplakia
OI	opportunistic infection
OPV	oral polio vaccine
ORS	oral rehydration solution
PaO$_2$	partial pressure of oxygen
PCP	*Pneumocystis jirovecii* pneumonia
PCR	polymerase chain reaction

PEM	protein energy malnutrition
PEP	post-exposure prophylaxis
PI	protease inhibitor
PID	pelvic inflammatory disease
PMLE	progressive multifocal leucoencephalopathy
PMTCT	prevention of mother-to-child transmission
PORN	progressive outer retinal necrosis
PPH	primary pulmonary hypertension
PPM	Pretoria pasteurization method
PsA	psoriatic arthritis
PTSD	post-traumatic stress disorder
PWA	person with AIDS
PY	patient years
PZA	pyrazinamide
RA	rheumatoid arthritis
RANTES	regulated-on-activation, normal T-cell-expressed and -excreted
RAPD	relative afferent pupil defect
RAU	recurrent aphthous ulcers
RBC	red blood cell
RCT	randomized clinical trial
RDA	recommended daily allowance
rEPO	recombinant erythropoietin
RMP	rifampicin
RPI	reticulocyte production index
RPR	rapid plasma reagin
RSV	respiratory syncytial virus
RT	reverse transcriptase
SAMA	South African Medical Association
SaO_2	oxygen saturation
SDF	stromal derived factor
SI	syncitium-inducing
SIADH	syndrome of inappropriate ADH secretion

SIV	simian immunodeficiency virus
SLE	systemic lupus erythematosus
SPECT	single positron emission computed tomography
SQV	saquinavir
SSRI	selective serotonin re-uptake inhibitors
STI	sexually transmitted infection
STS	short-term survivors
TB	tuberculosis
TBB	transbronchial biopsy
TBM	tuberculous meningitis
TDF	tenofovir
TEN	toxic epidermal necrolysis
TENS	transcutaneous electrical nerve stimulation
TLC	total lymphocyte count
TMP-SMX	trimethorprim-sulphamethoxazole
TNF	tumour necrosis factor
TNM	tumour-node-metastases
TPHA	*Treponema pallidum* haemagglutination
TST	tuberculin skin test
TTP	thrombotic thrombocytopenic purpura
US/S	ultrasound scan
UTI	urinary tract infection
VCT	voluntary counselling and testing
VDRL	Venereal Disease Research Laboratory
VL	viral load
VM	vacuolar myelopathy
VLBW	very low birth weight
VZIg	varicella-zoster immunoglobulin
VZV	varicella-zoster virus
WBC	white blood cell count
WHO	World Health Organization
WMA	World Medical Association
WR	Wasserman reaction

PART I

General introduction to HIV medicine

1 Epidemiology 3
2 Virology 16
3 The immune system and HIV infection 23
4 Interactions between HIV and tuberculosis 36
5 Laboratory investigations 41
6 HIV transmission and natural history 53
7 Counselling 69
8 Sex and sexuality 79
9 Preventing HIV infection: individuals and populations 84

Epidemiology

Understanding the epidemiology of HIV infection in South Africa – including the distribution of HIV in the country and the risk factors for HIV infection – is a critical first step in any attempt to address the epidemic. While an extensive array of numbers and statistics have been presented on the state of the epidemic, these all point towards a number of incontrovertible facts. First, the HIV epidemic is large, and touches on almost every aspect of South African society. Second, the epidemic is unevenly distributed in the population, with particular patterns of age, gender, socioeconomic status and geography that are important to understand to target prevention and treatment interventions. Third, the HIV epidemic is having a tremendous impact on morbidity and mortality in South Africa, and this will continue for the foreseeable future.

The HIV epidemic in South Africa

Sources of data

There are two general sources of information on the state of the HIV epidemic in South Africa. First, the results of epidemiological research studies provide empirical insights into the occurrence of HIV in certain populations. This includes studies of both HIV prevalence and HIV incidence (see Box 1 for definitions of prevalence and incidence). While these studies are invaluable, they can be costly and complex to conduct on a large scale (such as at a provincial or national level). Smaller studies, such as a study measuring HIV prevalence in a certain community, are more common, and provide useful snapshots of how the HIV epidemic operates at a local level. Second, mathematical models can be used to generate estimates of the distribution of HIV/AIDS in the population, including the incidence and prevalence of HIV as well as AIDS-related mortality. These kinds of models are particularly important in providing general predictions regarding the future course of the HIV epidemic, including how the future of the epidemic may vary with different prevention and treatment scenarios. Mathematical models are valuable for planning for health and other services. When viewed together, the results of empirical research and mathematical modelling present a clear picture of the dynamics of the HIV epidemic in South Africa, past, present and future.

Box 1: Definitions of prevalence and incidence

HIV prevalence $= \dfrac{\text{(the total number of HIV infections in a population)}}{\text{(the total number of individuals in that population)}}$

This is a measure of the proportion of individuals in a population who are HIV-infected.

HIV incidence $= \dfrac{\text{(the total number of } new \text{ HIV infections in a population)}}{\text{(the total number of individuals in that population)} \times \text{(the time period of observation)}}$

This is a measure of the rate of new HIV infections occurring in a population.

Trends in antenatal HIV seroprevalence

The best data on the occurrence of HIV in the South African population as a whole comes from annual surveys of HIV prevalence among pregnant women attending public sector antenatal care services at selected facilities across the country. These *sentinel surveys* (surveys conducted in a specific group for the purpose of surveillance) have been conducted since 1990, and provide a snapshot of how HIV has spread in the country, as well as the geographic distribution of HIV in the present. The greatest burden of HIV infection is seen in the eastern parts of South Africa, particulary KwaZulu-Natal, which has been the province with the highest prevalence of HIV among antenatal clinic attenders since the 1990s. Figure 1.1 shows the increase in national antenatal HIV seroprevalence from <1% in 1990 to 29.1% (95% confidence intervals, 28.3%–29.9%) in 2006. Table 1.1a shows the 2006 antenatal HIV seroprevalence by province, with the highest prevalences in KwaZulu-Natal and Mpumalanga, and the lowest prevalences observed in the Western Cape and Northern Cape. When the 2006 survey is analysed by age group (Table 1.1b), the highest HIV prevalence is among women ages 25–34 years.

Figure 1.1 Antenatal HIV seroprevalence in South Africa, 1990–2006

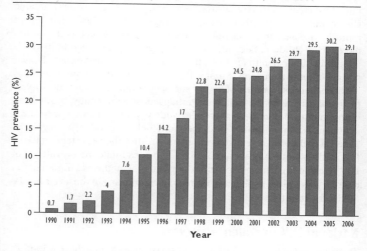

Table 1.1 HIV seroprevalence estimates, with 95% confidence intervals (CI), among women attending antenatal clinics in South Africa, 2006, according to (a) province and (b) age group. All values are percentages (%).

(a) Province	HIV prevalence (95% CI)	(b) Age group	HIV prevalence (95% CI)
KwaZulu-Natal	39.1 (37.5–40.7)	Less than 20 years	13.7 (12.8–14.6)
Mpumalanga	32.1 (29.8–34.4)	20–24 years	28.0 (26.9–29.1)
Free State	31.1 (29.2–33.1)	25–29 years	38.7 (37.3–40.2)
Gauteng	30.8 (29.6–32.1)	30–34 years	37.0 (35.5–38.5)
North West	29.0 (26.9–31.1)	35–39 years	29.3 (27.7–31.5)
Eastern Cape	28.6 (26.8–30.4)	40 years or older	21.3 (18.5–24.1)
Limpopo	20.6 (18.9–22.3)		
Northern Cape	15.6 (12.7–18.5)		
Western Cape	15.1 (11.6–18.7)		
Total	29.1 (28.3–29.9)	Total	29.1 (28.3–29.9)

SOURCE: Department of Health of South Africa. Report: National HIV and syphilis prevalence survey, South Africa, 2006. Pretoria: Department of Health, 2007.

While the antenatal HIV seroprevalence surveys provide valuable insights into the dynamics of HIV across the country, there are several notable shortcomings to this data. First, the survey only samples women of reproductive age, and does not include men or women too young or too old to have children. Second, by selecting participants from individuals attending public health facilities, these surveys focus on women of lower socioeconomic status, on average, than the South African population as a whole (because women of higher socioeconomic status are more likely to attend private health facilities). Perhaps most significantly, by focusing on pregnant women these surveys exclude women who are not sexually active, and women who use contraception (including condoms) regularly. Taken together, these considerations mean that the prevalence of HIV from annual antenatal surveys is likely to overestimate the prevalence of HIV in the South African population as a whole. Nonetheless, the antenatal care surveys are a valuable tool for regular monitoring of the levels of HIV across the country.

National HIV prevalence surveys

There have been few population-based surveys to examine the distribution of HIV infection among individuals of all ages, genders and backgrounds in South Africa. A national survey conducted in 2005 drew a representative sample of men and women two years of age and older; approximately 65% of those approached to participate agreed to be interviewed and provide specimens for HIV testing. This survey found the population HIV prevalence (across men and women of all ages) to be 10.8% (95% confidence intervals, 9.9%–11.8%). The breakdown of HIV prevalence according to age and sex is shown in Figure 1.2.

In keeping with the findings of the antenatal HIV prevalence surveys, the highest prevalence of HIV among women was observed in women 25-34 years of age. However the highest prevalence among men was observed among men 30-40 years of age. This pattern, with the highest prevalences of HIV seen at younger ages among women compared to men, is an important feature of the South African HIV epidemic. This finding strongly suggests that younger women are engaging in high-risk sexual partnerships with older men, and the increased risk conferred on younger women by having older male partners has been documented in several studies.

Figure 1.2. HIV prevalence in a national survey of women and men, aged 2 years and older, during 2005.

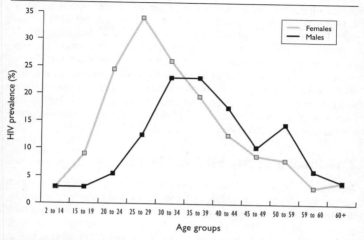

SOURCE: Shisana O, Rehle T, Simbayi LC, Parker W, Zuma K, Bhana A, Connolly C, Jooste S, Pillay V et al. South African National HIV prevalence, HIV incidence, behaviour and communication survey, 2005. Cape Town: HSRC Press, 2005.

Local studies of HIV prevalence and incidence

There have been hundreds of studies conducted over the past 15 years measuring the occurrence of HIV infection in specific populations within South Africa. Some of these studies have been based on individuals recruited at health facilities, such as those seeking treatment for sexually transmitted infections (STIs); others use population-based samples from particular communities. Such studies have shown the particularly high risk of HIV faced by women sex workers, demonstrated the high prevalence of HIV among hospital inpatients, and confirmed the unique age-gender distribution of HIV (discussed above) in specific communities.

In addition, these kinds of focused research studies are important because they allow us to quantify the incidence of HIV. Measuring HIV incidence requires *cohort studies* – following uninfected individuals through time to see how many become infected – which can be a complex and costly undertaking. Other methods based on the extrapolation of results from serological assays of prevalent infections remain controversial.

The long-term follow-up of one cohort of women sex workers in KwaZulu-Natal has demonstrated the sustained high incidence of HIV through time, with incidence rates of approximately 18 per 100 person-years (equivalent to 18 new infections observed among 100 women each followed for one year). Lower rates of new HIV infections have been observed in the general population, with HIV incidence rates in general population samples usually estimated between one and six new infections per 100 person years. The highest incidence of HIV is usually seen among sexually active adolescents and young adults, but substantial rates of new infection can be found in older age groups as well: one cohort study from Khayelitsha, Cape Town found an HIV incidence of two infections per 100 person-years among women ages 35–65 years.

The future of the HIV epidemic

The results of empirical studies provide important insights into the past and present distribution of HIV in South Africa, but provide little insight into the possible future of the epidemic. In addition, there are important statistics that are difficult to measure directly on a national scale, such as the numbers of individuals who have developed AIDS. Mathematical models have played a critical role in these areas by helping us to understand the likely course of the epidemic. The most prominent such model has been developed by the Actuarial Society of Southern Africa (ASSA), and is adjusted regularly to incorporate new empirical observations regarding the prevalence of HIV infection, the incidence of new infections, and the natural history of HIV/AIDS (with and without antiretroviral therapy). This model suggests that the numbers of new HIV infections in South Africa will continue to rise over the next decade, albeit at a diminishing rate, to a level of approximately six million infected individuals by 2015 (in a population of approximately 50 million, i.e, with approximately 12% of the population infected). The number of individuals developing AIDS (and thus the burden of HIV infection on the health care system, including the demand for antiretroviral therapy) will continue to increase steadily during the same time, with an estimated five million cumulative AIDS deaths occurring by 2015.

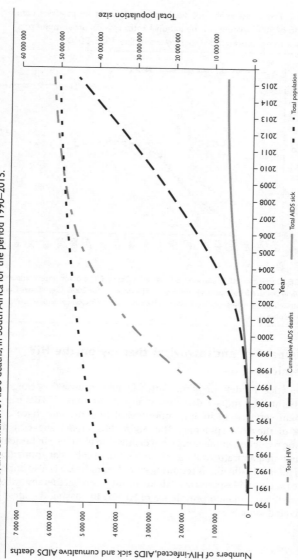

Figure 1.3. Estimates from the ASSA-2003 model of the projected population, number of HIV positive individuals, number of individuals with AIDS, and cumulative AIDS deaths, in South Africa for the period 1990–2015.

SOURCE: Dorrington RE, Johnson LF, Bradshaw D, Daniel T. The demographic impact of HIV/AIDS in South Africa. National and Provincial indicators for 2006. Cape Town: Centre for Actuarial Science Research, South African Medical Research Council and Actuarial Society of South Africa.

Figure 1.4. Projected number of deaths due to AIDS in South Africa, comparing a scenario of 90% coverage of the national antiretroviral programme to a scenario with no antiretroviral therapy availability, 1995–2010

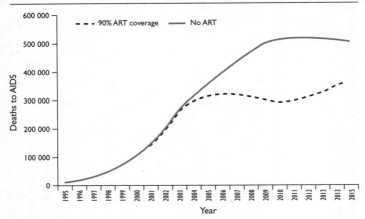

SOURCE: Dorrington RE, Johnson LF, Bradshaw D, Daniel T. The demographic impact of HIV/AIDS in South Africa. National and Provincial indicators for 2006. Cape Town: Centre for Actuarial Science Research, South African Medical Research Council and Actuarial Society of South Africa.

The impact of antiretroviral therapy on the HIV epidemic

Mathematical models are particularly valuable because they can provide insights into the impact that the large-scale delivery of HIV care and treatment services, including antiretroviral therapy, may have on the course of the HIV epidemic. The ASSA-2003 model suggests that a dramatic reduction in the number of deaths due to AIDS can be achieved if the national antiretroviral therapy programme can treat approximately 90% of infected individuals requiring care (Figure 1.4). It is also important to note that the widespread availability of antiretroviral therapy is likely to increase the population prevalence of HIV by increasing the lifespan of infected individuals.

Figure 1.5. A conceptual framework for thinking about the factors that influence the spread of the HIV epidemic in South Africa

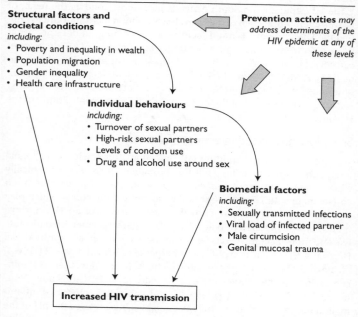

Structural factors and societal conditions
including:
- Poverty and inequality in wealth
- Population migration
- Gender inequality
- Health care infrastructure

Prevention activities *may address determinants of the HIV epidemic at any of these levels*

Individual behaviours
including:
- Turnover of sexual partners
- High-risk sexual partners
- Levels of condom use
- Drug and alcohol use around sex

Biomedical factors
including:
- Sexually transmitted infections
- Viral load of infected partner
- Male circumcision
- Genital mucosal trauma

Increased HIV transmission

Factors influencing the HIV epidemic in South Africa

Basic descriptive statistics regarding HIV prevalence and incidence (as discussed above) help us to understand the extent of the epidemic, but provide few insights into how HIV is spread, and in turn, why HIV is so common in South Africa. One general framework for thinking about the determinants of HIV in South Africa is presented in Figure 1.5. In this approach, the causes of the HIV epidemic can be understood as operating at several different levels of social and biological organization. The most immediate risk factors for HIV are biomedical conditions, such as the viral load of the infected partner, sexually transmitted infections or male circumcision. Another class of risk factors operates through individual behaviours, such as sexual partner selection, condom use, and alcohol consumption. Causes of HIV can also be thought of in terms of conditions regarding the structure of society, such as poverty, gender norms, and high levels of population migration.

The HIV epidemic in South Africa is best understood as the result of factors operating at each of these levels. In addition it is important to note that the HIV epidemic is multi-factorial in its aetiology: it does not result universally from a single cause, but from a combination of a wide range of causative factors. Although HIV is the necessary cause of AIDS, the extent of the HIV/AIDS epidemic in South Africa is best understood as the result of a range of biological, behavioural and societal factors. The following sections review several of the most important factors contributing to the HIV infection in South Africa.

Sexually transmitted infections (STI)

The probability of transmitting HIV infection in a single act of sexual intercourse is relatively low, but this probability increases dramatically when any of a number of co-factors is present. One of the most common co-factors in South Africa are sexually transmitted infections, which play a critical role in increasing both the infectiousness of an HIV-positive individual and the susceptibility of an HIV-negative partner. Both ulcerative and non-ulcerative STIs are extremely common in South Africa. Ulcerative STIs such as syphilis and herpes simplex virus type-2 (HSV-2) create direct portals for HIV to enter the body. In addition, there is significant evidence that HSV-2 increases shedding of HIV infection. Non-ulcerative STIs, including chlamydia and gonorrhoea, increase inflammation in the genital tract, while bacterial vaginosis raises the pH of the vagina, allowing the persistence of HIV. In addition, some STIs (including HSV-2) are more easily transmitted from an immune-suppressed individual, and all STIs share a major mode of transmission (sexual contact) with HIV. For these reasons, the STI and HIV epidemics can be thought of as in synergy, each fuelling the continued spread of the other.

Sexual behaviours

Since most new infections in South Africa take place through sexual contact, individual sexual behaviours play a critical role in the understanding of the epidemic. Average ages at first sexual intercourse (sexual debut) have been decreasing in South Africa, and in 2005 a national survey of sexual behaviours found that 84% of men and 91% of women were sexually active by the age of 24. Relevant aspects of sexual partnerships that are associated with increased spread of HIV at a population level include the numbers of sexual partners, the use of male or female condoms during sex, and drug and alcohol use.

Numbers of sexual partners

The more sexual partners an individual has, the greater the probability that they will have sex with someone who is HIV-infected. Among sexually active South Africans, 16.3% of men and 2.6% of women reported more than one sexual partner in the past 12 months during 2005. At a population level, the timing of sexual partnerships is a particularly important aspect of sexual networks: individuals with multiple partners at the same time (i.e. concurrent partnerships) may facilitate the spread of HIV through a population more than individuals with multiple partners spread over time (i.e. serial partnerships).

Condom use

Condoms can be highly effective in preventing the transmission of HIV during sex, but must be used consistently to afford protection. Levels of condom use vary widely across the country. A recent national survey of adolescents 15–24 years of age found that 57% and 48% of men and women, respectively reported condom use at their last sexual encounter. However, condom use among older adults is likely to be much lower; reported at 38%% and 32% among men and women, respectively. The practice of condom use is influenced by a wide range of factors, including accessibility, perceived risk of HIV, and partner attitudes. Condom use is also greatly reduced when either partner uses alcohol or other drugs.

An additional factor in the spread of HIV in South Africa is the role of coercion and violence in sexual relationships. While many studies assume that women and men freely choose who they have sex with, the high levels of rape in South Africa show that this often is not the case.

Structural determinants

In addition to the biomedical and behavioural risk factors, structural aspects of South African society have played an important role in facilitating the spread of HIV infection to its current levels. One example is the high levels of migration and population movement that take place across the country, usually between rural and urban areas. Recent research has suggested that migrancy contributes to the spread of HIV by separating stable partnerships and facilitating multiple sexual partners, with evidence that in partnerships where one member is a migrant both partners are more likely to have multiple sexual partners and be at increased risk of HIV infection. Similarly, individuals with mobile occupations, such as truck drivers, are likely to have a particularly high prevalence of infection.

Migrancy plays an important role in the geographic spread of HIV through the country; it is commonly found that the prevalence of HIV is greatest in urban centres and along transport routes.

Poverty is a more controversial structural determinant of the South African HIV epidemic. As elsewhere in the world, poverty plays an important role in increasing *vulnerability* to HIV/AIDS. Individuals of lower socioeconomic status are often at increased risk of becoming infected with HIV, for example through their increased exposure to high-risk situations (e.g. sexual partnerships where they are unable to negotiate condom use). Similarly, poverty may contribute to a worse prognosis for individuals who are already HIV-infected, for example by reducing access to appropriate health care services. In both cases, poverty is not the necessary cause of HIV or AIDS, but may be an important co-factor that contributes to placing individuals at increased risk of the infection and its sequelae.

Conclusion

Understanding the spread of HIV in South Africa and the current state of the epidemic is a critical first step in any attempt to mitigate the impact of the virus. The extent of the HIV epidemic is massive, making it the single most important public health issue in South Africa, and the factors influencing the spread of HIV are complex and multi-faceted. Insights into the distribution of HIV in the country and the factors that promote the spread of the virus play an important role in shaping interventions to prevent new infections as well as promoting the health of infected individuals.

References and further reading

Department of Health of South Africa. 2007 *Report: National HIV and syphilis prevalence survey, South Africa, 2006*. Pretoria: Department of Health.

Dorrington, R.E., Johnson, L.F., Bradshaw, D., Daniel, T. 2007. *The demographic impact of HIV/AIDS in South Africa. National and Provincial indicators for 2006*. Cape Town: Centre for Actuarial Science Research, South African Medical Research Council and Actuarial Society of South Africa.

Gouws, E. 'HIV incidence rates in South Africa. 2005' In: *HIV/AIDS in South Africa*. S.S. Abdool Karim and Q. Abdool Karim, eds. Cape Town: Cambridge University Press Southern Africa. Pages 67–78.

Hendriksen, E.S., Pettifor, A., Lee, S.J., Coates, T.J., Rees, H.V. 2007. 'Predictors of condom use among young adults in South Africa: the Reproductive Health and HIV Research Unit National Youth Survey.' *American Journal of Public Health*; 97(7):1241–8.

Jewkes, R., Levin, J., Mbananga, N., Bradshaw, D. 'Rape of girls in South Africa'. 2002. *Lancet*; 359(9303):319–20.

Johnson, L.F., Coetzee, D.J., Dorrington, R.E. 2005. 'Sentinel surveillance of sexually transmitted infections in South Africa: a review.' *Sexually Transmitted Infections*; 81(4):287–93.

Lurie, M.N., Williams, B.G., Zuma, K., Mkaya-Mwamburi, D., Garnett, G., Sturm, A.W. et al. 2003. 'The impact of migration on HIV-1 transmission in South Africa: a study of migrant and nonmigrant men and their partners.' *Sexually Transmitted Diseases*; 30(2):149–56.

Myer, L., Denny, L., de Souza, M., Wright, T.C. Jr, Kuhn, L. 2006. 'Distinguishing the temporal association between women's intravaginal practices and risk of human immunodeficiency virus infection: a prospective study of South African women.' *American Journal of Epidemiology*; 163(6):552–60.

Pettifor, A.E., Rees, H.V., Kleinschmidt, I., Steffenson, A.E., MacPhail, C., Hlongwa-Madikizela, L., Vermaak, K., Padian, N.S. 2005. 'Young people's sexual health in South Africa: HIV prevalence and sexual behaviors from a nationally representative household survey.' *AIDS*; 19(14):1525–34.

Ramjee, G. and E. Gouws. 2002. 'Prevalence of HIV among truck drivers visiting sex workers in KwaZulu-Natal, South Africa.' *Sexually Transmitted Diseases*; 29(1):44–9.

Shisana, O., Rehle, T., Simbayi, L.C., Parker, W., Zuma, K., Bhana, A., Connolly, C., Jooste, S., Pillay, V. et al. 2005. *South African National HIV prevalence, HIV incidence, behaviour and communication survey, 2005*. Cape Town: HSRC Press.

2 Virology

At the turn of the century, Africa contributed over 70% to the global burden of people living with human immunodeficiency virus (HIV) and acquired immune deficiency syndrome (AIDS). The success of this virus is based on the intrinsic molecular biological properties of the virus and the pathogenesis of infection.

Molecular biology of HIV

Classification

HIV belongs to the genus *Lentivirus* of the family *Retroviridae* and has been divided into two types:

- HIV Type 1 (HIV-1), responsible for the global pandemic; and
- HIV Type 2 (HIV-2), less pathogenic than HIV-1, and largely restricted to West Africa, with limited spread to other countries.

This chapter will focus only on HIV-1. HIV-1 is a highly variable virus and is further classified into three groups, based on sequence analysis of different regions of the genome:

- *Group M (major) viruses*: This group is further divided into subtypes or clades, referred to alphabetically. Subtypes are unevenly distributed around the world with subtypes A, C, D and G being most common in Africa and subtype B occurring in Europe and America. It is estimated that subtype C is responsible for over 90% of infections in southern Africa. Recombinant viruses, which are viruses with mosaic genomes made up of different subtypes, are becoming more common in regions where multiple subtypes are circulating. Numerous circulating recombinant forms (CRF) have been identified, e.g. CRF02_AG, which is a mixture of subtype A and G. This CRF is predominant in West Africa.
- *Group O (outlier) viruses*: These are largely restricted to the central African region.
- *Group N (non-M; non-O) viruses*: These are rare and have been identified in only a few individuals in Cameroon.

HIV-1 is a rapidly evolving virus, due to the error-prone nature of reverse transcriptase and the high viral turnover (see the section on viral dynamics in Chapter 6: HIV transmission and natural history). The ability of the virus to adapt rapidly and to diversify has serious implications:

- It enables rapid development of drug resistance.
- It enables the virus to escape detection by the immune system.
- It may affect vaccine efficiency.
- It may affect accurate diagnosis, especially pertaining to assays based on detection of the virus, such as viral load assays (see Chapter 5: Laboratory investigations).

Virus structure and function

General morphology

- The mature retrovirus particles are *spherical* with a diameter of 80–100 nm.
- Particles have an outer lipid bilayer that is host in origin.
- Embedded in the lipid bilayer is the surface glycoprotein (gp120) and transmembrane protein (TM, gp41).
- The viral core is conical in shape and made of p24 capsid protein (CA).
- Viral particles (virions) contain two identical pieces of viral RNA.
- Viral enzymes are packaged within virions including reverse transcriptase, protease, and integrase.
- The matrix protein (MA, p17) is located between the core and the outer lipid bilayer. (See Figure 2.1.)

Figure 2.1 Schematic diagram of an HIV virion (from R. Thomas, 2001)

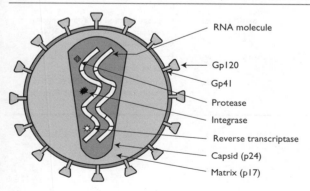

RNA molecule

Gp120

Gp41

Protease

Integrase

Reverse transcriptase

Capsid (p24)

Matrix (p17)

HIV genes, proteins, and their function

The HIV genes encode proteins, some of which are produced as polyprotein precursors and subsequently cleaved into functional proteins. Table 2.1 lists the functions of the different proteins.

Table 2.1 HIV-1 proteins and their function

Name		Size	Gene	Function
Structural proteins				
Gag	MA	p17	*gag*	Matrix protein, membrane anchoring, Env interaction, nuclear transport of viral core
	CA	p24	*gag*	Core capsid protein, protects genome
	NC	p7	*gag*	Nucleocapsid protein, binds RNA
		p6	*gag*	Binds Vpr
Env	SU	gp120	*env*	Surface glycoprotein, binds CD4 and co-receptors
	TM	gp41	*env*	Transmembrane protein, anchors the SU
Viral enzymes				
Protease		p15	*pol*	Cleavage of gag and gag-pol precursor, virus maturation
Reverse Transcriptase		p66; p51	*pol*	Reverse transcribes the viral RNA; also has RNAase H nuclease activity
Integrase		p31	*pol*	Integrates proviral DNA into cell genome
Regulatory and accessory proteins				
Tat		p14–16	*tat*	Activates HIV gene expression
Rev		p19	*rev*	Promotes expression of structural genes
Vif		p23	*vif*	Promotes virion maturation and infectivity
Vpr		p10-15	*vpr*	Proposed function to promote nuclear localization of preintegration complex, inhibits cell division
Vpu		p16	*vpu*	Promotes extracellular release of viral particles, degrades CD4
Nef		p27	*nef*	Downregulates CD4 and MHC Class I, increases viral Infectivity (See Chapter 3: immunology)

Cellular receptors and viral tropism

HIV enters cells via interaction between HIV envelope glycoproteins and cellular receptors and co-receptors (see Table 2.2). The receptors govern which cells HIV will infect. Receptors play an important role in HIV transmission and subsequent disease progression. (See Chapter 6: HIV transmission and natural history.)

- HIV-1 requires *two* receptors to enter cells, including CD4 and a second co-receptor belonging to the chemokine receptor family.
- The major co-receptors are CCR5 and CXCR4.
- These receptors are expressed on the surface of a subset of T-lymphocytes, monocytes, dendritic cells, and microglial cells in the brain.
- Viruses that use CCR5 receptor are referred to as R5 tropic, and are non-syncitium inducing (NSI) and macrophage tropic in tissue culture.
- Viruses that utilize the CXCR4 co-receptor are referred to as X4 tropic, and are syncitium inducing (SI) and T-cell tropic in tissue culture. Some viruses are dual tropic and are able to use both CCR5 and CXCR4 (R5X4 viruses).
- Some viruses can use other co-receptors in addition to CCR5 and CXCR4.

Naturally occurring chemokines block virus infection:
- The CC chemokines, which include RANTES (regulated-on-activation, normal T-cell-expressed and -secreted) (CC-chemokine ligand 5 or CCL5), MIP-1α (macrophage inflammatory protein) (CCL3), and MIP-1β (CCL4) are the ligands for CCR5 and inhibit viral entry of R5 isolates into cells.
- The CXC chemokine SDF-1 (stromal derived factor 1) (CXCL12) is the ligand for CXCR4 and blocks entry of X4 isolates into cells.

Table 2.2 Major HIV co-receptors used for viral entry

Co-receptors	Ligand	Expression Pattern	Comment
CCR5	CC chemokines: RANTES MIP-1α MIP-1β	Monocytes T-cells	Viruses that utilize CCR5 receptor are referred to as R5 and are NSI and macrophage tropic in tissue culture
CXCR4	CXC chemokine: SDF-1	Lymphocytes Macrophages Brain	Viruses that utilize the CXCR4 co-receptor are referred to as X4 tropic, and are SI and T-cell tropic in tissue culture

Virus life cycle

The virus life cycle can be divided into a number of steps (see Figure 2.2).

Binding, fusion, and virus entry

- HIV binds to cells via interaction between viral gp120 and the CD4 molecule.
- The gp120, which occurs as a trimer on the surface of the virus, undergoes conformational changes enabling interaction between gp120 and the co-receptor.
- The interaction between the virus and its receptors triggers the insertion of gp41 into the cell membrane and fusion of the virus with the cell.
- HIV fusion inhibitors are antiretroviral drugs that block HIV's ability to fuse and thus prevent infection of CD4 cells.
- The core is released into the cytoplasm, and the viral RNA released.
- Chemokine receptor blockers are drugs that inhibit viral binding (e.g. the CCR5 receptor antagonists).

Reverse transcription

- The viral RNA is reverse transcribed into double-stranded DNA.
- All these functions are fulfilled by the reverse transcriptase, which occurs as a dimer (p51; p66) with both reverse transcriptase and RNAase H nuclease activity.
- Reverse transcriptase has no proof-reading function and, on average, is one error is introduced per genome per replication cycle.
- The nucleoside reverse transcriptase inhibitors or NRTIs inhibit virus replication by directly blocking chain extension during reverse transcription using nucleoside analogues as chain terminators.
- The non-nucleoside reverse transcriptase inhibitors (NNRTIs) inhibit virus replication by binding directly to the reverse transcriptase and preventing reverse transcription.

Integration

- The pre-integration complex is transported to the nucleus.
- The viral enzyme, integrase, catalyses integration into the host chromosomal DNA.
- Integrated virus is referred to as provirus.
- Integrase inhibitors are drugs that block viral integration.

Figure 2.2 Life cycle of HIV (from R. Thomas, 2001)

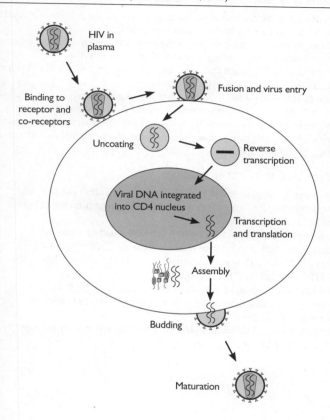

Transcription and translation

- Host enzymes transcribe proviral DNA using host cellular machinery.
- Viral RNA is either singly spliced or not spliced to make the structural proteins, or they are multiply spliced to generate RNAs to make the regulatory and accessory proteins.
- Full-length, unspliced RNA is shuttled to the membrane surface for inclusion into new virus particles.

Assembly, budding, and maturation

- Structural proteins, including the gag-pol precursor protein, aggregate at the cell surface for inclusion into new virions.
- Virus particles mature to form infectious viruses by cleavage of precursor gag-pol polyprotein by the viral protease enzyme.
- The virus buds through the membrane, taking the cellular lipid bilayer with it, to form mature virus particles.
- The gp160, embedded in the membrane of an infected cell, is cleaved by cellular enzymes to generate functional gp41 and gp120.
- Protease inhibitors inhibit formation of mature infectious virus particles by blocking protease activity and thereby preventing cleavage of the gag-pol polyprotein.

References and further reading

Hemelaar, J., Gouws, E., Ghys, P.D., Osmanov, S. 2006. 'Global and regional distribution of HIV-1 genetic subtypes and recombinants in 2004'. *AIDS*. 20(16):W13–23.

Johnston, M.I. and A.S. Fauci. 2007. 'An HIV vaccine-evolving concepts'. *New England Journal of Medicine*. 356(20):2073-81

Lusso, P. 2006. 'HIV and the chemokine system: 10 years later'. The EMBO Journal. 25(3):447–456.

Rambaut, A., Posada, D., Crandall, K.A., Holmes, E.C. 2004. 'The causes and consequences of HIV evolution'. *Nature Review of Genetics*. 5(1):52–61.

Thomas, R. 2001. Division of Medical Virology, University of Cape Town, unpublished.

The immune system and HIV infection

The immune system is a complex network of inter-related systems involving cells, cytokines and anatomical lymphoid structures that allow physical meeting points for dispersed T- and B-cells. These meeting points focus immune responses towards antigen and the removal of antigen. Once antigen has been removed, the immune response returns to a healthy state. If antigen cannot be removed, the immune system remains highly activated and in the process burns out. The degeneration of host immunity in response to HIV infection is a hallmark of AIDS. This chapter is split into three parts: part 1 explains some of the components of a normal functioning immune system; part 2 explains what happens to the immune system on HIV infection, introducing the notion that CD4-T cells in the gut associated lymphoid tissue are rapidly depleted and part 3 describes some of the treatment options that result in improved immunity. The important aspect of HIV infection is that it is a disease that 'eats' at the heart of the immune response and knowledge of how this occurs will provide an insight into a fuller clinical management of patients.

Part 1: The basics

What is the immune system?

The immune system protects the host from pathogenic insult after exposure and infection from bacteria, viruses, fungi, protozoa and allergens. Protection of the host occurs in a two-step process of innate immunity and then adaptive T-cell recognition of self versus non-self (invading organism), leading to the elimination of the organism and preservation of the internal body.

- Initial protection from invading organisms is the skin, and mucosal surfaces in the lung, genital and intestinal tract.
- The first line of defence are cells recruited as part of the innate immune response: natural killer cells and granulocytes, which release non-specific substances such as IL-2, IFN-γ and nitric oxide.
- The second line of defence is the adaptive (or acquired) immune response that involves T- and B-cells.
- There is a close link between innate and adaptive immunity via interaction with Toll-Like Receptors (TLR) and dendritic cells.

- B-cells produce antibodies. T-cells are divided into CD4 and CD8 cells and help to amplify the immune response (role of CD4) and/or destroy cells harbouring foreign organisms (role of CD8).
- B- and T-cells possess specific receptors that can bind antigens: B-cells express and release antibodies and T-cells express the T-cell receptor.

Antigens and receptors

Figure 3.1 Antigens and receptors

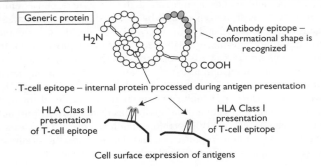

An antigen is a small part of a protein that makes up the invading organism that is recognized by a receptor expressed by T- and B-cells. T-and B-cells can successfully eliminate invading organisms because they can recognize or 'see' many antigens:
- B-cells recognize small parts of the tertiary (or conformational) structure of proteins. These are antigens that tend to be on the surface of protein structures.
- T-cells recognize small parts of digested proteins that are linear in nature. These antigens are always derived from deep inside protein structures.
- T-cells 'see' these inside antigens because the T-cell receptor only interacts with proteins that have been chopped up, or processed, by cellular enzymes.

Antigen processing and immune recognition

Antigens are presented to T-cells only after they have been processed by specialized antigen-presenting cells (APC). Antigen processing allows linear epitopes derived from the invading organism to be presented to the immune system.

- The initiation, or priming, of a new T-cell response involves presentation of epitopes by dendritic cells.
- Dendritic cells have the ability to move in an 'amoeba-like' fashion and 'patrol' the body for invading organisms.
- When a dendritic cell encounters an organism it will either engulf the organism and/or carry the organism to the secondary lymphoid organs.
- Dendritic cells ensure that invading organisms are digested and that epitopes are presented to the immune system within lymphoid tissue.
- Epitope presentation is determined by the genetic background of the host.

The role of human leukocyte antigen (HLA) and immune recognition

Epitopes are expressed on the surface of antigen-presenting cells by HLA molecules. The T-cell receptor recognizes the complex created by the epitope binding to the HLA molecule.

- All somatic cells express HLA class I molecules.
- HLA class II molecule expression is limited to antigen-presenting cells (macrophages, dendritic cells and B-cells for example).
- Naive resting T-cells do not express HLA class II molecules, but quickly upregulate class II expression once they have interacted with antigen.
- CD4 T-cells recognize epitopes presented by HLA class II.
- CD8 T-cells recognize epitopes presented by HLA class I.

Immune priming by antigens within lymphoid tissue

Initiation of T-cell and B-cell interactions with antigen occurs within secondary lymphoid tissue (lymph nodes). Antigen is carried by dendritic cells from non-lymphoid tissue to lymph nodes, where they provide the anatomical structures for T- and B-cell interaction with each other and with the antigen.

- T- and B-cells migrate through the lymph nodes via the lymphatic system and encounter antigen for the first time.

- B-cells interact with antigen that is presented by follicular dendritic cells within the germinal centres of the lymph nodes.
- T-cells interact with antigen that is presented by interdigitating dendritic cells within the paracortex of the lymph nodes.
- Both B- and T-cells rapidly undergo cell division after interacting with antigen and expand within the lymph nodes (clonal expansion) (Figure 3.2).
- The architecture of the lymph node provides an environment for close encounters between clonally expanded B- and T-cells.

Part 2: The immune system and HIV infection

Cell types infected by HIV

Through use of different receptors, primarily CD4 and chemokine receptors, HIV can infect many cell types distributed around the body both in lymphoid and non-lymphoid tissue.

HIV infects all cells expressing the CD4 receptor as well as chemokine receptors, most commonly CCR5 and CXCR4. The different cells that have been shown to be infected that express these receptors:

- CD4+ T-lymphocytes;
- monocytes/macrophages;

Figure 3.2 Clonal expression of CD4 T-cells

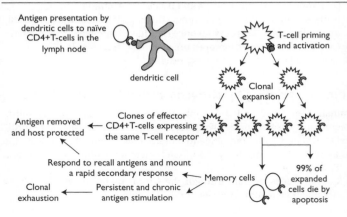

- microglial cells in the central nervous system;
- follicular dendritic cells.

Other cell types that have been reportedly infected by HIV, often under experimental conditions:
- Langerhans' cells of the skin;
- megakaryocytes;
- astrocytes and oligodendrocytes;
- endothelial cells;
- colorectal cells;
- cervical cells;
- retinal cells;
- renal epithelial cell;
- pulmonary macrophages.

Microglial cells are of monocyte/macrophage lineage and are CD4+. Infected blood monocytes may transport HIV infection to various tissues as cells migrate and differentiate into tissue macrophages.

General immune responses to HIV

A vigorous immune response occurs upon HIV infection involving cellular and humoral immunity but is unable to contain ongoing viral replication (see Figure 3.3).

The general immune response to HIV take place as follows:
- Antibodies to HIV usually appear within 2-12 weeks of primary infection and recognize Gag, Pol and Env viral proteins.
- Binding antibodies do not have a defined role in host defense.
- Potentially protective antibodies are neutralizing antibodies.
- CD8+ T-cells appear to play a major role in providing initial containment of virus replication.
- CD4+ T-cells appear to be important in providing initial help for CD8+ T-cell responses and for B-cells to produce binding and neutralizing antibodies.
- The viral set-point (see Chapter 6: HIV transmission and natural history) is thought to be determined by a balance between viral replication and a composite of host immunity.

Antibody responses during HIV-1 infection

Three types of antibodies develop during the host immune response to infection: binding antibodies, neutralizing antibodies and enhancing antibodies.

The main points to remember are:

- Binding antibodies to Gag have been useful for diagnosis, where anti-p24 antibodies can be used to determine seroconversion.
- Neutralizing antibodies are defined in vitro as antibodies that inhibit the infectivity of HIV by interacting with the viral envelope (Figure 3.3).
- Neutralizing antibodies emerge approximately eight to nine months after primary infection and are thought potentially to block viral entry and continued viral propagation within the host.
- Enhancing antibodies allow entry of virus into cells by an alternative receptor-mediated mechanism, such as Fc or complement receptors.
- It has also been proposed from experimental studies that these alternative receptors facilitate entry of virus into cells by shuttling bound virus to CD4/chemokine receptors for entry.

T-cell responses during HIV infection

Cellular activity is the earliest response that occurs as a result of HIV infection, most notably cytotoxic T-lymphocyte (CTL) activity.

Figure 3.3 Immune responses during primary HIV-1 infection

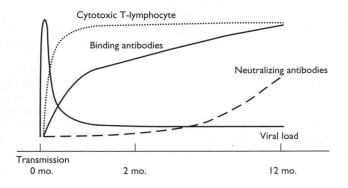

Cytotoxic T-lymphocyte

Binding antibodies

Neutralizing antibodies

Viral load

Transmission
0 mo.

2 mo.

12 mo.

- The first detectable cellular responses to be identified are CTL that target epitopes derived from any one of the nine gene regions of HIV-1 (Figure 3.3).
- These responses occur within hours of viral transmission and infection and prior to antibody formation (seroconversion) (Figure 3.3).
- The decline in plasma RNA copies/mL after primary infection is thought to be due to a concerted effect of a vigorous CTL response and sequestration of HIV to lymph nodes.
- CD4+ T-cell responses occur in parallel with class I HLA restricted CTL responses and there is some evidence that CTL activity depends on functionally competent CD4+ T-cell responses.
- As disease progresses, CD4+ T-cell numbers and function decline and CD8+ CTL no longer function adequately.
- CD8+ CTL have been demonstrated in vivo in peripheral blood, lung, and cerebrospinal fluid.

The role of lymphoid tissue in HIV infection

At the time of HIV-1 transmission into a host, the virus 'seeds' to secondary lymphoid tissues, for example the lymph nodes.

- After transmission of HIV from mucosal tissues (if acquired through sexual contact), the virus travels within the blood circulation and sequesters within lymphoid structures.
- Within a lymph node, the follicular dendritic cells (FDCs) play a major role in trapping virus within the germinal centers.
- HIV is thought to bind to FDCs through glycoprotein structures.
- CD4+ T-cells that pass through the germinal centers to the paracortical region will encounter HIV 'sitting' on FDC structures and potentially become infected.
- It has recently been found that CD4+ T-cells in lymph nodes around the gut and the colon are the main targets for SIV and HIV infection.
- CD4 memory cells (as marked by CCR5+ receptor expression) are depleted within days of infection before the noticeable CD4 count decline in the peripheral circulation.
- It is also thought that abnormal bacterial translocation occurs across the damaged gut lining (lamina propria) into the lymphatic and blood circulation causing non-specific T-cell activation.

The role of monocytes/macrophages in HIV infection

Monocyte/macrophage infection occurs via the CD4 and CCR5 receptors and persistence of virus is maintained in these cells.

- Infection of monocyte/macrophages does not cause cell lysis and results in viral persistence.
- Migration of monocytes from the blood into tissue and differentiation into tissue macrophages is thought to be one mechanism for transporting virus to various non-lymphoid tissues.

The following functions remain intact during HIV infection:

- phagocytosis;
- superoxide production;
- antimicrobial activity;
- antifungal activity;
- antitumour activity;
- TNF-α production;
- antibody-dependent cellular toxicity.

The following functions show defects during infection:

- chemotaxis;
- complement 3 receptor-mediated clearance;
- IL-1 production;
- antigen presentation.

Impairment of functional antimycobacterial activity has profound implications for protection against *Mycobacterium tuberculosis*, the most prevalent opportunistic infection in South Africa.

Immunopathology

Lymphoid tissue destruction during HIV infection

As the disease progresses, lymphoid architecture disintegrates and there is regression of germinal centers and an inability to initiate new immune responses. There is evidence that this occurs rapidly in gut associated lymphoid tissue.

- Early in disease there is intense immune activity that causes lymph node hyperplasia and lymphadenopathy associated with HIV infection.
- As disease progresses, there is gradual involution and destruction of lymphoid architecture.

- There is destruction of the FDC network.
- FDC destruction leads to loss of trapped HIV, which then 'spills' out into the circulation leading to increased viraemia.

CD4+ T-cell abnormalities during HIV infection

A decline in peripheral blood CD4 numbers is only one of many characteristics that defines the effect of HIV infection.

Table 3.1 shows the main defects within the CD4 T-cell compartment:

Table 3.1 Defects within the CD4 T-cell compartment

Characteristic	Function
CD4+ T-cell absolute count	Decreased proliferative responses to mitogens
	Decreased secretion of cytokines
CD4+ T-cell defects	
Early disease	Decreased response to recall antigens
Mid-disease (chronic stage)	Decreased response to alloantigens
Late disease	Decreased response to mitogens
Cytokine secretion	Decreased production of IFN-γ and IL-2
	Increased production of IL-4 and IL-10

HIV infection results in a number of defects, often occurring before cell numbers decline:

- These defects are functional and include a hierarchical loss of proliferative responses to antigen, alloantigen and mitogen over the course of the infection (Table 3.1).
- Cytokine secretion is severely disrupted.
- Th1 cytokine profiles (IL-2, IL-12, INF-γ, TNF-α) decline as disease progresses and Th2 cytokine profiles (IL-4, IL-5, IL-10) increase.
- Concomittant parasitic infections, common in South Africa, will further push cytokine profiles to Th2-type during disease progression.

CD8+ T-cell abnormalities during HIV infection

Loss of CD8+ T-cell function during infection has been attributed to lack of CD4+ T-cell help:

- It leads to loss of HLA class I restricted CTL functional killing capacity, and so to persistent activation, as measured by expression of HLA-DR and CD38.
- Interleukin-2 receptor expression is lost.
- Accelerated exhaustion of CD8+ T-cells leads to deleted antigen-specific clones.
- Cells are unable to respond to exogenous cytokines (IL-2, IL-7 or IL-15) and to expand into central memory T-cells.

B-cell abnormalities during HIV infection

B-cells are not infected by HIV in vivo, but the main functional abnormality is hypergammaglobulinaemia.

- Chronic B-cell activation results in spontaneous B-cell proliferation and polyclonal hypergammaglobulinaemia.
- Defects in antigen- and mitogen-induced B-cell proliferation occur.
- The number of circulating B-cells decreases.
- Epstein-Barr virus related B-cell lymphomas increase.
- B-cell abnormalities are mainly due to dysregulation of cytokines that stimulate B-cells (such as IL-4, IL-5, IL-6 and IL-10).

The proposed mechanisms for CD4+ T-cell depletion and dysfunction during HIV infection

There are multiple mechanisms that have been proposed to account for CD4+ T cell depletion and abnormal function, some of which have been extrapolated from *in vitro* studies. These include:

- direct destruction of CD4 cells due to HIV infection of the cell, which mainly occurs in gut associated lymphoid tissue;
- hyperactivation of cells, leading to deletion of specific T-cell-receptor bearing cells;
- programmed cell death (or apoptosis);
- cell killing by CTL;
- HIV infection of the thymus leading to abnormal thymic output.

Thymic dysfunction in HIV infection

It is now generally recognized that the thymus functions well into adult life to generate new (naive) CD4 and CD8+ T-cells by a process of negative and positive selection of cells able to interact with foreign antigen.

- T-cells from a human thymus have been shown *in vitro* to be infected by HIV, including CD4+/CD8+ double positive thymocytes, CD4+ and CD8+ single thymocytes and epithelial cells.
- Thymic destruction occurs, leading to impaired T-cell maturation and the inability of cells to adequately differentiate into distinct CD4 and CD8+ T-cell subsets.
- Thymic epithelial cell maturation and function is disrupted.
- The microenvironment and cellular architecture of the thymus is destroyed.

Autoimmune responses during HIV infection

The acute and chronic immune activation caused by the persistence of HIV and the inability of host immunity to clear virus precipitates a number of clinical immune abnormalities frequently found in infected individuals.

Clinical manifestations of autoimmunity

- systemic lupus erythematosus-like syndrome:
  o rash,
  o glomerulonephritis,
- arthritis:
  o Reiter's syndrome,
- anaemia;
- thrombocytopenia;
- coagulation pathology;
- neuropathies;
- polymyositis.

PART 3: Treatment options

Immunotherapies designed to restore immune competence

By knowing how HIV destroys the immune system, immune replacement therapies have been developed to restore immune competence. However, many of the approaches are often very experimental and clinically impractical. Table 3.2 summarises what is available.

Table 3.2 Summary of available immunotherapies

Aim of therapy	Implementation system
Increase CD4+ T-cell numbers	Inhibit apoptosis
	Restore glutathione levels
	Transplantation of stem cells
	Transfusion of peripheral blood cells
	Ex vivo expansion of CD4+ T-cells
Restore deficient cytokines	IL-2 therapy
Supplement T-cell immunity	IL-12 or IL-15
Boost anti-HIV immune responses	Immunization with vaccines

Preventative and therapeutic vaccines

Although a preventative vaccine is sought to blunt and prevent new infections in southern Africa, a therapeutic vaccine that would redirect immunity and lower viral load in infected individuals is highly desirable:

- A preventative vaccine would need to elicit both CTL and neutralizing antibodies; both arms of immunity thought to provide protective immunity.
- A new generation of candidate vaccines use HIV genes inserted into vectors that allow endogenous processing of HIV proteins and expression of class I and II HLA restricted epitopes.
- Current trends are to use a prime (usually DNA) and a heterologous boost (either Modified Vaccinia Ankara or Adenovirus 5) containing 3-5 HIV genes.
- Provision of a single vectored vaccine (without a prime or a boost) has been shown to provide no efficacy.
- Other approaches in clinical trials are recombinant HIV proteins, such as gp120 and whole killed HIV.
- It is widely thought that to redirect host immunity with a vaccine during HIV infection, suppression of viral replication by use of antiretroviral drugs is a prerequisite.

Immune restoration and antiretroviral therapy

There is a significant body of data to show that suppression of HIV replication through antiretroviral therapy allows host immunity to return to a more normal state:

- It will be apparent from the information in this chapter that high levels of viral replication lead to destruction of most facets of the immune system, ranging from lower CD4 numbers and function to lymph node destruction.
- It has been shown that HIV infected individuals provided with highly active antiretroviral therapy have:
  o increased CD4 counts,
  o increased numbers of new (naive) CD4+ and CD8+ T-cells,
  o improved antigen recall responses,
  o improved CTL competence,
  o regenerated lymphoid structures.
- Viral suppression is important so that immunity can be restored.
- The immune system has enough plasticity, prior to AIDS, to show a degree of self-regeneration.
- Implementation of a vaccine during viral suppression may allow the immune system to respond to the vaccine.
- Immune restoration after the initiation of antiretroviral therapy may lead to manifestations of the immune reconstitution inflammatory syndrome and clinicians should be aware of this (see Chapter 50: Immune-constitution inflammatory syndrome).

References and further reading

Walker, B.D. and D.R. Burton. 2008. 'Toward an AIDS vaccine'. *Science* 320:764.

4 Interactions between HIV and tuberculosis

Epidemiology

While tuberculosis (TB) notification rates continue to decrease in many parts of the world, rates have increased more than three-fold in many countries in sub-Saharan Africa since 1990, fuelling a 1% annual increase in global TB incidence. In 2005 the African continent, with just 11% of world's population, accounted for 27% of the global burden of TB and 30% of TB-related deaths. Over two million new TB cases and over 500 000 TB-related deaths were estimated to occur in the region annually.

Among individuals with latent *Mycobacterium tuberculosis* (MTB) infection, the lifetime risk of developing active TB is approximately 10% in non-HIV-infected people; in those with HIV infection however, the risk is greatly increased to around 10% per year. Disease caused by the relatively non-virulent non-tuberculous mycobacteria, such as *Mycobacterium avium* complex, tends to affect only those with very low blood CD4 lymphocyte counts. In contrast, the risk of TB increases after HIV seroconversion and is elevated across the full spectrum of immunodeficiency, increasing steeply as the CD4 cell count declines.

HIV-infected persons not only have high rates of reactivation TB, but also have a heightened susceptibility to new exogenous infection and rapidly progressive primary disease. Genetic fingerprinting studies have shown that high TB recurrence rates are fuelled by a high rate of exogenous reinfection. Nosocomial transmission of TB among HIV-infected individuals is a major hazard as was illustrated by the outbreak of extensively drug resistant (XDR) TB in KwaZulu-Natal, South Africa, in 2006.

Clinical features of TB infection in HIV

The features of TB in HIV-infected individuals with well-preserved CD4 lymphocyte counts are indistinguishable from those of non-HIV-infected individuals with TB. However, in HIV-infected persons, progression of immunodeficiency is associated with an increasing frequency of cutaneous anergy to purified protein derivative and an increased risk of extrapulmonary, miliary and disseminated forms of the disease.

Radiographic appearances of pulmonary TB in patients with HIV coinfection reflect impairment of the host inflammatory response, with reduced likelihood of cavitation, fibrosis and classical apical disease. Mediastinal lymphadenopathy and non-specific patterns of consolidation are more common. In view of the high frequency of non-cavitatory pulmonary disease and extrapulmonary forms of TB, sputum smear microscopy has a low sensitivity for diagnosis. Sensitivity is substantially increased by sputum culture, but this is slow and expensive and the necessary infrastructure is not available over much of Africa.

Impairment of cell-mediated immunity to TB and increased susceptibility to other opportunistic pathogens contribute to increased mortality rates among patients with TB and HIV coinfection. Acute sepsis, for example, is a common cause of death among these patients. Autopsy specimens from patients who died of TB and AIDS show a high frequency of extrapulmonary and disseminated disease with multi-organ involvement. However, TB in such patients with advanced HIV is often under-diagnosed; occult disseminated TB is a frequent finding in post-mortem studies of people from sub-Saharan Africa who died with AIDS.

Immunopathological mechanisms in TB/HIV coinfection

HIV critically impairs cell-mediated host responses to *Mycobacterium tuberculosis*. Examination of bronchoalveolar lavage fluid from tuberculous lung segments in HIV-infected patients reveals failure of recruitment and activation of CD4 lymphocytes. Numeric depletion and functional impairment of these cells and disruption of CD4-lymphocyte-macrophage interactions results in impaired granuloma formation. This ultimately results in failure of mycobacterial restriction.

Histologically, a spectrum of appearances is seen, with increasing immunodeficiency being associated with progressive failure of granuloma formation and increasing mycobacterial burden. This is similar to the histological spectrum seen between tuberculoid and lepromatous forms of leprosy. Three histological stages of cellular immune response that correlate with depletion of the peripheral blood CD4 lymphocyte count have been described. First, in immunocompetent individuals with HIV infection, TB granulomas are characterized by abundant epithelioid macrophages, Langerhans giant cells, peripherally located CD4 lymphocytes, and a paucity of bacteria. Secondly, in individuals with moderate HIV-associated immunodeficiency, Langerhans giant cells are not seen, epithelioid differentiation and activation of macrophages are absent, there is CD4 lymphocytopenia, and acid-fast bacilli (AFB) are more numerous. Finally, in individuals with advanced HIV-associated immunosuppression and AIDS, there is a striking paucity of granuloma formation with little cellular recruitment, very few CD4 lymphocytes, and even larger numbers of AFB.

The interaction between TB and HIV is bi-directional because activation of mononuclear cells during the host response to TB augments HIV replication. Immune activation increases the susceptibility of mononuclear cells to infection with HIV and causes accelerated HIV replication within infected cells. HIV load is therefore increased both at sites of TB disease and within the systemic circulation. Via these mechanisms, TB is thought to lead to accelerated decline in immune function in HIV-infected individuals.

Tuberculosis and antiretroviral treatment

Between 10–25% of patients enrolling in antiretroviral treatment programmes in sub-Saharan Africa are either receiving antituberculosis treatment or have previously undiagnosed active TB. Diagnosis of TB among highly immunocompromised patients is difficult due to atypical presentations and a high index of suspicion is needed. Antiretroviral therapy reduces the risk of TB by 70–90% in the first one to two years of treatment. However, in the longer term, rates do not decrease to the levels seen among non-HIV-infected patients probably due to incomplete immune recovery and possibly fuelled by nosocomial TB transmission. Despite pharmacokinetic interactions (see Chapter 49: Drug-drug interactions) and high pill burden and potential for co-toxicity, patients receiving concurrent non-nucleoside reverse transcriptase inhibitors (NNRTI)-based antiretroviral therapy and rifampicin-containing antituberculosis treatment have good immunological and virological responses to antiretroviral therapy.

Immune reconstitution disease is a common complication during the initial weeks of antiretroviral therapy among patients who had TB at the time such treatment was initiated. Rapid restoration of TB-specific immune responses may lead to an exacerbation of the host inflammatory response to residual mycobacterial antigen. This manifests as the clinical deterioration of TB at the original disease site or the appearance of new TB lesions at another site. Immune reconstitution disease commonly presents with recurrence of fever, systemic symptoms and pulmonary, intra-abdominal or peripheral lymph node disease. This most commonly occurs among patients with CD4 cell counts <100 cells/μl who initiate antiretrovirals within the first one to two months of antituberculosis treatment. Most cases of TB immune reconstitution disease are mild and self-limiting. However, manifestations are sometimes severe and occasionally life-threatening, requiring systemic steroid therapy and possibly discontinuation of antiretrovirals. Immune reconstitution during antiretroviral therapy may also contribute to the high TB rate during the initial weeks of treatment by 'unmasking' previously sub-clinical disease.

The optimal time to initiate antiretroviral therapy in patients with TB is unclear. The complexities of pharmacokinetic interactions, pill burden, co-toxicity and immune reconstitution disease all favour delaying anti-retroviral therapy at least for the first two months of antituberculosis treatment. However, early mortality rates are exceptionally high in antiretroviral programmes in Africa, especially among those with WHO stage 4 disease or with CD4 cell counts <100 cells/μl. In view of this mortality risk, such patients should probably start antiretroviral therapy within a few weeks, as soon as the TB treatment is tolerated.

TB control in high HIV prevalence communities

The World Health Organisation (WHO) DOTS strategy remains the central component of global TB control strategies. However, while successful in low HIV prevalence settings, this strategy alone has proven insufficient to contain the African TB epidemic in high HIV prevalence countries. Additional strategies are needed. These might include intensified or active case-finding in patient populations at high risk of TB. Isoniazid prophylaxis may be used among HIV-infected patients, and causes a time-limited reduction in TB risk of approximately 40%. Although antiretroviral therapy dramatically reduces TB rates, patients nevertheless have a greatly increased lifespan. Since risk of TB long-term remains higher than the background rate, life-time risk of TB may not be substantially affected by antiretroviral therapy. Scale-up of antiretroviral therapy may therefore make little or no contribution to TB control at the community level. Ultimately, control of the HIV epidemic is needed to stem the TB epidemic in the countries of southern Africa.

References and further reading

Corbett, E.L., Watt, C.J., Walker, N. et al. 2003. 'The growing burden of tuberculosis: global trends and interactions with the HIV epidemic'. *Archives of Internal Medicine* 163: 1009–1021.

De Cock, K.M. and R.E. Chaisson. 1999. 'Will DOTS do it? A reappraisal of tuberculosis control in countries with high rates of

HIV infection'. *International Journal of Tuberculous Lung Disease* 3: 457–465.

Lawn, S.D., Butera, S.T., Shinnick, T.M. 2002. 'Tuberculosis unleashed: the impact of human immunodeficiency virus type 1 infection on the host granulomatous response to *Mycobacterium tuberculosis*'. *Microbes and Infection* 4: 635–46.

Lawn, S.D., Bekker, L.G., Middelkoop, K., Myer, L., Wood, R. 2006. 'Impact of HIV on epidemiology of tuberculosis in a peri-urban community in South Africa: the need for age-specific interventions'. *Clinical Infectious Diseases* 42:1040–1047.

Lawn, S.D., Myer, L., Bekker, L.G., Wood, R. 2006. 'Burden of tuberculosis (TB) in an antiretroviral treatment (ART) service in sub-Saharan Africa: impact on ART outcomes and implications for TB control'. *AIDS* 20:1605–1612.

Lawn, S.D., Bekker, L.G., Miller, R.F. 2005. 'Immune reconstitution disease associated with mycobacterial infections in HIV-infected individuals receiving antiretrovirals'. *Lancet Infectious Diseases* 5:361–373.

Lawn, S.D., Bekker, L.G., Wood, R. 2005. 'How effectively does HAART restore immune responses to *Mycobacterium tuberculosis*? Implications for tuberculosis control'. *AIDS* 19:1113–1124.

5 Laboratory investigations

Diagnosing HIV infection

HIV screening is recommended for patients in all health-care settings after the patient is notified that testing will be performed unless the patient declines (opt out screening).

In most contexts, antibody tests are sufficient to make an accurate diagnosis of HIV infection. The use of two different enzyme-linked immunosorbent assay (ELISA) tests or two different rapid tests (on site) to confirm HIV infection meets the World Health Organization (WHO) testing recommendations for regions where HIV prevalence exceeds 10%. At lower HIV prevalence, a three-test strategy is recommended. Almost all ELISA and rapid tests are designed to detect both HIV-1 and HIV-2 antibodies.

For laboratory-based antibody testing, send at least 1 mL of clotted blood. For rapid testing, between 10 and 50 μl of blood is typically required;

Figure 5.1 A simple HIV testing algorithm. (A first line test should be extremely sensitive. A second line or 'confirmatory' test should be selected for its high specificity.)

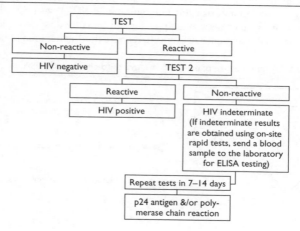

a fingerprick (<2 drops) is adequate to collect this volume. If you are performing a rapid test yourself, make sure that you check the expiratory date of the test kit and follow the instructions very carefully. Consult your laboratory or a virologist if you encounter diagnostic problems.

Diagnostic tests for HIV

Table 5.1 summarizes the utility of available diagnostic HIV tests.

Enzyme-linked immunosorbent assay

ELISA is an acronym for enzyme-linked immunosorbent assay. This is the most widely used serological technique today, and is used to detect antibodies against antigen from many infectious agents including HIV.

The third-generation ELISA tests for HIV antibody have a sensitivity approaching 100% and specificity >99%. These tests have been in use since the early 1990s. Unlike earlier versions, the third generation ELISA tests detect both IgM and IgG antibody classes, and so detect HIV infection from a very early stage (see 'The window period').

An ELISA for HIV antibody uses HIV antigen to capture HIV antibodies in a blood sample. HIV antigen is fixed to a 'solid-phase', e.g. a plastic well in a multi-well plate.

A second step is required to detect any captured antibody. This step commonly utilizes an enzyme-substrate colour reaction. The intensity (optical density) of the resulting colour can be measured, and the antibody levels can be adjudged as low or high, relative to control sera.

Today, large laboratories run fully automated ELISA systems. Blood tubes are given bar codes and sampled directly by a robotic system. Figure 5.2 illustrates the sequence of events in reactive third-generation ELISA.

Figure 5.2 The sequence of events in reactive third-generation ELISA

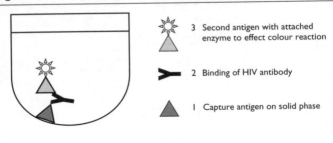

3 Second antigen with attached enzyme to effect colour reaction

2 Binding of HIV antibody

1 Capture antigen on solid phase

Table 5.1 A summary of the available diagnostic HIV tests

Tests that detect HIV antibody

Test	Target	Sensitivity	Specificity	Use	Comment	Blood sample	Lab time	Cost*
ELISA†	Specific HIV antibodies	Very high	Very high	Adult diagnosis, Infant screening	Best test in most contexts	Clotted tube	40–150 min.	R90
Rapid test devices	Specific HIV antibodies	High (variable)	High (variable)	Adult diagnosis, Infant screening	Immediate on-site results	Clotted tube, fingerprick	±10 min.	R35
Western blot	All HIV antibodies	High	High, but depends on interpretation	Low or indeterminate ELISA results Confirmation of HIV-2 countries	Seldom used in developing	Clotted tube	4 h.	R500

Tests that detect HIV itself

Test	Target	Sensitivity	Specificity	Use	Comment	Blood sample	Lab time	Cost*
PCR‡	Viral nucleic acid	Very high	Very high	Very early diagnosis Low or indeterminate ELISA results Definitive diagnosis in infants	Requires technical expertise	EDTA tube (Take minimum 0.5 mL)	8 h.	R370 (diagnostic) R570 (viral load)
Culture	Viable virus	High	Very high	Research	Will detect novel strains of HIV	EDTA or heparin tube (Take minimum 5 mL)	21–28 d.	R1000

* Approximate ZAR, public sector, 2008.   † Enzyme-linked immunosorbent assay.   ‡ Polymerase chain reaction.

Rapid test devices

Rapid HIV testing can play an important role by expanding access to testing in both clinical and non-clinical settings and overcoming some of the barriers to early diagnosis and improved linkage to care for infected persons. Rapid tests are primarily easy to perform, and require minimal equipment and user expertise. The majority of rapid tests are immunochromatographic, somewhat like an ELISA reaction in a simplified format. Others are latex agglutination tests. Even the simplest test must be performed with absolute attention to both the expiratory date and test instructions, without short cuts and user innovations. The better tests include a control to validate the result. Used correctly, the best rapid tests have an accuracy closely approaching that of ELISA tests. However, lack of regulatory legislation may allow lesser quality tests to be imported.

A note on non-invasive HIV ELISA and rapid tests

Although immunoglobulin levels in saliva and urine are approximately 1 000-fold lower than in plasma, there have been technical advances allowing the increasingly accurate detection of HIV antibody in these body fluids. At present, such non-invasive tests are largely used for surveillance, but they may in future be increasingly used as diagnostic tests.

The Western blot test

HIV antibodies are not homogenous, but are a population of antibodies to many of the protein components of the virus. A Western blot has the advantage of distinguishing these different antibodies, so that the patient's exact antibody profile can be visualized. The basis of the Western blot is a strip of cellulose membrane embedded with the different HIV proteins, arranged according to their molecular weights. A person's serum is incubated with the strip. A second phase reveals the 'bands' where the antibodies have bound. Empirically, certain antibody bands have more diagnostic significance than others. Criteria for a positive blot can vary slightly. The Centers for Disease Control and Prevention (CDC), Atlanta, require the presence of any two of the p24, gp41, and gp120/160 bands for a positive blot. A negative blot shows no bands, or only an isolated p18 band. Any other pattern of bands is regarded as an indeterminate result. Indeterminate results are common (up to 20% of uninfected persons). With the advent of excellent ELISA tests, a Western blot is no longer regarded as essential for confirmation of HIV infection. However, an HIV-2 specific Western blot remains the most reliable confirmatory test for infection with HIV-2.

The p24 antigen

The p24 protein is a core HIV protein (see Chapter 2: Virology). At times of high viral replication, p24 protein is directly detectable in the blood. This occurs during primary HIV infection and again in the late stages of acquired immune deficiency syndrome (AIDS). Notably, p24 is detectable in <10% of people in the asymptomatic phase of HIV infection. The p24 antigen test should, therefore, not be used instead of an antibody test, only as a supplementary test (see 'The window period'). The p24 antigen is usually measured by the ELISA technique. The sensitivity of the test may be increased if it is preceded by a dissociation step to break up complexes of the p24 antigen and its antibody.

Polymerase chain reaction

In the polymerase chain reaction (PCR), 'primers' target a specific DNA sequence, in this case a portion of the HIV genome. Primers are short sequences of synthetic DNA that are complementary to one end of a gene sequence of interest. Primers prime a DNA polymerase enzyme to make copies of the DNA to which they are bound. Temperature shifts initiate different steps in the reaction. The final result is an exponential increase in copies of the targeted DNA fragment. This DNA is then readily detectable. The technique can potentially detect a single intact copy of HIV nucleic acid in a blood sample. Good laboratory technique is required to avoid cross-contamination of samples. Despite technical and logistical factors, as well as costs, this test has become increasingly utilised. The blood transfusion services have moved towards this type of testing in place of antibody and antigen tests for HIV.

Culture

HIV can be grown in cell culture, just like many other viruses. Fresh peripheral blood mononuclear cells from an uninfected donor are incubated with the sample for testing. The addition of the cytokine interleukin-2 is necessary to stimulate the cells. Growth of HIV is visible microscopically by cytopathic effect in the cells, and the detection of p24 antigen or reverse transcriptase activity in the culture. Culture is largely a research technology available in reference laboratories.

The window period

Following HIV infection, there is a delay before HIV antibodies become detectable in the blood. This diagnostic 'window period' is approximately four weeks (see Figure 5.3). Tests for the virus itself will reveal the infection somewhat earlier. The p24 antigen test is positive in the majority of patients a week before antibody ELISA tests become reactive. PCR testing can detect HIV in the blood from approximately two weeks after infection.

Figure 5.3 The sequence of events following HIV infection

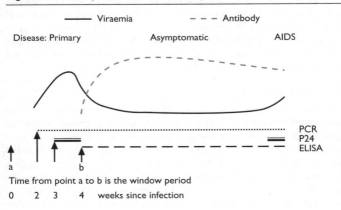

Time from point a to b is the window period

0   2   3   4   weeks since infection

Should a patient present with a suspected primary HIV illness and HIV-antibody tests are negative or indeterminate, a p24 antigen or a qualitative viral load test may confirm infection. In addition, do follow-up antibody testing one to two weeks later. While there is variation in the timing, seroconversion more than three months after infection is extremely unusual.

Blood donors, organ donors, and needle-stick injury source patients should be routinely tested for PCR and p24 antigens when HIV antibody tests are negative. Combined p24 and antibody ELISA tests are available, sometimes known as fourth-generation HIV tests.

The p24 antigen test has been largely superseded by nucleic acid amplification technologies because it has approximately 75% sensitivity relative to PCR in identifying infectious persons in the window period.

HIV diagnosis in babies

Between 0 and 30% of babies are vertically infected by the mother:
- *in utero*;
- perinatally; or
- by breastfeeding.

The risk is determined primarily by maternal viral load and the use of prophylactic antiretrovirals.

All babies newly born to HIV-positive women will test HIV-antibody-positive because of the transfer of maternal antibodies to the baby across the placenta. Uninfected babies will serorevert to HIV-negative at 11 months on average, but may have detectable maternal antibody for up to 18 months. Infected babies will be persistently seropositive beyond 18 months of age.

To discriminate between infected and uninfected babies before the age of 18 months, it is necessary to utilize tests that detect the virus itself.

Nucleic acid testing (usually PCR) has the highest sensitivity and specificity in this context. Standard p24 antigen testing is insensitive and will detect approximately 40% of infected babies. Therefore, a positive p24 antigen test indicates infection, but a negative result does not exclude infection.

Timing HIV diagnosis in babies

- PCR testing at birth will detect only those babies infected *in utero*.
- PCR testing from two weeks of age will detect babies infected *in utero* or perinatally.
- The recommended age for reliable HIV PCR testing in babies is (less than or equal to) four weeks.

Bear in mind that there is a significant, ongoing risk of infection while breastfeeding.

Tests for HIV: Monitoring the disease

The bread-and-butter tests are the viral load and the CD4 count. The information that these tests give has been compared to the parameters of a train journey: The viral load measures the speed of travel of the train, the CD4 count indicates the distance from the crash, while the crash indicates the onset of AIDS. In other words, viral load predicts the rate of disease progression (rate of loss of CD4 cells) and the CD4 count indicates the stage of disease that the patient has already reached. (See also Chapter 6: HIV transmission and natural history.)

Viral load

HIV viral load is the concentration of free virus in the blood plasma. In its free form, HIV is an RNA virus and all the commercially available viral load tests measure HIV RNA. Note that commercial viral load assays are only available for HIV-1.

There are three main types of viral load test:

- quantitative PCR;
- nucleic acid sequence based amplification (NASBA); and
- branch-chain DNA assay.

All of these tests can measure free HIV in the range of 50 to 1 000 000 copies/mL. For practical purposes, any of these tests give reliable results. The less common HIV-1 subtypes may be quantified sub-optimally or not at all, but HIV-1 subtype C (the predominant HIV-1 clade in southern Africa) does not present problems in viral load testing. Although results obtained with different tests are comparable, it is best to remain with one type of test for ongoing monitoring of a particular patient.

The viral load should not be measured during an acute illness or within several weeks of a vaccination.

The viral load is expressed as copies/mL or as a $\log_{10}$ value. The viral load fluctuates by a factor of two ($\log_{10} 0.3$) in otherwise stable patients. Converting the viral load to the $\log_{10}$ value makes it easier to detect clinically meaningful changes over time: *only viral load changes of >0.5 $\log_{10}$ which represents a three-fold change are significant.* (See Table 5.2). These changes are used when deciding to initiate therapy, and to monitor the response to therapy. (See Chapter 44: Adult antiretroviral therapy and Chapter 45: Paediatric antiretroviral therapy.) Ideally, when monitoring the effect of antiretroviral therapy, a patient's viral load should be <50 or <400 copies/mL (depending on the test) after four to six months of treatment. However, in the present national antiretroviral programme, a confirmed viral load >5 000 copies/mL after addressing possible poor adherence is used as a threshold for switching from first to second line therapy.

Table 5.2 Log_{10} values of viral load changes

Fold change in viral load	Log_{10} change
2	0.3
3	0.5
5	0.7
10	1.0
100	2.0
1 000	3.0

For example: a patient has a viral load of 5.8 log_{10} (631 000 copies/mL) before starting antiretroviral therapy, a viral load of 4.3 log_{10} (21 400 copies/mL) after one month of treatment (~30 fold reduction), and 1.7 log_{10} (50 copies/mL) after four months of treatment (~400 fold reduction). The log_{10} viral load change (5.8–4.3 = 1.5 and 4.3–1.7 = 2.6) is >0.5 log_{10} in both cases and therefore represents an appropriate response to antiretroviral therapy.

CD4 count

All T-lymphocytes have T-cell receptors that are also identified as CD3 molecules. CD4 is a molecule found on the surface of helper T-lymphocytes. CD8 is yet another molecule found on cytotoxic T-lymphocytes. CD4 and CD8 molecules play a subsidiary role in the binding of CD3 to MHC-II and MHC-I respectively, during antigen presentation.

CD4 is also the major receptor for HIV, and CD4+ T-lymphocytes are the main target of HIV infection. CD4+ T-lymphocytes are directly and indirectly destroyed by HIV. While these cells are initially replaced as quickly as they are destroyed, over time the regenerative capacity of the immune system is exhausted, and the CD4+ cell numbers fall. Since these cells play a central stimulatory role in the immune system, their falling numbers correlate with an increasing degree of immune suppression. CD4+ cells are detected using monoclonal antibodies to the CD4 molecule. A fluorescent-activated cell sorter (FACS) machine is commonly used to count them, but other options are available. The cost of performing a CD4 cell count is determined by the cost of the specific monoclonal antibodies , the capital costs of the machine and technician time. The locally developed panleucogate assay (PLG) is widely used for monitoring in the national antiretroviral programme as cost-savings have been made by using a generic CD45 antibody.

Table 5.3 provides a rough guide to the relationship between the CD4 count and immune suppression.

Table 5.3 CD4 counts and immune suppression

CD4 count	Degree of immune suppression
±1 000 cells/µl	Normal immune function (adults)
200–500 µl	Moderate immune suppression
<200 µl	Advanced immune suppression (Institute prophylaxis against OIs)
<50 µl	Severe immune suppression

In children, normal CD4 counts are age dependent and vary widely. Therefore, CD4 counts are often expressed as a percentage of normal, rather than an absolute number. (See Chapter 10: Clinical assessment (paediatric).)

A CD4:CD8 ratio is sometimes reported. In a normal immune system, CD4 cells are in slight excess of CD8 cells so the ratio is slightly >1. As CD4 cells are lost and some compensatory increase in CD8 cells occurs, the ratio falls to <1.

Drug resistance testing

In patients receiving antiretroviral therapy, an elevated viral load indicates possible drug failure or poor adherence. A confirmed viral load >5 000 copies after addressing adherence issues is an indication in the national antiretroviral programme for switching from first to second line therapy. For those patients failing second-line therapy, and who have further therapeutic options, drug sensitivity testing may help further management. The two main laboratory procedures used to assess susceptibility to antiretroviral drugs are the genotypic and phenotypic assays.

Genotype assays

Genotypic analysis identifies mutations of the HIV-*pol* gene sequences, encoding reverse transcriptase (*rt*) and protease enzymes (*pr*), which are associated with phenotypic resistance to antiretrovirals. Following reverse transcription of the *pol* gene, DNA sequencing of the amplicons is compared with a consensus reference sequence. The genotype report is given in a 'letter-number-letter' format. Where the initial letter indicates the amino acid of wild type consensus virus; the number, the codon of interest; and the final letter indicates the substituted amino acid at this codon. For example, 'M184V' indicates that valine has been substituted for methionine at codon number 184 of the *rt* gene

Table 5.4 Amino acid-letter code used in genotype reports.

A	Alanine	I	Isoleucine	R	Arginine
C	Cytosine	K	Lysine	S	Serine
D	Aspartic acid	L	Leucine	T	Threonine
E	Glutamic acid	M	Methionine	V	Valine
F	Phenylalanine	N	Asparagine	W	Tryptophan
G	Glycine	P	Proline	Y	Tyrosine
H	Histidine	Q	Glutamine		

Indications for genotype analyses include antiretroviral naïve patients if prevalence of resistant virus in the area or risk group >10% and for optimising new regimens for those with viral failure on antiretroviral therapy.

Limitations of the genotypic assays are:

- that they are expensive >R700;
- that they can only be performed when viral load is high enough to be amplified (>1 000 copies/mL);
- that they only identify mutations present in >20% of circulating virions;
- that they should be performed while patients are taking a failing anti-retrovial regimen; and that they should be interpreted in conjunction with a knowledge of prior antiretroviral usage.

Genotypic assays most reliably identify those drugs that should be avoided and are less reliable for identifying drugs likely to be active.

Therapeutic drug monitoring (TDM)

Although treatment failure is usually a result of poor adherence the combination of unexplained treatment failures and the potential for drug-drug interactions (DDI) has led to an interest in monitoring antiretro-viral drug concentrations. Assays are available for non-nucleoside RT inhibitors (NNRTI) and protease inhibitors (PI) as there is a recognized association between trough plasma concentrations and virological response. In contrast virological effect of nucleoside reverse transcriptase inhibitors (NRTI) is due to the intracellular concentration of the triphosphorylated pro-drug which is not easily measured. The present cost of TDM is approximately R80.

References and further reading

Centers for Disease Control and Prevention. 2006. 'Revised recommendations for HIV testing of adults, adolescents and pregnant women in health-care settings'. *Mortality and Morbidity Weekly Report*; 55(RR14); 1–14.

Greenwald, J.L., Burnstein, G.R., Pincus, J., Branson, B. 2006. 'A rapid review of rapid HIV antibody tests'. *Current Infectious Disease Reports*; 8:125–131.

Martin, D., and Sim, J. 2000. 'The laboratory diagnosis of HIV infection.' *South African Medical Journal*; 90 (2): 105–9.

6 HIV transmission and natural history

The demographics of southern African countries have been profoundly altered by the spread of HIV through young adult populations. The majority of adult infections are transmitted by heterosexual contact, with homosexual contact and intravenous recreational drug use playing relatively minor roles.

Biological factors affecting transmission

Sexual transmission of HIV usually occurs after the exposure of non-keratinised genital surfaces to infected genital secretions or blood. Biological factors influencing the risk of sexual HIV transmission are:

- viral load – a higher viral load is associated with increased transmission risk;
- acute HIV infection – increased risk of HIV transmission due to very high viral load (especially clade (sub-type) C virus – see below);
- stage of HIV infection – low CD4 count associated with increased risk of transmission;
- untreated sexually transmitted infections (STIs) – ulcerative and non-ulcerative in either partner – increased HIV transmission risk;
- herpes simplex type 2 infection – recurrences associated with increased HIV viral load in genital secretions and increased HIV transmission;
- bacterial vaginosis in young women increases transmission risk;
- cervical ectopy in young women – increased risk of HIV infection;
- circumcision – halves the risk of HIV transmission to HIV-uninfected men, but increases the risk of transmission from HIV-infected men to uninfected partners if there is unprotected sex before the wound has fully healed;
- rare inherited mutations of chemokine receptors (e.g. homozygous CCR5 delta 32 mutation) or chemokine ligands (e.g. stromal derived factor SDF-3'A ligand for CXCR4) reduce risk of transmission.

Unusual protective immunological responses reduce HIV transmission, including cellular responses and local IgA responses, and may be linked to certain human leukocyte antigen alleles.

The probability of HIV transmission is determined by a variety of factors. The following behaviours increase the risk of HIV transmission:

- Frequent sexual intercourse without barrier protection (e.g. the male condom).
- More than one current sexual partner (concurrent partnerships).
- Working as a migrant labourer (men) or being married to a migrant labourer (women).
- Non-disclosure of HIV status to the partner (women may be afraid to disclose due to risk of intimate partner violence).
- Young women having sex with older men, because of sexual coercion and inability to negotiate condom use, or in exchange for material benefits (transactional sex).
- Sexual activity at a young age (early age of coital debut).
- Usual sexual partner HIV infected (discordant relationship).
- HIV infected partner not taking antiretroviral therapy.
- Specific sexual practices that damage genital mucosa and increase genital blood exposure, e.g. anal sex, dry sex, traumatic sex with genital bleeding, sex during menstruation.
- Regular alcohol abuse (associated with increased number of partners, concurrent STIs and condom failure).

Several risk factors may be present in any individual, and may be especially important in young women: for example in some studies HIV prevalence is 33% in women and 12% in men between the ages of 25 and 29 years. Sexual HIV transmission in southern Africa is incompletely understood and future studies may define other important risk factors.

HIV can also be transmitted:

- to children infected *in utero*, during labour, or during breastfeeding (discussed further in Chapter 46: Prevention of mother-to-child transmission of HIV);
- by occupational exposure, usually following needle-stick injury (discussed further in Chapter 52: Occupational post-exposure prophylaxis);
- through infusion of infected blood products: Risk can be substantially reduced through selecting blood donors with low HIV risk profile, and screening the donated blood for HIV antibodies, for P24 antigen, and viral RNA (recently implemented in South Africa).

Acute HIV infection following sexual exposure

HIV-infected genital secretions are produced by the vaginal and cervical mucosa in women, and by the seminal vesicles, prostate and urethral glands in men (pre-ejaculate and semen). HIV is found in genital secretions:

- as free virions suspended in the genital fluid;
- associated with infected inflammatory cells;
- attached to spermatozoa.

Non-keratinised genital epithelium that is vulnerable to infection with HIV occurs:

- in the vagina, cervix and endocervix;
- on the undersurface of the foreskin and in the urethral meatus;
- in the rectum and colon;
- on the base of ulcers in penile and vulval skin.

The probability of HIV transmission occurring after a single exposure is in the range of one in 200 to one in 1 000. Therefore the vast majority of exposures do not result in infection. In these circumstances HIV remains trapped in the genital mucous lining and on the surface of the epithelium, without penetrating beneath the most external epithelial cell layers. Adhesion to the epithelial layer may be facilitated by fibronectin in semen that links viral gp120 to β1-integrin expressed on epithelial surfaces.

In order for infection to become established HIV needs to come into contact with CD4+ immune cells with CCR5 or CXCR4 chemokine receptors. HIV can cross the epithelial barrier by:

- transcytosis from the apical to the basal membrane of epithelial cells;
- infection of dendritic cells that span the epithelial layer;
- infection of superficial CD4 cells that migrate back into sub-epithelial tissue.

Genital trauma, genital ulceration and inflammation disrupt the external epithelial surface and cause inflammatory cells to localise to within the superficial epithelial layer. The commonest immune cells found in genital epithelium are dendritic cells (DC) that express the CD4 receptor, the CCR5 chemokine receptor and C-type lectin receptors, for example DC-SIGN. R5-trophic HIV enters DC via CD4 and CCR5 receptors, and begins replication. The infected DC expresses and presents viral proteins to T-cells that form DC-T-cell conjugates, which permit the rapid infection of the T-cells by HIV. The virus can also bind to the surface of DC using the C-type lectin receptors. These DC can migrate to inguinal lymph-nodes where the virus is brought into intimate contact with follicular DC and CD4 T-cells. Immune cell infection and viral replication increases exponentially and virions enter the blood-stream by lymphatic drainage through the thoracic duct. Disseminated HIV infection is established within days. X4 trophic virus is less likely to be transmitted due to the paucity of immune cells expressing the CXCR4 receptor in the epithelium.

About 60% of all CD4 cells are located in gut-associated lymphoid tissue (GALT). Importantly most of the GALT CD4 cells are CCR5+ memory cells and are vulnerable to HIV infection in both the activated and resting states, possibly due to a favourable cytokine milieu. Clade C virus is especially well adapted to infect GALT CD4 cells and clade C viral load during acute infection is markedly higher than that associated with other HIV clades. Therefore individuals acutely infected by clade C HIV are highly infectious. This important observation could partially explain the rapid spread of clade C HIV infection through southern Africa.

Within 14 to 21 days the viral load begins to fall because of profound depletion of GALT CD4 cells and a partially effective adaptive immune response involving both cytotoxic CD8 cell and HIV-specific antibodies.

Importantly the widespread destruction of CD4 memory cells handicaps the immune response against the acute infection. Other CD4 cells, dendritic cells and macrophages located in lymph-nodes, spleen, tonsils and bone marrow are also rapidly infected during the acute stage of the infection. Loss of GALT CD4 cells permits translocation of bacteria across the bowel wall, which drives ongoing immune activation and CD4 infection by HIV.

HIV seroconversion syndrome

The onset of the adaptive immune response occurs at the same time as the HIV seroconversion syndrome, which occurs in about half to two thirds of infected individuals. The severity of the syndrome ranges from mild non-specific 'viral' or 'flu-like' symptoms to a severe infectious mononuleosis-like illness with immune dysregulation and transient profound CD4 depletion.

Common features include:

- malaise, anorexia, fevers, sweats, myalgia;
- generalised lymphadenopathy, hepatosplenomegaly;
- non-exudative pharyngitis and apthous ulceration;
- truncal rash – either maculopapular or urticarial (skin biopsy shows perivascular lymphocytic and dermal mononuclear cell infiltrates);
- headache, photophobia, meningism and meningoencephalitis (CSF analysis is compatible with viral meningitis);
- lymphopenia and thrombocytopenia;
- elevated transaminases and alkaline phosphatase.

More severe manifestations include:

- ascending demyelinating motor neuropathy (Guillian-Barré syndrome);
- *Pneumocystis* pneumonia, cryptococcal meningitis and oesophageal candidiasis.

Acute HIV infection is diagnosed by demonstrating positive HIV PCR (qualitative test) or HIV p24 antigen (ultrasensitive test) in blood and negative or indeterminate assay for HIV antibodies.

Management of the acute HIV seroconversion syndrome remains controversial. There is evidence that severe seroconversion illness predicts rapid HIV disease progression due to a high viral load set point (see below). Early initiation of antiretroviral therapy may preserve long-term immune competence, but needs to be weighed against the risks of drug side-effects and adherence issues causing antiretoviral resistance. Cases should be managed by an expert HIV clinician and ideally patients should be enrolled into acute seroconversion illness cohort studies.

Chronic HIV infection in adults

The natural history of HIV infection is summarised in Figure 6.1.

During recovery from the acute seroconversion illness the total lymphocyte count recovers, but the ratio of CD4 to CD8 cells inverts due to increased anti-HIV CD8 cell production and ongoing depletion of CD4 cells. CD4 cell depletion can be attributed to:

Figure 6.1 The natural history of HIV infection (adapted from Fauci, A.S. et al. 1996).

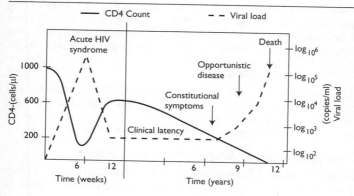

- HIV infection of activated anti-HIV CD4 cells;
- HIV-mediated cytopathic effect;
- CD4 cell apoptosis;
- destruction of infected CD4 cells by anti-HIV cytotoxic CD8 cells;
- impaired development of CD4 cells from lymphocyte stem cells.

Steady state viral dynamics

The viral set point represents the dynamic equilibrium between the production and clearance of viral particles by the immune system. Up to 10 billion viral particles are produced and cleared every day, even during the asymptomatic (clinically latent) phase of HIV infection. The half-life of viral particles in the circulation is estimated to be a few minutes, indicating that there is continual viral turnover. Most virions are produced by short-lived CD4 cells, which also show enhanced destruction and turnover of up to two billion cells/day. In addition long-lived cell populations of memory T-cells and macrophages also contribute to the viral pool. Some of these cells are latent and serve as viral reservoirs that pose an obstacle to viral eradication by antiretroviral therapy.

Profiles of disease progression

Figure 6.2 illustrates the role of HIV viral load in disease progression and transmission.

Rapid progressors

A small proportion of individuals develop AIDS within one to two years following HIV infection. This is associated with high levels of viral replication and a precipitous decline in CD4 numbers. Most of these individuals are unable to mount an effective immune response because of the depletion of CD4 cells, and are not able to control viral replication.

Intermediate progressors

The majority of HIV-infected individuals are able to regulate viral replication for many years because of an effective immune response. However, over time there is a steady decline of CD4 T-cell numbers and a slow erosion and eventual destruction of the immune system.

Slow progressors or long-term non-progressors

A small proportion of individuals are able to control HIV viral load very effectively without the assistance of antiretroviral therapy. Long-term

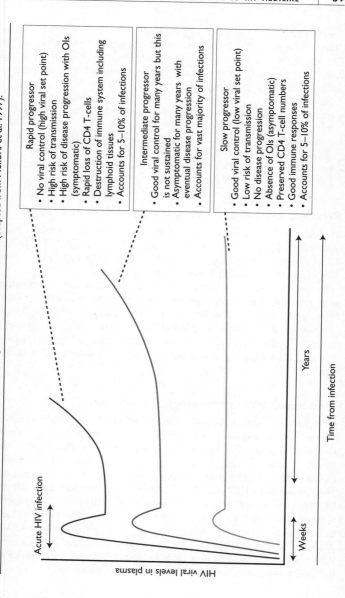

Figure 6.2 The central role of HIV viral load in prognosis and risk of infection (adapted from Mellors et al. 1997).

Rapid progressor
- No viral control (high viral set point)
- High risk of transmission
- High risk of disease progression with OIs (symptomatic)
- Rapid loss of CD4 T-cells
- Destruction of immune system including lymphoid tissues
- Accounts for 5–10% of infections

Intermediate progressor
- Good viral control for many years but this is not sustained
- Asymptomatic for many years with eventual disease progression
- Accounts for vast majority of infections

Slow progressor
- Good viral control (low viral set point)
- Low risk of transmission
- No disease progression
- Absence of OIs (asymptomatic)
- Preserved CD4 T-cell numbers
- Good immune responses
- Accounts for 5–10% of infections

Acute HIV infection

HIV viral levels in plasma

Weeks

Years

Time from infection

non-progressors (LTNPs) have low, and in many cases undetectable, plasma viral loads, with high CD4 counts and robust immune systems (see Chapter 3: The immune system and HIV infection). Many such individuals have been infected for more than 20 years. The reasons for slow disease progression appear to be multiple.

They include:

- genetic factors, such as a 32 base-pair (32 bp) deletion in CCR5 resulting in non-functional CCR5 receptors;
- virological factors, e.g. some people have been infected with replication-defective viruses; and
- immunological factors, i.e. strong immune responses, including neutralizing antibodies and cytotoxic T-cell responses.

Relationship between viral load and CD4 cell loss

Traditionally CD4 cell loss has been thought to be largely attributable to the viral load, with a higher viral load causing a more rapid CD4 decline. This concept holds for large cohorts of patients (Figure 6.3) but cannot fully explain CD4 cell loss in individuals (Figure 6.4).

An explanation for the phenomenon of rapid CD4 loss in individuals with low viral load could be increased immune activation (causing increased numbers of vulnerable CD4 cells) and abundant HIV replication in lymphoid tissue that is not reflected in the plasma viral load. Therefore the utility of the HIV viral load in determining the need for antiretroviral therapy is limited, and needs to be used with clinical data and serial CD4 counts.

Virological and immunological evolution

The viral set point represents the net effect of viral replication and immunological response. Once the viral set point has been established HIV evolves to evade cell-mediated and antibody mediated attack. HIV mutations are exceedingly common due to the lack of proof-reading capability in the reverse transcriptase enzyme and high rate of replication. Mutations in the V1, V2 and V3 regions of gp120 permit HIV to switch from CCR5 tropism to CXCR4 tropism (i.e. using the CXCR4 chemokine receptor to enter CD4 cells). This receptor switch from R5 to X4 virus (previously called syncitium-forming virus) is associated with more rapid CD4 depletion and occurs in about 50% of individuals. Reasons for the receptor switch are controversial and seem to be associated with the complex and dynamic relationship between HIV and the immune system.

Figure 6.3 Estimated annual CD4 cell count loss in untreated HIV-infected patients according to plasma HIV RNA level (adapted from Rodríguez, B. et al 2006).

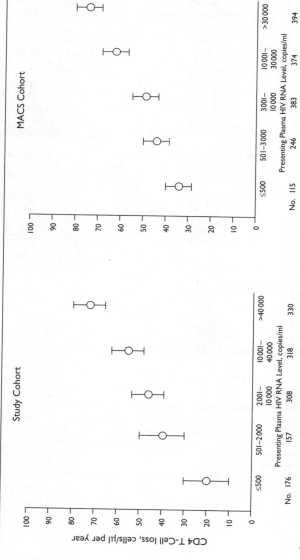

Data are presented as estimates of CD4 cell loss from random-effects models for each stratum with their associated 95% confidence intervals. HIV indicates human immunodeficiency virus; MACS, Multicenter AIDS Cohort Study.

Figure 6.4 Histograms of CD4 cell count change by categories of presenting plasma HIV RNA level among all patients in study cohort (adapted from Rodríguez, B. et al. 2006).

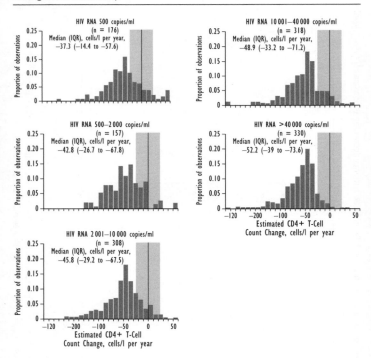

Data are model-based individual estimates of yearly CD4 cell decline obtained from random-effects modelling. The light-tinted region represents the −25 to 25 cells/μl per year range, an arbitrary reference to emphasise the slight increase in CD4 cell decline with increasing plasma HIV RNA levels. Note the extensive overlap across these frequency distributions. HIV indicates human immunodeficiency virus; IQR interquartile range.

Clinical progression of HIV disease

A period of good health lasting about six to eight years usually follows HIV seroconversion. During this time the integrity of the immune system is steadily eroded by qualitative and quantitative CD4 cell decline. Median survival from the time of HIV infection is about 10 years, and is similar in sub-Saharan Africa and the developed world. Importantly, patients over the age of 45 years tend to progress more rapidly and have shorter survival times. The progression of HIV disease in cohorts of individuals is represented by the revised 2006 WHO HIV staging system. Higher WHO stage reflects increasingly severe immune deficiency and risk of death (See Figure 6.5). The 2006 WHO staging system for HIV-infected adolescents and adults is shown in Appendix 1.

The incidence of common HIV-associated opportunistic infection in sub-Saharan African countries is shown in Table 6.1.

Figure 6.5 Survival of a cohort of South African HIV-infected patients stratified by WHO clinical stage, using 1990 WHO staging criteria (from Maartens, G. 1999).

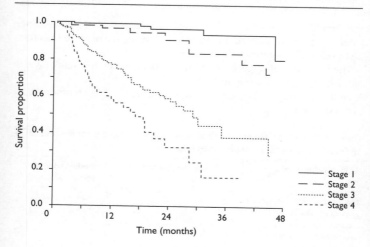

Table 6.1 Incidence of common HIV-associated conditions in sub-Saharan African countries

Infection	Incidence per 100 PY
Sepsis	16.2
Pneumonia	4.3–16.5
Tuberculosis	8.5–10 .4
Oral candidiasis	3.8–36.7
Malaria	5.7–33.8
Herpes zoster	7.3
Kaposi's sarcoma	5
Cryptococcal disease	2.2–4.0
Oesophageal candidiasis	3.5
Pneumocystis pneumonia	0.5–1.2
Toxoplasmosis	1.2
Non-Hodgkin's lymphoma	0.9

Importantly, the incidence of tuberculosis and malaria in HIV-infected adults varies in relation to the background incidence of these infections in the general community.

The incidence of opportunistic infections increases substantially with advanced HIV disease (Figure 6.6).

Table 6.2 shows the average CD4 count and prognosis of common AIDS-defining conditions.

Table 6.2 Median CD4 count and survival in months for the commonest AIDS-defining illnesses without antiretroviral therapy

AIDS-defining illness	Median CD4 count	Median survival (months)
Extra-pulmonary tuberculosis	111	> 24
Herpes simplex (chronic)	114	> 24
Kaposis's sarcoma	118	12
Oesophageal candidiasis	76	9
Pneumocystis pneumonia	39	7
Cryptococcal meningitis	32	7
HIV encephalopathy	121	3
HIV-wasting syndrome	45	1

Figure 6.6 Trends in the incidence of opportunistic infections by CD4 count strata (adapted from Holmes, C.B. et al. 2006).

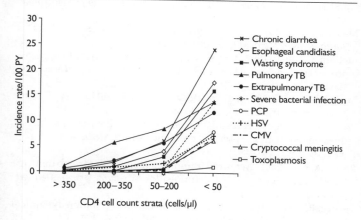

The natural history and prognosis of HIV-infection has been substantially improved by combination antiretroviral therapy (see Chapter 44: Adult antiretroviral therapy). However the incidence of tuberculosis remains high (3.5 per 100 person years after one year of antiretroviral therapy), and virological failure on antiretroviral therapy is associated with an increased risk of opportunistic infections. The epidemiology of HIV is continually changing and developing and the impact of widespread access to antiretroviral therapy remains to be assessed.

References and further reading:

Beyrer, C. 2007. 'HIV Epidemiology Update and Transmission Factors: Risks and Risk Contexts – 16th International AIDS Conference Epidemiology Plenary.' *Clinical Infectious Diseases*; 44: 981–987.

Centlivre, M. et al. 2007. 'In HIV-1 pathogenesis the die is cast during primary infection.' *AIDS*; 21:1–11.

Fauci, A.S. et al. 1996. 'Immunopathogenic mechanisms of HIV infection'. *Annals of Internal Medicine*; 124:654-63.

Holmes, C.B. et al. 2003. 'Review of Human Immunodeficiency Virus Type 1–Related Opportunistic Infections in Sub-Saharan Africa.' *Clinical Infectious Diseases*; 36:652–662.

Holmes, C.B. et al. 2006. 'CD4 Decline and Incidence of Opportunistic Infections in Cape Town, South Africa: Implications for Prophylaxis and Treatment.' *Journal of Acquired Immune Deficiency Syndrome*; 42:464–469

Maartens, G. 1999. 'Clinical progression of HIV infection in adults.' *South African Medical Journal*; 89:1255–1258.

Mellors, J.W. et al. 1997. 'Plasma viral load and CD4+ lymphocytes as prognostic markers of HIV-1 infection.' *Annals of Internal Medicine*; 126:946–54.

Morgan, D., and J.A.G. Whitworth, 2001. 'The natural history of HIV-1 infection in Africa.' *Nature Medicine*; 7 (2): 143–145.

Pope, M. et al. 2003. 'Transmission, acute HIV-1 infection and the quest for strategies to prevent infection.' *Nature Medicine*; 9:847–852.

Post, F.A. et al. 2001. 'Acquired immunodeficiency syndrome in Africa: Survival according to AIDS defining illness.' *South African Medical Journal*; 91:583–586.

Regoes, R.R. et al.'The HIV coreceptor switch: a population dynamical perspective.' *Trends in Microbiology*; 2005; 13:269–277.

Rodríguez, B. et al. 2006. 'Predictive Value of Plasma HIV RNA Level on Rate of CD4 T-Cell Decline in Untreated HIV Infection.' *Journal of the American Medical Association*; 296:1498–1506.

Van Oosterhout, J. J. G. et al. 2005. 'A Community-Based Study of the Incidence of Trimethoprim-Sulfamethoxazole–Preventable Infections in Malawian Adults Living With HIV.' *Journal of Acquired Immune Deficiency Syndrome*; 39:626–631.

World Health Organization. 2006. 'WHO case definitions of HIV for surveillance and revised clinical staging and immunological classification of HIV-related disease in adults and children.' Available: http://www.who.int/hiv/pub/guidelines/hivstaging/en/index.html (accessed 7 September 2007).

Appendix 6.1 WHO clinical staging of HIV/AIDS for adults and adolescents with confirmed HIV infection (reproduced with permission)

STAGE 1
- Asymptomatic
- Persistent generalized lymphadenopathy

STAGE 2
- Unexplained moderate weight loss (<10% of presumed or measured body weight)[1]
- Recurrent respiratory tract infections (sinusitis, tonsillitis, otitis media and pharyngitis)
- Herpes zoster
- Angular cheilitis
- Recurrent oral ulceration
- Papular pruritic eruptions
- Seborrhoeic dermatitis
- Fungal nail infections

STAGE 3
- Unexplained severe weight loss[2] (>10% of presumed or measured body weight)
- Unexplained chronic diarrhoea for longer than one month
- Unexplained persistent fever (above 37.5 °C intermittent or constant, for longer than one month)
- Persistent oral candidiasis
- Oral hairy leukoplakia
- Pulmonary tuberculosis
- Severe bacterial infections (such as pneumonia, empyema, pyomyositis, bone or joint infection, meningitis or bacteraemia)
- Acute necrotizing ulcerative stomatitis, gingivitis or periodontitis
- Unexplained anaemia (<8 g/dl), neutropenia (<0.5 × 109 per litre) and/or chronic thrombocytopenia (<50 × 109 per litre)

STAGE 4 (AIDS)[3]
- HIV wasting syndrome
- *Pneumocystis* pneumonia
- Recurrent severe bacterial pneumonia

- Chronic herpes simplex infection (orolabial, genital or anorectal of more than one month's duration or visceral at any site)
- Oesophageal candidiasis (or candidiasis of trachea, bronchi or lungs)
- Extrapulmonary tuberculosis
- Kaposi's sarcoma
- Cytomegalovirus infection (retinitis or infection of other organs)
- Central nervous system toxoplasmosis
- HIV encephalopathy
- Extrapulmonary cryptococcosis including meningitis
- Disseminated non-tuberculous mycobacterial infection
- Progressive multifocal leukoencephalopathy
- Chronic cryptosporidiosis
- Chronic isosporiasis
- Disseminated mycosis (extrapulmonary histoplasmosis or coccidio-mycosis)
- Recurrent septicaemia (including non-typhoidal *Salmonella*)
- Lymphoma (cerebral or B-cell non-Hodgkin)
- Invasive cervical carcinoma
- Atypical disseminated leishmaniasis
- Symptomatic HIV-associated nephropathy or symptomatic HIV-associated cardiomyopathy

Notes:

1 Assessment of body weight in pregnant woman needs to consider the expected weight gain of pregnancy.
2 Unexplained refers to where the condition is not explained by other causes.
3 Some additional specific conditions can also be included in regional classifications (such as reactivation of American trypanosomiasis [meningoencephalitis and/or myocarditis]) in the WHO Region of the Americas and penicilliosis in Asia).

The WHO's presumptive and clinical criteria for recognising HIV-related clinical events are given in http://www.who.int/hiv/pub/guidelines/hivstaging/en/index.html.

7 Counselling

Indigenous or traditional healers and Western counsellors and psychotherapists often operate in isolation from one another in southern Africa. While both see themselves as looking after the health of their clients, their background experience, training and worldviews may be very different. Yet it is necessary to work with both if HIV is to be contained in our society. Counsellors who have been trained in Western approaches need to develop an awareness of the differences in cultural traditions if they are to help clients from different backgrounds in a meaningful way. This involves familiarising themselves with, and being sympathetic to, their clients' beliefs. A basic premise for building rapport and demonstrating empathy for another person – a core counselling skill – is the ability to enter the client's world and to see the world through his or her eyes. If this is not done the counsellor may lack connection with the client, misunderstanding him or her, and a poor therapeutic relationship results. Counselling should always be based on the client's needs. One of the most effective ways to get people to work toward their own healing is to utilize what makes sense to them. People with deep traditional values and trust in indigenous healers may need to be encouraged to honour their beliefs while considering Western alternatives.

Why is counselling necessary?

A person who has tested HIV-positive may never have the same quality of life again. HIV-positive individuals who have positive and helpful experiences at the time of testing deal with their situations more satisfactorily and are better able to talk about their fears and feelings, and to plan for the future. Emotional and psychological support from the counsellor, family, and friends can help HIV-infected individuals live constructive and rewarding lives.

The aims of counselling

HIV counselling aims to:
- provide a supportive environment;
- help clients manage their problems and issues;

- explore coping skills that clients have used before and help them to develop new ones;
- empower clients to become self-sufficient in dealing with emerging issues and problems;
- counsel HIV-negative clients so that they know how to remain negative;
- counsel HIV-positive clients on how to avoid re-infection and how to prevent infecting others; and
- explore options with clients that will help them to bring about necessary changes in behaviour.

These options should include abstinence, monogamy (mutual faithfulness), and the correct use of condoms.

HIV testing

Every client who contemplates HIV testing should ideally be fully counselled by a professionally trained counsellor. However, in many situations this is neither possible nor practical. In most cases, the HIV test will be offered for medical reasons and so the immediate consent procedure will be carried out by the person ordering the test. The person doing the test must ensure that the patient is able to give informed consent. Wherever possible, this same person should give the result and ensure adequate post-test counselling. (See Appendix 7.1. for the counselling checklist.)

Both pre- and post-test counselling are very important. It is dangerous to compromise the counselling process and to take short cuts in the counselling room.

Pre-test counselling

The best counselling approach is client centred, where the focus is on what the client is feeling and experiencing. Again, in busy clinics this may be very difficult, but all reasonable efforts should be made to ensure a private session, free of interruptions, where confidentiality can be assured. The practitioner should be able to set aside adequate time.

When giving pre-test counselling, ensure that you do the following:

- Assure clients that both counselling and testing are confidential procedures.
- Discuss possible referral to a trained counsellor in the event of a positive result. Discuss the possibility of follow-up sessions.

- Provide information about HIV infection and transmission and its links to AIDS, sexually transmitted infections, and tuberculosis.
- Provide information on the technical aspects of testing, i.e. the window period and its implications and what the terms 'positive' and 'negative' mean.
- Discuss the implications of a positive or negative diagnosis.
- Clients should consider whom to tell (sexual partner/s) and whom not to tell (e.g. their employer, or third parties). Clients are not obliged to tell anyone apart from their sexual partners.
- Determine whether clients have coping resources and support systems in the event of a positive result.
- Help clients to contain their emotions as they deal with relationship issues.
- Provide clients with a sense of support and hope.
- It is advisable to document the patient's consent.

Always ask clients, during or following counselling, whether they have any questions about what has been discussed.

Issues that may arise during pre-test counselling

The following issues may arise during pre-test counselling:
- trust (e.g 'Is my partner faithful?');
- facts versus myths (e.g. many people still believe that you can become infected through casual contact, either socially or at work; clients often feel that they would somehow intuitively 'know' if their partner were HIV-positive);
- lack of empowerment and assertiveness;
- relationships, sexual and social problems, loneliness; and
- guilt or anger over past infidelity, and fantasies of punishment.

Post-test counselling, including giving results

Post-test counselling helps clients to work through the initial crisis and any other issues that may arise as a result of learning their HIV status.

Giving the results

- Give the results as soon as they arrive. Do not prolong the suspense with inane conversation.
- Give the results face to face, never telephonically and never through third parties.
- The person who conducted the pre-test counselling should, if at all possible, also give the result and post-test counselling. This is the person that the client trusts.
- If the result is positive, do not give it unless you can see the client again or have adequate referral resources. Delaying the next session makes your job more diffcult. The client may already have become depressed, and decisions such as not to inform the partner, or not to use condoms, may already have become entrenched.

HIV-negative result

If the HIV result is *negative*:

- Discuss the window period.
- Reinforce the message of prevention and safer sexual practices.
- Evaluate risk behaviour. This is an important opportunity for risk reduction counselling. This should be interactive and tailor made to the clients' experiences and reports.
- Discuss referral if necessary.

Ongoing counselling or referral may be recommended if the client:

- is disenfranchised or in an abusive relationship, and is in danger of becoming HIV-positive (in this type of situation help clients to review their options);
- indulges in risky behaviour and needs ongoing support;
- needs to be counselled for anxiety or depression; or
- requires assertiveness training.

This may be the only time that the counsellor can intervene to save another person's life.

HIV-positive result

First priority: Containment

In the first session the following should be addressed:

- Concentrate on managing the resultant crisis and addressing the client's immediate concerns.
- Discuss how the client will manage until the next follow-up appointment, which should ideally take place the next day to prevent depression.
- Once the client's emotions have been contained, reiterate information given in the pre-test counselling session, but be careful of information overload. At this point, clients often do not remember much besides the fact that they are HIV-positive and that there is at least one person to whom they can talk, namely their counsellor.
- If it is more practical to refer the patient for formal counselling at this point, introduce the concept to the client, obtain permission, and, if at all possible, introduce the client either personally, or by letter. Again, reinforce the fact that confidentiality will be maintained.

Second priority: Questions and concerns

This session should take place the day after the first session or soon after, if at all possible. Practitioners who cannot do this themselves should be aware of other counselling resources (i.e. other counsellors, social workers, support groups and so on) and know how to refer to them. *It would be useful to explore the clients' options for support that they could draw on during this time and the counsellor could work with this.*

Remember that:

- Clients will be feeling devastation and grief. Continue to contain these emotions.
- Answer any questions that clients may have, including the inevitable 'What do I do now?'
- Reassure them that you will be there for them, and will answer any questions or explain any procedures or terminology that they may not understand.
- Remind clients that they need to notify their partners. Remember that they will still be in shock and may not be ready to do this yet. Be sensitive to their emotional state. If necessary, plan a third session.

Next priority: Integration

The client should now be more receptive to information (repeated and new). Discuss some or all of the following:

- safer sex;
- the cost and availability of antiretroviral therapy;
- the importance of a well-balanced diet, rest, and exercise; and
- the need to eliminate alcohol, smoking, and drugs.

Ongoing counselling

Ongoing counselling helps the client to deal with issues such as partner notification, relationship difficulties, queries about health and treatment, and disclosure to others. With written permission, the counsellor may liaise with other caregivers. Develop a good working relationship, because you may be able to share contacts and referral sources.

The counsellor is a crucial source of support, because clients often feel that they cannot share the diagnosis with other people and they are initially very vulnerable.

The following issues need to be discussed with women who are, or plan to become, pregnant:
- the risk of transmitting HIV to the fetus during pregnancy and labour (see Chapter 46: Prevention of mother-to-child transmission of HIV);
- strategies to prevent mother-to-child transmission, including antiretroviral therapy for mother and infant, and elective Caesarean section;
- breastfeeding vs. formula feeding and the supply of formula postnatally (see Chapter 12: Infant feeding);
- testing the baby to ascertain its HIV status; and
- future contraception (see Chapter 27: Contraception).

Referral after testing

All HIV-positive clients should be informed of all available treatment choices and referred appropriately into HIV care. While not everyone will need antiretroviral therapy immediately, getting onto a care programme with regular monitoring and CD4 testing will ensure that antiretroviral and prophylactic medication is started at the correct time.

Issues that may arise in post-test counselling

Crisis situations

A crisis is an event that upsets the balance of your daily routine and causes trauma that has a negative impact on you and on your ability to function normally.

Receiving an HIV-positive diagnosis is very traumatic and places the client in a crisis situation. This may be compounded by earlier trauma, such as discovering a partner's infidelity or realising that an intimate experience has resulted in HIV infection.

Post-traumatic stress disorder

Post-traumatic stress disorder occurs as a result of major psychological trauma. The individual typically experiences intrusive, recurring thoughts and distressing dreams. Increased arousal results in insomnia and poor concentration. The individual may avoid stimuli associated with the trauma and block certain aspects of the experience from memory. The symptoms last for at least a month and may require referral for more specialised help.

Rage reaction

If clients have not been prepared emotionally and psychologically, they may feel intense rage when they receive a positive result. This may result in the following behaviour patterns:

- The client discloses the result prematurely and is stigmatised and ostracised.
- The client becomes depressed and decides to commit suicide or to injure the person believed to have transmitted the infection.
- The client decides 'If I'm going down I'll take others with me,' and sets out to infect others.

Rage reaction is a risk unless proper emotional and psychological support is given. Simply providing the client with information and numerous facts, while extracting information, may make rage reaction more likely. A client needs to be reassured that these emotional reactions are normal and the counsellor's capacity to contain this will be very important. It is useful to go through the various stages of the grieving process with a client – if they are stable enough to hear this – as it prepares them in the anticipation of various shifts in their emotional states.

Denial

Some clients come to believe that the doctors 'made a mistake' and that they are, in fact, HIV-negative. Destructive behaviour may result, such as 'shopping around' different practitioners.

Further counselling options

Couple counselling

HIV infection invariably involves couples and throws couples into crisis. When counselling a couple you should do the following:

- Help the couple to take stock of their relationship and to build up trust and honesty.
- Contain emotions related to infidelity and betrayal.
- Help the couple to support each other and to work as a unit so that they can face the extended family and make decisions about issues such as disclosure, infant feeding, and condom use.

Family counselling

Family counselling helps family members to remain united in a crisis, rather than each tackling the problem alone, or fighting with each other:

- Allow all family members to give their opinions openly without attacking or being attacked.
- Questions should be asked and answered without recrimination.
- The process of family counselling could be a liberating and positive experience for all.

If family members cannot be reconciled, it may be necessary to remove the person with HIV/AIDS to a safer environment. Again, recognize the need and know what resources are available.

Support groups

These groups are often run in the community by non-governmental organizations or self-help groups:

- A support group should provide a safe and caring environment in which people with HIV/AIDS can support and encourage each other, share ideas and experiences, and empower themselves.

- The group facilitator helps the group to generate a programme that should include a variety of structured activities, and should facilitate the discussion of personal problems.
- If members are at various stages of HIV infection, those at more advanced stages are able to empathize with, and support, those at earlier stages.
- The members of the support group are sometimes the only people, apart from the counsellor, who know an individual's status. Confidentiality must be assured.

Counselling and the healthcare worker

Regardless of how experienced a counsellor you are, you never become comfortable with telling someone that he or she is HIV-positive. This process does not get better with time. When a health care worker is required to give three or more positive results a day, the stress is extreme. For this reason, among others, any practitioner or counsellor should have support. Practitioners should know when, and to whom, they can appeal for help when a counselling situation is difficult, and they should be able to recognize the symptoms of stress related to this type of counselling. (See Chapter 60: Healthcare worker burnout.)

References and further reading

Bor, M. et al. 1993. *Theory and practice of HIV counselling: A systematic approach*. New York: Brunner/Mazel.

Castle, C. rev. by K. Attawell, and S. Long. 1999. *HIV testing: A practical approach*. London: Healthlink Worldwide.

Green, J., and A. McCreaner. eds. 1989. *Counselling in HIV infection and AIDS*. London: Blackwell Scientific.

UNAIDS. 1999. *Counselling and voluntary HIV testing for pregnant women in high HIV prevalence countries: Elements and issues*. Geneva: UNAIDS.

Van Dyk, A. 2001. *HIV/AIDS care and counselling: A multidisciplinary approach*. Cape Town: Maskew Miller Longman.

Appendix 7.1 Checklist for pre- and post-test counselling

Pre-test counselling checklist

- Reassure the client about the confidential nature of the exchange.
- Provide general information about HIV and discuss the transmission routes.
- Explain what the test is, how long it takes, and the blood-drawing procedure.
- Discuss the 'window period'.
- Differentiate between a 'positive' and a 'negative' result.
- Explain the advantages and disadvantages of knowing one's HIV status.
- Discuss the implications of a positive test (e.g. pregnancy, work, etc.).
- Discuss the implications of a negative test.
- Explain the risk factors for HIV infection.
- Answer questions and clarify issues.

Post-test counselling checklist

- Give the results face to face.
- Encourage the client to attend with a close relative, friend, or partner.

Negative result

- Discuss the window period.
- Discuss risk reduction.
- Offer follow-up testing.

Positive result

- Contain emotions.
- Give support.
- Reassure.
- Reiterate HIV facts.
- Discuss safer sex and risk reduction.
- Discuss partner notification.
- Provide information on access to medical care.
- Provide information on the availability of antiretroviral therapy.
- Discuss lifestyle changes (e.g. diet, exercise, alcohol, smoking).

8 Sex and sexuality

Before looking at the very important subject of sex and sexuality, there are a few key messages that must be remembered:

- Most HIV-positive patients will want to have a sex life.
- HIV-positive patients are often overlooked during HIV prevention programme planning.
- Do not avoid taking a sexual history.
- Discussing sex is not just about fertility choices.

Sexuality

Sex is a basic human need. In southern Africa, the vast majority of adult infections are acquired sexually. Health care workers often find the topic difficult and embarrassing to broach with patients, but as HIV is largely sexually transmitted, this is essential. Focused HIV prevention interventions in HIV-positive patients ('prevention with positives') are one of the neglected areas of prevention, and health care workers should aim to integrate knowledge of safe sex into broader health messages aimed at HIV-positive patients in the clinic.

Sexual history taking, orientation, terminology and culture

This aspect of history taking is often neglected in clinical training. Taking a sexual history may be awkward, as HIV status is often known by the clinician, and the clinical utility of a detailed sexual history is seen as unimportant. Furthermore, cultural, age disparities and language difficulties between patients and health care providers can make obtaining this history very time-consuming. Indeed, some aspects of a sexual history may not be relevant, and common sense with a directed intelligent history is always more useful than set questions. As mentioned above, a directed sexual history may allow for effective counselling about safe sex.

Identification of sexual orientation is complex, especially as individual self-identification of orientation may not fit classical classifications. For instance, in the US, the 'down-low' phenomenon, where men who have sex with men and are often married to women, characterize themselves as 'heterosexual', is well described. There are anecdotal reports of similar self-characterization among southern African men in certain situations.

Terminology should be used carefully when discussing issues with people from different cultures. Healthcare workers should be mindful that a term as simple as 'faithful' was found to mean 'primary partner' rather than implying exclusivity in one South African study. Similarly, discussion about different safe sex practices may require careful and explicit exploration as certain topics, such as masturbation and even use of condoms may be misunderstood.

Professionalism on the part of the health care provider allows patients to feel more comfortable. Patients are likely to pick up on health care worker discomfort, and this may compromise effective history taking. Health-care workers should be very conscious of their own values and prejudices when taking a history.

Practical tips include:

- Try to speak to the patient alone – this can be impossible when inter-preters are used, which may compromise history taking. Ensure interruptions are kept to a minimum.
- Gentle introductory questions that set the scene for more probing questions – a question on the desire for children may lead to a discussion on current sexual partners and sexual practices; inquiring about the use of condoms may lead to an understanding of sexual orientation.
- Questions that allow the patient to qualify issues – 'Do you use condoms for both women and men?', or 'Is there something about your sex life you would like to change?' may also be useful.
- Avoid making assumptions about patients' sex lives.

A history specific to a patient's sex life, along with the usual attention to sexually transmitted infections (STIs), gynaecological, obstetric or urological history, should include:

- Sexual orientation.
- Relationship status – including plans for finding new partners.
- Sexual activity – ill patients often are not sexually active, and this may change.
- Fertility decisions – it is important that this aspect is addressed sub-sequently, as decisions on the part of the patient may change.
- Contraceptive use – explore consistency, especially in the use of condoms.
- Alcohol and substance use during sex – see below.

Sexual risk taking

The decision to have sex is seldom rational or considered. Education campaigns about sexual risk have yielded often disappointing results, with poor correlation between knowledge of risk and actual behaviour change. Health care workers, in particular doctors, appear to have a high impact in terms of other risky behaviours, such as smoking, inactivity and poor diet. Recently, research on issuing a behaviour 'prescription', e.g. – agreeing not to have sex when intoxicated, insisting on condom use during sex – has been found to help patients to target specific high risk behaviours.

HIV testing and 'know your status' campaigns have been a central part of HIV prevention programmes. Sexual risk-taking appears to significantly decrease once patients are made aware that they are HIV positive. However, paradoxically, several studies have suggested that testing HIV-negative usually does not improve risk taking, and may even lead to behavioural disinhibition. Health care workers are well placed in HIV services to intervene in terms of improved risk reduction counselling, and should be mindful that patients testing HIV negative may need additional attention.

Alcohol use is strongly associated with disinhibition and greater sexual risk taking. Casual sex, non-use of condoms and higher rates of risky sex are directly correlated with alcohol use. In addition, sexual assault appears to be more likely if alcohol is involved, possibly due to disinhibition in the assailant, and because the person assaulted may be less aware of potentially dangerous circumstances. Similarly, other recreational drugs, such as cocaine and crystal methamphetamine (tik), may lead to increased disinhibition and risk taking.

Sexual networks have received much attention recently, pointing to a complex system of sexual relations and behaviours within southern African communities. Practically, this has bearing on prevention programmes. HIV is rarely (although commonly assumed to be) spread via contact with sex workers. Transmission appears to be a function of the number of concurrent sexual relationships within a community. This means that married couples and people in long term relationships, often presumed to have single partners by health care workers, often have other stable partners. This understanding, coupled with newer understandings that HIV is very infectious in the first few months of infection, allows us to understand how HIV can rapidly spread if introduced into a stable sexual network. Practically, partner reduction and consistent condom use with partners appears to be an important message.

Special issues

- Discordant couples: Health care workers often view discordant couples as a problem purely from a fertility standpoint, where desire to fall pregnant may involve unprotected sex. However, sex between discordant couples may be understandably stressful, and may need directed interventions and counselling regarding safer forms of sex, as well as emphasis on consistent condom use (which is difficult and uncommon in long-term relationships).

- Children should not be neglected. Increasingly, children born with HIV are entering puberty and adulthood, as antiretroviral therapy becomes widely available. Sexual debut may be very complex in these patients, and careful discussion regarding prevention, dating and disclosure should be initiated by the health care worker, noting that care givers may not be comfortable or prepared to do this.

- Changes when on antiretrovirals. Patients should be counselled about the series of events that occur on initiation of antiretrovirals, which may have an impact on their sex lives. Libido, especially in patients with profound immunosuppression, may return unexpectedly, accompanied by weight gain, improved skin condition, and improved self image, giving the patient added sexual confidence. Change in body shape on antiretrovirals, specifically lipoatrophy and lipodystrophy, may have significant negative impacts on self-image.

- Finding a sexual partner. Sex is a basic human need. Finding a sexual partner is complex for HIV-positive people, especially where serosorting (indirectly or directly signifying one's HIV status with a view to having a relationship and/or sex with someone with the same HIV status) does not occur. Patients may find partners through clinics, support groups or even specialist websites. Ideally, barrier contraception should be encouraged between concordant couples to prevent infection with different HIV strains, and to prevent transmission of antiretroviral resistance.

- Attitudes to condom usage when one or both partners are on antiretrovirals. These couples often presume that they do not require condoms due to low risk of transmission. Risk of resistant viruses should be discussed.

- Sexual violence and assault: This is very common in southern Africa, although links to HIV risk are not clear. Post-exposure prophylaxis, where appropriate, should be accompanied by supportive counselling.

- Depression: This is common in any chronic illness, and has been shown to be linked to added sexual risk taking, decreased adherence, erectile dysfunction and poor quality of life.

References and further reading

Tomlinson, J. 1998. 'ABC of sexual health: Taking a sexual history'. *British Medical Journal* 317:1573–1576

Faulder, G.S., Riley, S.C., Stone, N., Glasier, A. 2004. 'Teaching sex education improves medical students' confidence in dealing with sexual health issues'. *Contraception* 70:135–139

Andrews, W.C. 2000. 'Approaches to Taking a Sexual History'. *Journal of Women's Health and Gender-Based Medicine*; 9 (supplement 1).

Kripke, C.C. and L. Vaias. 1994. 'The importance of taking a sensitive sexual history.' *Journal of the American Medical Association*; 271: 713.

9 Preventing HIV infection: individuals and populations

Sub-Saharan Africa and especially southern Africa bears the brunt of this pandemic. Although the picture in sub-Saharan Africa is largely one of a 'stable' epidemic where AIDS related mortality is matched by the incidence of new infections, some countries in the southern regions have continued to see increasing HIV prevalence. In this light, there is an urgent need for new approaches to HIV prevention. The focus here is on interventions that address sexually transmitted HIV, since the vast majority of new HIV infections in Africa are through heterosexual contact, and other important HIV prevention interventions (such as blood safety interventions and the prevention of mother-to-child transmission) are not included.

Prevention lessons from HIV epidemiology in Africa

Our understanding of prevention interventions can be framed by two general principles from infectious diseases epidemiology. First, the transmission dynamics of HIV can be described in terms of the basic reproductive number (R_o), which represents the number of secondary infections emanating from a single infectious individual (i.e. a primary case) introduced into a population of susceptible individuals. The equation: $R_o = \beta c D$ shows how the basic reproduction number R_o is influenced by the probability of HIV transmission between individuals (β, a function of both the infectiousness of the primary case and the susceptibility of uninfected individuals), as well as the number of sexual partners (c) and the duration of infectiousness (D) of the primary case. Evidence from different parts of Africa suggests that variability in both the transmission probablility and sexual partner changes are important in explaining the variable course of HIV epidemics in different regions.

The second key HIV prevention principle suggested by infectious diseases epidemiology is that reductions in transmission risk among the most sexually active members of the population can have a disproportionately large impact on the HIV epidemic. In other words, the most efficient and effective prevention strategies should be targeted at specific population groups where HIV acquisition risk is high.

Epidemiological data on the distribution and causes of HIV/AIDS in South Africa indicate the scope of interventions that are needed to stem the spread of the epidemic. Just as the causes of the epidemic can be thought of in biomedical, behavioural and structural terms, the interventions to address the epidemic can also be conceptualized at each of these levels.

Biomedical interventions

Most scientific research on HIV prevention is focused on biomedical interventions that reduce the transmission of HIV. A number of interventions with a biological basis for preventing the transmission of HIV infection have been shown to be effective in reducing HIV transmission, including antiretroviral drugs for reducing mother-to-child transmission of the virus, treatment of bacterial sexually transmitted infections (STIs) such as syphilis, gonorrhoea, chlamydia, and post-exposure prophylaxis using antiretrovirals. Each of these interventions should be available through the public sector, and each is likely to play a role in reducing the transmission of HIV in areas where they are widely available and accessible. For instance, there is preliminary evidence that the prevalence of paediatric HIV infection has declined in recent years, probably due to the success of prevention of mother-to-child transmission (PMTCT) programmes within antenatal care. Convincing evidence now exists for the benefit of needle exchange and clean syringes in methadone clinics, called 'harm reduction' where HIV transmission risk is related to shared intravenous drug use equipment. In addition, the supply of HIV free blood and blood products as well as sterile needles and syringes for injections and universal precautions in hospitals has much reduced nosocomial transmission of HIV.

Male circumcision

The role of male circumcision in the prevention of HIV and STI acquisition has been shown in a number of cross sectional studies from different parts of Africa, supported by more recent data suggesting reductions in HIV transmission among HIV serodiscordant couples where the man is circumcised. In addition to this epidemiologic data, there are biologically plausible mechanisms for the observed reduction in HIV acquisiton among circumcised males. The inner mucosa of the foreskin is rich in HIV target cells, e.g. dendritic cells, CD4+ T- cells, and macrophages that express relevant HIV binding receptors such as chemokine receptors (CCR5) and DC-SIGN. By contrast the external foreskin is keratinized and much less vulnerable to HIV infection. After circumcision, the only exposed mucosa is in the urethral meatus. Removal of the foreskin's target cells and receptors can represent a direct biological mechanism of protection.

Three randomized control trials (RCTs) have recently been initiated in sub-Saharan Africa to explore the efficacy of male circumcision. The results of the RCT conducted in Orange Farm, South Africa demonstrated a 60% reduction in the risk of acquiring HIV infection over 21 months of follow-up in newly circumcised, 18-24-year-old males. The implementation of this modality in the general population will still require further investigation of a range of issues including acceptability, rates and types of adverse events of the procedure, cost and logistics of introduction, and importantly the long term effect of circumcision on behaviours such as partner reduction and condom use .

Vaccines

An effective preventive HIV vaccine would provide the best method for controlling the HIV pandemic, especially in under resourced countries and so any successful vaccine will need to be applicable to all regions regardless of virus subtype and be licensed for use in all age groups, including older children and adolescents. After almost 20 years of HIV vaccine clinical trials, and numerous phase 1 and 2 studies, there are a variety of vaccine strategies.

For a number of years the vaccine pipeline was limited to simple gp 120 or gp 160 proteins based on laboratory strains of the virus, synthetic peptides and simple pox virus HIV recombinant vectors. The constructs currently in the pipeline include gp 120 constructs based on clinical HIV isolates, bird virus vectors and other vectors such as modified vaccinia Ankara and Venezuelan Equine Encephalitis virus replicon expressing multiple HIV genes, and different constructs of naked DNA. Other strategies have included live-attenuated vectors containing a variety of HIV genes. These attenuated vectors include adenovirus, associated adenovirus and sindbis.

The lack of an immune correlate of protection (clear type of immune response needed to provide protection against HIV) and the lack of an adequate animal model that can mimic human disease infection poses significant scientific challenges to developing a successful vaccine. In addition HIV-1 genetic diversity may complicate the development of a globally relevant HIV vaccine. Diversity may be addressed by the development of vaccine candidates comprised of cocktails of proteins of regional variants with the assumption that the immune responses elicited by a multiclade, multigene vaccine will be of sufficient cross-reactivity to protect against a range of wild type strains.

Current HIV vaccine candidates elicit reasonably potent cellular immune responses, but very low levels of neutralizing antibodies. Cytotoxic T-lymphocytes are part of the cellular immune response that controls viral replication. Used as preventive vaccines they may thus control viral replication and modify disease in an individual who has breakthrough infection leading to less morbidity, longer time to AIDS and possibly less HIV transmission. Antibodies provide the first line to the immune system defense and neutralizing antibodies inactivate or prevent the virus making contact with target cells, providing the best possibility to abort or prevent infection. Neutralizing antibody stimulation would thus be a highly sought after characteristic in a preventive vaccine but has, to date, been very difficult to achieve.

Prime-boosting is a new combination strategy that seeks to enhance vaccine responses by invoking various types of immunity. A typical strategy would involve priming with a naked DNA vaccine, which would be expected to do little more than stimulate production of memory T-cells, followed by boosting with a live vector/protein, which would then stimulate a strong cellular response as well as neutralizing antibodies.

Microbicides

In view of the problems associated with male condoms, developing HIV prevention technologies that are under the control of women is an important avenue for HIV prevention. One of the most promising technologies currently in large scale human trials is vaginal microbicides. A microbicide is a substance formulated significantly to reduce transmission of HIV and other STIs when applied topically to the vagina or rectum. They can be formulated as gels, creams, films, suppositories, sponges or vaginal rings, or used in conjunction with other barrier methods such as the diaphragm or cervical cap. The modes of action of microbicides include antiviral activities, barrier action between the pathogens and vaginal and rectal tissue, or modification of vaginal or rectal milieu that makes HIV infection less likely. Compared to male or female condoms, microbicides are expected to interfere less with intimacy and sexual pleasure and be more discrete.

Although microbicides are primarily being developed for use by women, it is possible that they may have a bidirectional protective effect for men as well as women. As women's reproductive intentions alter throughout their lives, both contraceptive and non-contraceptive microbicides are being developed. A microbicide that is protective for partners practising anal sex is also in development, as such a product could be used for both heterosexual and MSM sex. Importantly a microbicide shown to be safe and effective should be easily available over the counter.

Barrier methods

Currently, the most widely available tool for prevention of HIV infection during sexual intercourse is the male condom. Male condoms afford a high degree of protection: consistent and correct male condom use reduces HIV transmission by 80%-97%. However, in many parts of Africa, condoms are not acceptable as they act as a contraceptive and may also interfere with sexual pleasure and reduce intimacy. Men predominantly control use of male condoms during sexual intercourse, and many women do not have the power to negotiate condom use in their relationships. As a result, there have been significant recent developments in other types of barrier methods to prevent the sexual transmission of HIV.

The female condom

Numerous studies have shown that the female condom is an acceptable method for many women and men, and is a valuable alternative for women whose partners refuse to use male condoms. Unlike the male condom, the female condom can be inserted some time before sex, and does not depend on the same degree of male cooperation for its successful use. The female condom is a soft, loose fitting polyurethane sheath that covers the vagina, cervix and external genitalia. Laboratory studies have shown that the female condom is effective at preventing the transmission of viruses and bacteria. While there is less clinical data available than for the male condom, the WHO has agreed that the female condom is effective in preventing HIV and other STIs.

Cervical barrier methods

In the last few years, interest has grown in cervical barrier methods as potential technologies for HIV prevention. The cervix is covered by a single cell layer of columnar epithelium compared to the stratified squamous epithelium of the vagina. As a result cervical columnar epithelium is more friable than the stratified squamous epithelium of the vaginal walls, making it more susceptible to mechanical disruption. This anatomical vulnerability is compounded by the increased presence around the cervix of surface receptors targeted by HIV as well as inflammatory cytokines, both of which may also facilitate HIV infection. Additional evidence from primate experiments has shown that cervical epithelium is the first site of infection after vaginal exposure to Simian Immunodeficiency Virus.

Based on this evidence, barrier methods that protect the cervix specifically (such as the diaphragm, the sponge and the cervical cap) may be useful tools for HIV prevention, and there are a number of trials of this topic underway in southern Africa.

Herpetic genital ulcer disease control

The role of bacterial STIs (including syphilis, chlamydia and gonorrhoea) in increasing the risk of HIV infection are well-established. HSV-2 is also an important risk factor for heterosexually-transmitted HIV. HSV-2 is the most common STI worldwide, typically causing recurrent episodes of genital ulcers, although a large proportion of infected individuals are asymptomatic.

Genital ulcers act as a portal of entry or exit for HIV and activated lymphocytes, including CD4 cells, are frequently recruited to these sites of inflammation and are primed to receive or present HIV at the site of ulceration. A recent meta-analysis of 19 epidemiological studies showed that prevalent HSV-2 may increase the risk of HIV acquisition in men and in women by as much as three-fold even after adjustment for sexual behaviour, and that HSV-2 may account for as many as 38%–60% of new HIV infections in women, and 8%-49% in men in the general population.

Controlling HSV-2 may have an important impact on HIV incidence, particularly in settings where HSV-2 prevalence is high. Currently the options for herpes control are limited to a few strategies: primary prevention through condom use and behavioural modification will be useful in those populations that are uninfected, e.g. young people. Treatment of HSV-2, primarily with aciclovir, may also have an effect on HIV and randomised control trials are currently underway to investigate this.

Sociobehavioural interventions

In addition to the biomedically-focused interventions discussed above, behavioural interventions remain a valuable strategy for reducing new infections. We know what specific behaviours contribute to the spread of HIV in South Africa (large numbers of new sexual partners and unprotected sexual contacts) and yet the virus continues to spread. Two sets of theories have been used to explain and predict the spread of HIV and attempts to curb this spread.

The first set focuses on individual behaviour and behaviour change, and discusses the ways in which intentions, attitudes and beliefs affect health behaviour. The second set involves understanding the broader social issues that affect the epidemic. For example, it seems clear that an important part of what drives the epidemic is not individual intentions and behaviours but broader social, economic and cultural conditions. Women, for example, may find themselves in a situation in which, for reasons of immediate survival, they may be forced into transactional sexual relationships with men that involve unprotected sex. A key challenge for those wishing to reduce the spread of HIV through behaviour change is to design interventions that bridge the divide between individual models of behaviour change and those that focus on broader social issues. Health practitioners, by virtue of their training, are often better at thinking about individual level issues and interventions than in intervening and assessing interventions at a broad social level.

However, the need for both levels does remain. At a practical level, voluntary counselling and testing (VCT) represents an important strategy for changing sexual behaviors. There is substantial evidence that appropriate risk reduction messages provided during VCT can have a significant impact in reducing high risk behaviours among individuals who wish to be tested for HIV. In one multi-country trial, including sites in Kenya and Tanzania, there was a more than 30% reduction in unprotected intercourse among individuals receiving VCT, compared to individuals who received health promotion messages only. This study and related research has contributed to what some policy makers have called a 'serostatus approach' to addressing the HIV epidemic, in which HIV testing is a critical first step that can be used to target services for HIV prevention (for HIV-negative individuals) or care and treatment (for HIV-positive individuals).

Conclusion

Although prevention efforts need to be redoubled in sub-Saharan Africa where prevalence rates are so high, there is at least some hope for success. The most recent UNAIDS report on the Global AIDS epidemic states: 'Among the notable new trends are the recent declines in national HIV prevalence in two sub-Saharan African countries (Kenya and Zimbabwe), urban areas of Burkina Faso, and similarly in Haiti, in the Caribbean, alongside indications of significant behavioural change – including increased condom use, fewer partners and delayed sexual debut.' However, there are indications that in regions where HIV rates have declined, a resurgence in new infections, particularly among specific risk groups, for example young MSM populations is occurring. Furthermore, we do not yet know the potential impact on transmission and prevalence that increasing global access to antiretroviral therapy may have, particularly in sub-Saharan Africa.

References and further reading

Asamoah-Odei, E., Garcia Calleja, J.M., Boerma, J.T. 2004. 'HIV prevalence and trends in sub-Saharan Africa: no decline and large subregional differences'. *Lancet* 364: 35.

Anderson, R. M. and R.M. May. 1991. *Infectious Diseases of Humans: Dynamics and control*. Oxford: Oxford University Press.

Gregson, S., Garnett, G.P., Nyamukapa, C.A. et al. 2006. 'HIV decline associated with behaviour change in eastern Zimbabwe'. *Science* 311 (5761):664–6.

Buve, A., Weiss, H.A., Laga, M. et al. 2001. 'The epidemiology of trichomoniasis in women in four African cities'. *AIDS* 15 (Suppl 4): S89–96.

Auvert, B., Taljaard, D., Lagarde, E., Sobngwi-Tambekou, J., Sitta, R., Puren, A. 2005. 'Randomized, Controlled Intervention Trial of Male Circumcision for Reduction of HIV Infection Risk: The ANRS 1265 Trial'. *PLoS Medicine* 2(11):e298.

McMichael, A.J. 2006.'HIV vaccines'. *Annual Review of Immunology*; 24:227–55.

Abdool-Karim, S.S. and Q. Abdool-Karim (Eds) 2005. *HIV/AIDS in South Africa*. Cape Town. Cambridge University Press.

D'Cruz, O.J. and F.M. Uckun. 2006. 'Dawn of non-nucleoside inhibitor-based anti-HIV microbicides'. *Journal of Antimicrobial Chemotherapy*; 57(3):411–23.

Minnis, A.M. and N.S. Padian. 2005. 'Effectiveness of female controlled barrier methods in preventing sexually transmitted infections and HIV: current evidence and future research directions'. *Sexually Transmitted Infections*; 81(3):193–200.

Stone, A. 2002. 'Microbicides: A new approach to preventing HIV and other sexually transmitted infections'. *Nature review*; 1:977–985.

Freeman, E.E., Weiss, H.A., Glynn, J.R. 2006. 'Herpes simplex virus 2 infection increases HIV acquisition in men and women: systematic review and meta-analysis of longitudinal studies'. *AIDS*; 20(1):73-83.

Wasserheit, J. 1992. 'Epidemiologic synergy : interrelationships between human immunodeficiency virus infection and other sexually transmiited diseases'. *Sexually transmitted diseases*; 19:61–77.

PART 2

Approach to HIV infection in children

10 Clinical assessment (paediatric) 95
11 Childhood vaccination 109
12 HIV and infant feeding 121
13 Expressed breastfeeding in hospital 130
14 Nutrition 145
15 Diarrhoea 152
16 Paediatric tuberculosis 160
17 Sexual abuse 174
18 Setting up an HIV/AIDS clinic for children 178

Clinical assessment (paediatric)

In 1983, Rubinstein et al from the Albert Einstein College of Medicine, the Bronx, New York, described acquired immunodeficiency and reversed T4/T8 ratios in infants born to drug-addicted mothers, three of whom had AIDS. They invoked mother-to-child transmission (MTCT) of an unidentified transmissible agent. Since then, HIV has been identified and has become a major cause of mortality and morbidity throughout the world, especially in resource-poor areas.

Epidemiology

In 2009 the seroprevalence of HIV among antenatal clinic attendees of public institutions in South Africa was 29.4%, showing a persistent annual increase from 0.7% in 1990 until 2004 and then stabilising at this high level. With approximately one million births per year, this translates into 330 000 'at risk' deliveries per year. An actuarial model predicted 41 000 infants infected during the first six weeks of life and an additional 28 000 through breastfeeding in 2004 (www.assa.org.za). The perinatal transmission rate from mother to infant, in the absence of intervention, varies between 20% and 30%. Breastfeeding, especially when given as part of mixed feeding, contributes an additional 10 to 15%.

Programmes to reduce transmission have been implemented in South Africa since 2003, with variable success. Under the best circumstances, transmission can be reduced to between 2% and 3%. Because of the high seroprevalence of HIV in antenatal clinic attendees, even with access to effective programmes, relatively large numbers of HIV-infected children will still be born. A 2% transmission rate translates into approximately 6 000 HIV-infected infants per year.

Natural history and prognosis

In the absence of antiretroviral therapy, HIV infection is usually fatal. Even in the absence of antiretroviral therapy, outcome is far better in resource-rich than in resource-poor countries. For example, in the pre-antiretroviral era, the median survival in Florida was 38 months from the time of diagnosis (usually under the age of two years). In a meta-analysis of cohorts from nine African vertical transmission prevention studies, 60%

of infected infants had died by two years of age. Without antiretroviral therapy, extended survival is possible with supportive therapy and prevention of opportunistic infections even in relatively resource-poor communities. Recent data shows extremely high HIV-related mortality in the first year of life, most notable, however, in the first four months in the absence of antiretroviral therapy.

Pathogenesis – differences between children and adults

The immune system reaches maturity between two and six years of age, explaining why children have more rapid disease progression than adults. In adults plasma HIV RNA declines to set point within four months. The process may take as long as five years in children. Thymic infection, defined by a CD4 count below 1 814 or CD8 below 904 cells μl, in the first six months of age carries a severe prognosis. Differences in disease presentation between adults and children are shown in Figure 10.1. In the infant, age is the most important determinant of HIV-related disease.

Modes of transmission

- MTCT: This accounts for by far the majority of infections in children (>95%) either *in utero*, perinatally or through breastfeeding.
- Sexual abuse: Approximately 1% of children attending the 'Family Clinic for HIV' at Tygerberg Academic Hospital, Cape Town have been infected through sexual abuse.
- Transfusion of blood and related products: This route has been virtually eliminated through the improved screening of donors. Nevertheless, a small number of individuals may be infected due to failure of detection of viraemic donors prior to antibody production. With the recent introduction of nucleic acid testing and combined antigen-antibody detection assays, this route should be eliminated.
- Horizontal: A small number of infants with seronegative parents have been identified. One should consider that the infant may not be the offspring of the parents. Poorly labelled expressed breast milk from HIV-infected mothers can inadvertently be given to uninfected hospitalized infants. Surrogate breastfeeding is also possible. Nosocomial transmission through contaminated medical equipment is possible. 'Single-use' razor blades are necessary for shaving the scalps of infants prior to insertion of intravenous infusions. It is incorrect practice to re-use the blades after casual attempts at disinfection with

Figure 10.1 Relationship between CD4 depletion over time and onset of HIV-induced pathology and concomitant infections in (A) adults and (B) children

ADULT

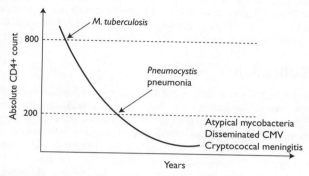

CHILDREN

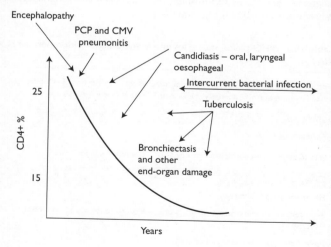

an antiseptic solution. Therefore, a history of a scalp vein infusion or other 'minor' surgical procedures should be sought. Sterilization of endoscopes is a complex procedure, requiring specific training. Although seldom documented, syringes may be used on more than one occasion, especially when giving the same medication to more than one patient at a time. Sterile fluids retained for multi-use, such as heparin-saline used in ICUs to flush indwelling lines, may become contaminated with HIV and other blood-borne viruses when a syringe connected to a patient's line is used to draw saline. Pre-mastication of food by parents and caregivers for weaning toddlers has been linked to HIV infection of children. Poor oral hygiene exacerbates the risk.

Classification

The World Health Organization (WHO) developed a classification system in 2005, after consultation with clinicians and researchers from mid-developed and developing countries. It addresses chronic lung disease, failure to thrive, prolonged diarrhoea, pulmonary tuberculosis and recto-vaginal or -vesical fistulae. The classification also provides criteria for presumptive diagnosis of HIV in infants below 18 months of age who require urgent antiretroviral therapy in the absence of virological diagnosis. (See Tables 10.1 through 10.2). It is useful for prognosis and for decisions regarding antiretroviral therapy.

Table 10.1 WHO clinical staging for infants and children with confirmed HIV infection

(For use in those under 15 years with confirmed laboratory evidence of HIV infection; HIV antibody where age >18 months, virological or P24 Ag testing if age <18 months)

STAGE 1
Asymptomatic
Persistent generalised lymphadenopathy (2 or more non-contiguous sites)

STAGE 2
Hepatomegaly/splenomegaly/ both
Recurrent or chronic upper respiratory tract infections (otitis media, otorrhoea, sinusitis)
Parotid enlargement (assympt.,bilateral)
Seborrhoeic dermatitis
Papillary pruritic eruptions
Extensive molluscum contagiosum (facial, >5% body area or disfiguring)
Herpes zoster

Fungal nail infections

Extensive human papilloma virus (facial, >5% body area or disfiguring)

Recurrent oral ulcerations (≥2 in 6 months)

Lineal gingival erythema (LGE)

Angular chelitis

STAGE 3

Conditions where a presumptive diagnosis can be made using clinical signs or simple investigations:

Unexplained moderate malnutrition not adequately responding to 2 weeks of standard treatment (very low Wt for age, Wt for Ht of −2SD)

Unexplained persistent diarrhoea (≥14 days)

Unexplained persistent fever (intermittent or constant, for ≥ 1 month)

Oral candidiasis (outside neonatal period)

Oral hairy leukoplakia

Acute necrotizing ulcerative gingivitis/periodontitis

Pulmonary tuberculosis

Severe recurrent presumed bacterial pneumonia

Conditions where confirmatory diagnosis testing is necessary:

LIP

Unexplained anaemia (<8 g/dl), neutropenia (<1 000/mm³) or thrombocytopenia (50 000/mm³) for ≥1 month

Chronic HIV associated lung disease including bronchiectasis

STAGE 4

Conditions where a presumptive diagnosis can be made using clinical signs or simple investigations:

Unexplained severe wasting or severe malnutrition not adequately responding to 2 weeks standard treatment (severe wasting of muscles, with/without oedema, and/or Wt for Ht of −3SD)

PCP

Recurrent severe presumed bacterial infections (e.g. empyema, pyomyositis, bone or joint infection, meningitis, but excluding pneumonia)(≥2 episodes in 1 year)

Chronic Herpes simplex infection (orolabial or cutanous ≥1 month, visceral of any duration)

Extrapulmonary TB

Kaposi's sarcoma

Oesophageal candidiasis

CNS toxoplasmosis (outside neonatal period)

HIV encephalopathy

Conditions where confirmatory diagnostic testing is necessary:

CMV infection (CMV retinitis or infection of organs other than liver, spleen or lymphnodes onset at age 1 month or more)

Cryptococcal meningitis (or other extrapulmonary disease)

Any disseminated endemic mycosis (e.g. extra-pulmonary histoplasmosis, coccidiomycosis, penicilliosis)

Cryptosporidiosis (with diarrhoea>1 month)

Isosporiosis

Disseminated non-tuberculous mycobacterial infection

Candida of trachea, bronchi or lungs

Visceral herpes simplex infection

Acquired HIV-related rectal fistula

Cerebral or B cell non-Hodgkin's lymphoma

PMLE

HIV-related cardiomyopathy

HIV-related nephropathy

See http://www.who.int/hiv/pub/guidelines/HIVstaging150307.pdf for diagnosis of staging criteria.

For circumstances where virological diagnosis is not possible in infants below 18 months of age:

- HIV antibody positive; and
- any AIDS diagnosis; or
- symptomatic with two or more of the following:
  o oral thrush
  o severe pneumonia
  o severe sepsis.

Other factors of note:

- recent maternal death of HIV-related causes or advanced HIV disease;
- CD4 <20%.

Because of the high risk of mortality in the first four months of life, in the presence of any of the following signs, serious consideration should be given to initiating antiretroviral therapy, while awaiting laboratory confirmation:

- oral candidiasis, any lymphadenopathy, hepatomegaly (>1cm below right costal margin);
- splenomegaly;
- weight for age below 10th centile and clinical gastro-oesophageal reflux (cough and vomit associated with feeds).

A meta-analysis of data for 3 941 children from eight cohort studies and nine randomised trials in Europe and the USA, either not on antiretrovirals or only monotherapy provides useful data for CD4 percentages and counts in children as a prognostic tool for disease severity (Table 10.2). The CD4+ count declines with age in healthy children until adult levels are reached at between five and six years of age. In contrast, the CD4+ percentage remains constant.

Higher CD4 counts or percentages at younger ages carry a worse prognosis than lower values in older children.

Table 10.2 Immunological categories by CD4% and absolute CD4 count for paediatric HIV infection

Immune status	Age up to 12 months	Age 13 months or over	6 years or over
No significant immunosuppression	>35 %	>25%	>500 cells/µl
Mild immunosuppression	25–34%	20–24%	350–499 cells/µl
Advanced immunosuppression	20–24%	15–19%	200–349 cells/µl
Severe immunosuppression	<20%	<15%	<200 cells/µl

Hidden effects of HIV

HIV infection in children is a family disease. Because the majority of paediatric infection is through vertical transmission, the mother, and usually also the father, are infected. Uninfected spouses and children are affected by HIV.

The hidden effects of HIV include:
- chronic illness;
- multiple hospital visits;
- economic impacts – caregivers may need to stop working, the cumulative costs of care can be immense;
- travel costs to health care centres; and
- emotional burden and guilt.

Diagnosis

There are two diagnosis scenarios:
- an infected infant can be identified through post natal testing; or
- infants and children may present with suggestive clinical symptoms and signs. The infant is the index patient for the family, who may be unaware of HIV. There may be a history of the mother not wishing to pursue a diagnosis of HIV, suggesting incomplete and inadequate counselling.

DNA polymerase chain reaction (PCR) is the diagnostic test of choice in infants under 18 months of age. (RNA PCR is equivalent.) Although

Figure 10.2 Relationship between HIV and poverty

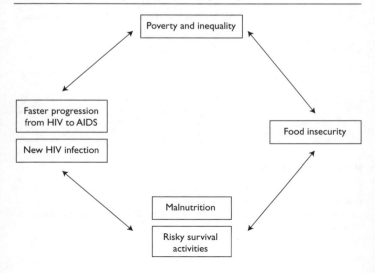

maternal antibodies may persist for up to 18 months, the older the infant, the more likely it is that HIV antibodies reflect infection rather than maternal antibodies. For example, above 15 months of age, HIV antibodies imply HIV infection in almost 100% of children. The ELISA test becomes negative in more than 50% of seroreverters by nine months of age. (See also Chapter 5: Laboratory investigations.) 'Rapid testing' may be used to confirm HIV exposure in children. A positive test confirms infection, but a negative test may not be sensitive enough in young infants or after recent exposure. It must be performed by a trained person. A negative test should be repeated with a test from another manufacturer or submitted to a laboratory for formal ELISA.

Currently, in the South African public sector, a single PCR is advised at four to six weeks. This, together with clinical findings of HIV, indicates that the child is infected. A baseline viral load will confirm a positive diagnosis. If the clinical and laboratory results are contradictory, the PCR should be repeated and the laboratory informed to check its quality assurance.

Where vertical transmission prevention has been sub-optimal e.g. an unbooked mother, or maternal viral load >1 000 copies near term or with prematurity, the PCR should be done in the first 48 hours of life (some elect two weeks of age). The first PCR should be done immediately in any symptomatic infants. If negative, the PCR should be repeated at six to eight weeks of age.

For breastfed infants, the PCR should be repeated, at a minimum of six weeks after cessation of breastfeeding and six monthly for prolonged breastfeeding. Above the age of 18 months a rapid test is probably sufficient, but should be repeated after three months.

In a recent study of HIV-exposed and infected infants at a median of 42 days of age, if any one of oral thrush, hepatomegaly, splenomegaly, lymphadenopathy, diaper dermatitis, or weight <50th centile were present, sensitivity for HIV infection was 86%. Sepsis and clinical gastro-esophageal reflux are also highly specific for HIV infection in young infants. Any of these signs or symptoms should precipitate a diagnostic PCR, with rapid turn-around time for the result.

The HIV exposed uninfected infant and child

These children should be retained in care as they are more vulnerable than unexposed uninfected children. The long term outcome of exposure to antiretrovirals is not known.

Higher risk of mortality and morbidity than unexposed uninfected infants has been described. PCP has also been noted in the first six months of life. Subtle neurodevelopmental impairment, especially for language delay, has been observed.

An approach to outpatient care for HIV-exposed and infected children

The HIV-exposed infant: First visit (usually from two weeks)

- Find out the perinatal details, i.e. birth weight, gestational age, mode of delivery, maternal RPR status and Hepatitis B status. If a caesarean section was done, was it elective? Get detailed information on the mother's antiretroviral history and strategies to prevent vertical transmission.
- When was HIV diagnosed in the mother? Has there been disclosure to the father? Does the mother have support systems? Disclosure is VITAL for successful antiretroviral therapy in the infant.
- Does anyone in the household or any visitor have active TB or suggestive symptoms or signs (cough, weight loss, fever)? TB can present at any age, even in neonates.
- Already prepare the mother for rapid initiation of antiretroviral therapy if the infant is infected.
- What is the mother's CD4 count? Was a viral load done close to delivery?
- What is the antenatal and perinatal antiretroviral history? Is the mother on antiretroviral therapy for her own health? Which drugs were given for prevention of vertical transmission and for how long?
- Did the neonate receive postnatal zidovudine, nevirapine or other antiretrovirals? If so, when was it initiated and for how long?
- Check the feeding history, i.e. breast milk, formula, or both? (See Chapter 12: Infant feeding.) Does the mother prepare formula feed correctly? Is she aware of the need for sterility? (hand washing, use of sterilizing solutions such as 'Milton'). Does she use a cup or a bottle? (cups are preferable).
- Measure head circumference, weight and length and plot on percentile charts.
- Check the infant for oral candidiasis, lymphadenopathy, or hepato-splenomegaly.
- Check the right upper arm for a BCG ulcer and right axilla for asymmetrically enlarged lymph nodes.

- Measure the respiratory and heart rate:
  - tachypnoea (>50/min) and tachycardia (>150/min) may be the first manifestation of PCP. Check O_2 saturation (should be >92% on coast and 90% at altitude)
  - other causes of unexplained tachypnoea include anaemia, myocarditis and metabolic acidosis.
- Commence co-trimoxazole prophylaxis from four weeks of age. In the absence of neonatal jaundice, it can be commenced from two weeks as PCP may occur in the first four weeks of life.
- Prescribe a vitamin A-containing multivitamin preparation.

Start education about antiretroviral therapy and provide counselling support and education at all subsequent visits.

First visit of HIV-infected infant or child

- Obtain the perinatal history and MTCT details.
- Examine the 'Road to Health' booklet, widely used in southern Africa, for perinatal, immunization, and growth details.
- Check on the health and infection status of other family members.
- Specifically ask about possible TB infection in caregivers or household contacts.
- Offer referral to a social worker.
- Check the infant's height, weight, and head circumference.
- Perform a full physical examination.
- Prepare for rapid initiation of antiretroviral therapy. Antiretroviral therapy can be initiated at that visit with subsequent preparedness sessions taking place in the next few days. Antiretroviral therapy can also be initiated while awaiting confirmatory plasma HIV RNA result (or confirmatory DNA PCR) and baseline CD4 count, full blood count and transaminases.

Special investigations

Confirm the HIV infection status if necessary, and do the following tests:
- full blood count (FBC) and differential;
- ALT;
- CD4 percentage and count;
- urine dipstick – exclude proteinuria and haematuria; and
- chest radiograph (useful as a baseline, as chronic lung disease and TB are common);

- for young infants infected despite vertical transmission prophylaxis, resistance testing should be performed if possible, especially where the mother was on antiretroviral therapy and where either a NNRTI or lamivudine were used.

Second visit

This should be done after two weeks and affords the opportunity to review the diagnosis and special investigations with the parent or caregiver. Remember to praise the parent or caregiver for positive aspects of the child's health, such as good dental hygiene, good weight gain, and general appearance. Do not admonish parents or caregivers about factors beyond their control, but rather help them find ways to overcome difficulties. Check adherence and antiretroviral knowledge. Are the parents caring for themselves adequately? Adjust antiretroviral dosages according to weight.

Frequency of visits

For neonates, see frequently, as early signs of deterioration may be subtle. See monthly or weekly or two-weekly if necessary for the first six months.

Regular out-patient visits

- Enquire about the health of the child, recent symptoms, or hospitalization since your previous encounter.
- Check on the health status of the other family members. Always ask about the possibility of TB exposure.
- Always check the 'Road to Health' booklet.

Special investigations

- There is little point in performing excessive investigations.
- The FBC and CD4 count should be repeated if there is clinical deterioration, or six to 12-monthly.
- The chest radiograph should not be repeated unless clinically indicated.

Medication

- multivitamin preparation containing vitamin A (3 000 to 5 000 IU per day);

- elemental iron 1 mg/kg/day (prophylaxis) if the child's diet is likely to be deficient in iron;
- give an anti-helminthic agent every six months (either mebendazole or albendazole);
- folic acid (2.5 mg per day) may be beneficial in 'symptomatic' patients and chronic diarrhoea;
- co-trimoxazole prophylaxis should be given (see Table 10.2) at a dose of 5 mg/kg/day daily.

For all exposed infants in the first year of life, unless two negative PCRs have been obtained at least three months after the last breastfeed:

- Continue co-trimoxazole until child demonstrates a good CD4 recovery on antiretroviral therapy; CD4 at least >15% on two consecutive occasions.
- For co-trimoxazole intolerant patients, use dapsone 2 mg/kg/day or 4 mg/kg/week.

Disclosure

While not easy for the child or parent, a disclosure process is essential, preferably before the onset of adolescence, but when the child is mature enough to understand the importance of privacy (probably from eight to nine years of age). Disclosure is a process that may take a number of months (or even years) to complete. The assistance of the primary care-giver and colleagues skilled in counselling should be sought. The need to disclose should be discussed with the caregiver in a planned way, when considered appropriate by the caregiver. Even in a newly diagnosed infant, the need for disclosure in a number of years time should be mentioned. The disclosure process should include:

- The process should be discussed with the caregiver.
- Discussions with the child should be undertaken to determine his or her current knowledge status, with the permission of the caregiver.
- The best setting for disclosure is not known but is probably best under-taken by the caregiver in a setting of his or her choice.
- Both caregiver and child require post-disclosure support.

References and further reading

Mandell, L. et al. Eds. 2000. *Principles and practice of infectious diseases*, 5th edition. Philadelphia: Churchill Livingstone.

Pickering, L.K. Ed. 2006. *Red Book: Report of the Committee on Infectious Diseases*, 26th edition. Elk Grove Village: American Academy of Pediatrics.

HIV Paediatric Prognostic Markers Collaborative Study Group. 2003. 'Short-term risk of disease progression in HIV-1-infected children receiving no antiretroviral therapy or zidovudine monotherapy: a meta-analysis.' *Lancet*; 362: 1605–1611.

Health Systems trust. Available: www.hst.org.za

Interim WHO Clinical Staging of HIV/AIDS and HIV/AIDS Case Definitions For Surveillance African Region. 2005. Available: whqlibdoc.who.int/hq/2005/WHO_HIV_2005.02.pdf [Accessed 18th September 2005].

Jaspan, H.B., Myer, L., Madhi, S.A. et al. 2011. Utility of clinical parameters to identify HIV infection in infants below ten weeks of age in South Africa: A prospective cohort study. *BMC paediatrics*; 11: 104.

World Health Organization. 2010. *Antiretroviral therapy for HIV infection in infants and children: towards universal access. Recommendations for a public health approach*. 2010 revision. Geneva: WHO.

Violari, A., Cotton, M.F., Gibb, D. et al. 2007. 'Antiretroviral therapy initiated before 12 weeks of age reduces early mortality in young HIV-infected infants: evidence from the Children with HIV Early Antiretroviral Therapy (CHER) Study.' In: 4th IAS conference on pathogenesis, treatment and prevention Sydney, Australia: International AIDS Society; 2007.

Childhood vaccination

General principles

Vaccine schedule

- Vaccine schedules for HIV-1 exposed/infected children are identical to those for HIV-1-uninfected children. (Table 11.1)
- There is no need to test for HIV infection before starting immunization.
- Many new vaccines have been included in the expanded programme for immunization (EPI).

Immune responses

- HIV infection is associated with a multifaceted suppression of both humoral and cell mediated immune responses.
- Immunosupression, particularly if severe (CD4+ lymphocyte count <15%), is associated with impaired immune responses to both live-attenuated and sub-unit/toxoid/killed vaccines.
- HIV-infected children not on antiretroviral therapy are more likely to have rapid decline in antibody levels and loss of anamnestic responses, possibly shortening the duration of protection.
- Antibody concentrations to most vaccine antigens are lower in newborns of HIV-infected women.
- The functionality of antibodies induced by conjugate *Haemophilus influenzae* type b and *Streptococcus pneumoniae* vaccines is impaired among antiretroviral naive HIV-infected children.
- Immunocompetent HIV-infected children on effective antiretroviral therapy have similar quantitative antibody responses compared to HIV-uninfected children.
- 20% of HIV-infected children will have severely decreased CD4+ lymphocyte counts (<25%) at six weeks of age when immunization, other than that given at birth, is administered. The majority should respond adequately, especially if on antiretroviral therapy.
- Revaccination of HIV-infected children following immune reconstitution after initiating antiretroviral therapy and response thereto remains to be determined. Current data however supports re-immunization.

Vaccine safety

- There are isolated case reports of severe adverse events following vaccination, especially with the live-attenuated vaccines (see below for individual vaccines).
- The transient increase in HIV plasma levels following immunization, especially with the sub-unit influenza and pneumococcal poly-saccharide vaccines, are not clinically important. The conjugate pneumococcal vaccine is not associated with an increase in HIV viral load post-vaccination.
- Adverse events with the live-attenuated vaccines are theoretically less likely if given when HIV-infected children are still immunocompetent.
- Heightened suspicion of vaccine–related complications is important in all immunocompromised children, especially if the live-attenuated vaccines are given (e.g. hospitalizations occurring within 14–30 days of vaccination), and should be notified and appropriately investigated.
- Adverse events should be considered in all HIV-infected children hospitalised, within one month after vaccination, especially for live-attenuated vaccines. Adverse events have been reported up to one year following vaccination.

Specific vaccine issues

BCG vaccine in HIV-infected children

Bacille Calmette-Guérin (BCG) is a live-attenuated *Mycobacterium bovis* vaccine. BCG is effective in preventing disseminated tuberculosis (miliary tuberculosis and tuberculous meningitis) in young children. In South Africa, intradermal vaccination with Danish strain BCG is routinely administered in the right deltoid region at birth. There is concern regarding the safety of BCG in HIV-infected infants, based on several cases of local and disseminated BCG disease reported in HIV-infected infants. The Global Advisory Committee of the WHO states that BCG is contra-indicated in HIV-infected infants. The benefits of BCG in HIV-exposed uninfected infants is considerable. Care must be taken that programmes act carefully to consider the best approach for BCG administration. Current South African policy still recommends routine vaccination at birth in HIV-exposed infants.

What is a normal reaction and what is a BCG adverse event?

Normal: at three weeks, a small area of redness, then at six weeks to 10 weeks a raised papule with slight redness, and at 14 weeks a shallow ulceration with crusting.

BCG *adverse events* are classified as local/regional, or systemic.

Local BCG complications: an injection site abscess of ≥10 mm × 10 mm diameter, a severe BCG scar ulceration or persistent ulceration beyond 20 weeks.

Regional BCG complications: BCG adenitis ≥15 × 15 mm diameter beyond the vaccination site in the right-sided axillary, supraclavicular, cervical or upper arm area. Lymph node involvement may include enlargement, suppuration and fistula formation. With lymphadenopathy in the cervical or supraclavicular region, exclude conditions like tuberculosis. BCG immune reconstitution inflammatory syndrome (BCG-IRIS) usually manifests as acute onset right-sided axillary adenitis within three months of initiation of antiretroviral therapy.

Systemic or disseminated disease

Disseminated BCG disease will usually cause severe systemic illness, which may mimic septicaemia or severe end-organ disease, e.g. pulmonary disease. The isolation of *M. bovis* BCG in a distant site beyond the vaccination area, e.g. gastric aspirates, blood culture, bone marrow biopsy or cerebrospinal fluid indicates disseminated BCG disease. Pulmonary BCG disease may be identical to pulmonary tuberculosis on chest radiography.

The following children should be investigated in hospital:

- All HIV-infected children with a BCG adverse event – there is a risk of BCG dissemination beyond the lymph node.
- All children with lymphadenopathy complicated by inflammation/ fluctuation, enlargement, or discharge may need surgery.
- Any other systemically ill child with a BCG adverse event with a history suggestive of immune suppression, (e.g. poor growth, recurrent infections or hospitalizations). Remember to check HIV status. Children with B-cell abnormalities may be unable to make antibodies to HIV.
- There are limited data on optimal treatment regimens, but the high mortality of systemic BCG disease in immune-compromised children warrants aggressive management.

See Appendix 11.1 for the diagnostic workup and management of BCG adverse events in children.

Polio vaccines

- Inactivated Salk and the live-attenuated Sabin vaccines include polio-viruses types 1, 2 and 3. Currently, live-attenuated oral polio trivalent vaccine is provided at birth and six weeks of age and inactivated trivalent polio vaccine, in combination with DTPa-HibCV, at 6, 10, and 14 weeks and a booster dose at 15 to 18 months of age.
- In South Africa, no documented cases of wild-type polio have occurred since 1989.
- Approximately one million HIV-1-infected children have received oral polio vaccine (OPV). However, only one case of vaccine associated flaccid paralysis in an HIV-infected child has been reported. This may be due to under-recognition. Consider OPV associated adverse event in all HIV-infected children with motor regression, particularly if vaccinated in previous six months.
- OPV may be transmitted to susceptible immunocompromised HIV-infected adults who may develop neurological signs, including Guillain-Barré syndrome.
- Inactivated vaccine is recommended in developed countries for HIV exposed/infected children.
- It is important for health workers to be aggressive in evaluating all cases of flaccid paralysis both in HIV-infected children and adults for possible vaccine-related events. Submission of at least two stool samples within 14 days of onset of the signs is vital if the safety of the vaccine is to be confirmed.

Diphtheria-tetanus-pertussis

- Diphtheria and tetanus toxoids produce a favourable antibody response in HIV-infected African children with no increase in either local or systemic adverse events.
- Acellular pertussis vaccines have fewer adverse events than the whole-cell killed pertussis vaccines and are now routinely used in the South African EPI.
- The immunogenicity of the acellular vaccine is reasonable in older HIV-infected children.
- Many of the new-generation combination vaccines include acellular pertussis vaccine together with diphtheria and tetanus toxoid as well

as *Haemophilus influenzae* type b conjugate vaccine and some also include hepatitis B vaccine.

- Revaccination with DTP in HIV-infected children aged two to nine years following immune reconstitution after the initiation of anti-retroviral therapy although associated with a booster response is also associated with limited durability.

Measles

- HIV-infected children are predisposed to more severe measles (28–40% mortality rates) than uninfected children.
- Children born to HIV-infected mothers and children in home-care facilities appear to be susceptible to measles at a very young age (<9 months).
- Wild-type and vaccine-associated measles may be atypical in HIV-infected children, making the diagnosis difficult and facilitating noso-comial spread.
- One case of vaccine-related death due to pneumonia has been reported in a vaccinated HIV-infected adult.
- Empirical evidence suggests that vaccination is safe in HIV-infected individuals. This may however represent both under-recognition and -reporting.
- Approximately 80% of HIV-infected children, in the absence of antiretroviral treatment, would be immunocompromised and have stigmata of AIDS at the time of their measles vaccination at nine months of age.
- 'Routine' immunization for hospitalized children in the absence of proof of immunization is not indicated and may predispose to further immunosuppression, but may be required during measles epidemics.
- All HIV-infected children irrespective of immunization status should receive immunoglobulin prophylaxis if exposed to wild-type measles virus.
- In developed countries, measles vaccination is recommended for all HIV-infected children at the routine age of immunization except for those children with severe immunosupression (defined as a CD4+ lymphocyte count <15%).
- In South Africa, in keeping with the WHO recommendations, routine immunization is advocated without distinguishing levels of immuno-supression. Reporting of adverse events is essential to define the safety of the vaccine.

Mumps and rubella

- These vaccines are not included in the EPI schedule.
- Both vaccines appear to be safe in HIV-infected children.
- They are recommended in some industrialized countries for HIV-1-infected children.

Varicella vaccine

- This is not included in the EPI schedule.
- The vaccine is safe and immunogenic in immunocompetent HIV-infected children.
- It is recommended for HIV-infected children at 18–24 months of age if immunocompetent or stable and controlled on antiretroviral therapy.

Hepatitis B vaccine

- Routine hepatitis B vaccination is included in the EPI in South Africa.
- Being a subunit vaccine, the vaccine poses little added risk of serious adverse events.
- Vaccination of the infant may need to be augmented by administering hepatitis B immunoglobulin at birth if the mother is an active carrier (HbsAg positive), since dual infection is likely given the similarity in acquisition of both pathogens.
- A lower proportion of HIV-infected children (80% versus 97%) generate protective levels of antibody following a primary series of hepatitis B vaccines and HIV-infected children also have less durable antibody concentrations following vaccination.

Rotavirus vaccine

- This live-attenuated vaccine (Rotarix®) was introduced into the South African EPI in April 2009.
- Studies in Africa have confirmed safety, immunogenicity and efficacy in preventing severe and mild rotavirus illness, including in settings with a high prevalence of paediatric HIV-infection.
- Two doses of rotavirus vaccine are provided at 6 and 14 weeks of age in the EPI schedule.
- Rotavirus vaccine is safe and immunogenic in HIV-infected children, both in the presence and absence of antiretroviral treatment.

Haemophilus influenzae type b (Hib) conjugate vaccine (HibCV)

- Hib conjugate vaccines have been included in the EPI schedule in South Africa since July 1999.
- In children receiving antiretroviral treatment the vaccine is immunogenic, although the mean antibody titres is lower than in HIV-uninfected children and there is a more rapid decline in antibody titre.
- HIV-infected children not receiving antiretroviral drugs have lower antibody concentrations, less functional antibody and less durable antibody following a primary series of HibCV.
- South African data show diminished efficacy in reducing invasive Hib disease in HIV-infected children (48%, $CI_{95\%}$ – 54.7% to 80.3%) compared to HIV-uninfected children (98% effectiveness).
- HIV-infected children probably require booster doses of HibCV, although the frequency thereof and immune responses thereto need to be determined.

Streptococcus pneumoniae vaccination

- *Streptococcus pneumoniae* is the most common bacterial cause of invasive disease (IPD) including bacteraemia, pneumonia and meningitis in HIV-infected children. The risk is 40-fold greater in the absence of antiretroviral treatment and 20-fold greater on antiretroviral treatment than HIV-uninfected children.
- Polysaccharide pneumococcal vaccine is not useful in children under five years of age. The vaccine is associated with a negative outcome, especially an increase in pneumonia, in HIV-infected African adults in Uganda, albeit associated with a 16% reduction in mortality.
- A new-generation vaccine, pneumococal polysaccharide-protein conjugate vaccine (PCV), is immunogenic in children from six weeks of age onwards.
- HIV-infected children receiving antiretroviral drugs have similar antibody concentrations to PCV compared to the general population.
- HIV-infected children not receiving antiretroviral drugs have lower antibody concentrations, less functional antibody and less durable antibody concentrations following a primary series of three doses of PCV during infancy.
- PCV is associated with a 65% reduction in invasive pneumococcal disease due to vaccine serotypes and a 15% reduction in all-cause lower respiratory tract infections following a primary series of PCV

during infancy among HIV-infected children. There is, however, loss of protection against IPD in the absence of a booster dose of vaccine.

- Currently, 13-valent PCV (Prevenar®) is included in the EPI and provided at 6, 14 and 40 weeks (booster dose) of age in South Africa. Two doses of PCV, spaced two months apart, are recommended for HIV-infected children not immunized during infancy.
- The safety and immunogenicity of PCV in HIV-infected children on antiretrovirals is similar to that of HIV-uninfected children.
- Vaccination of HIV-infected children on antiretroviral therapy, between two to19 years of age, with two doses of PCV followed by a single dose of pneumococcal polysaccharide vaccine, has reasonable immunogenicity and is indicated even if the child has been previously vaccinated with the pneumococcal polysaccharide vaccine.

Influenza vaccine

- This is not included in the South African EPI programme.
- HIV-infected children have an eight-fold increased risk of being hospitalised with influenza-associated severe lower respiratory tract infections.
- Currently only the subunit influenza vaccine is licensed for use.
- The current recommendation in the USA is to vaccinate all HIV-infected individuals on antiretroviral therapy, preferably when the plasma HIV RNA levels have been stable.
- HIV-infected children older than six months of age should receive two doses one month apart during the first season and then single doses before the start of subsequent influenza seasons. Initial studies from South Africa have, however, found that trivalent inactivated influenza vaccine is only modestly immunogenic and lacks efficacy in HIV-infected children.
- The live-attenuated vaccines that are administered intranasally are currently being evaluated. Although safe in HIV-infected adults, they should probably not be used in HIV-infected individuals, since prolonged shedding may predispose to mutation and virulence.
- Vaccination of HIV-infected children is recommended in South Africa.

Other vaccines

- Other vaccines not evaluated in HIV-infected children, or where there are limited indications for use, include yellow fever and hepatitis A. Hepatitis A vaccine is likely to be useful in patients stable on anti-

retroviral therapy. Hepatitis A infection can mimic drug-related hepatotoxicity.
- Yellow fever vaccine is not indicated in HIV-infected children and travel to yellow-fever endemic areas is not recommended for HIV-infected individuals.

Conclusion

- Immunizing as per routine EPI programme is recommended for HIV-infected children.
- Vaccine related adverse events should always be considered in HIV-infected children requiring medical treatment, particularly in the month following vaccination and possibly thereafter.
- Reporting of all suspected vaccine-related adverse events and vaccine failures is mandatory.
- New vaccines that could benefit HIV-infected children should be introduced into the EPI programme and there needs to be advocacy for this.

Reference and further reading

Lane, H.C., Depper, J.M., Greene, W.C., Whalen, G., Waldmann, T.A., Fauci, A.S. 1985. 'Qualitative analysis of immune function in patients with the acquired immunodeficiency syndrome.' *New England Journal of Medicine*; 313:79–84.

Lotte, A., Wasz-Hockert, O., Poisson, N., Dumitrescu, N., Verron, M., Couvet, E. 1984. 'A bibliography of the complications of BCG vaccination. A comprehensive list of the world literature since the introduction of BCG up to July 1982, supplemented by over 100 personal communications.' *Advances in Tuberculosis Research*; 21:194–245.

Katz, S.L. 1998. 'Immunizations for HIV-infected children.' In Pizzo, P.A. and Wilfert, C.M. (Ed) *Paediatric AIDS – The challenge of HIV infection in infants, children, and adolescents.* Third edition. Chapter 32:543–552. Williams and Wilkins, Baltimore, Maryland, USA.

Table 11.1 Childhood programme for immunization schedule

Age at vaccination	Vaccine	Vaccine characteristic
Birth/ Newborn	Bacille Calmette-Guérin (BCG)	Live-attenuated vaccine
	Oral polio vaccine (OPV)	Live-attenuated vaccine
6, 10 and 14 weeks (spaced 4 weeks apart)	Diphtheria-Tetanus-Acellular Pertussis Inactivated trivalent polio Haemophilus influenzae type b (DTa-IPV-Hib)	Diptheria and tetanus are toxoid (inactive) vaccines Pertussis bi-valent acellular vaccine, Haemophilus influenzae type b conjugate vaccine and trivalent inactivated polio vaccine
	OPV	Live attenuated
6 and 14 weeks	Pneumococcal conjugate vaccine[1]	Polysaccharide of specific pneumococcal serotypes conjugated to protein antigen (13-valent vaccine currently in South Africa)
	Rotavirus vaccine[2]	Live-attenuated monovalent vaccine (Rotarix®)
9 months	Measles	Live-attenuated vaccine
	Pneumococcal conjugate vaccine	Polysaccharide of specific pneumococcal serotypes conjugated to protein antigen (13-valent vaccine currently in South Africa)
15–18 months	Measles	Live-attenuated vaccine
	Acellular Pertussis-inactivated trivalent polio Haemophilus influenzae type b (DTPa-IPV-Hib)	Diptheria and tetanus are toxoid (inactive) vaccines Pertussis bi-valent acellular vaccine, Haemophilus influenzae type b conjugate vaccine and trivalent inactivated polio vaccine

[1] Recommended for all HIV-infected children less than 9 years of age. Children less than 7 months of age require dosing as above. Children 7 months–two years of age require two doses one month apart and a booster dose at 15–18 months of age. Children older than two years of age require two doses two months apart.

[2] Recommended as two dose schedule at 10 and 14 weeks of age. Safety studies in HIV-infected children underway.

Appendix 11.1 Suggested diagnostic workup and management of BCG adverse events in children

A. All children

- Full history and clinical assessment, including documentation of size and location of local and regional BCG lesions. Note the presence or absence of a BCG scar and whether BCG was given.
- Fine needle aspirate for mycobacterial culture.
- HIV testing.

B. All HIV-infected children or other suspected/proven immune deficiency

- chest radiography (antero-posterior and lateral);
- minimum two gastric washings for mycobacterial culture;
- mycobacterial blood culture if febrile (TB Bactec);
- CD4+ T-lymphocyte count and viral load, if applicable and not done in prior two months;
- full blood and differential count;
- baseline liver function tests for monitoring of toxicity;
- refer to infectious diseases service.

Note: all positive cultures require confirmation by PCR to distinguish BCG from *Mycobacterium tuberculosis*.

C. Additional investigations for HIV-related and other immune deficiencies with suspected distant or disseminated BCG disease

As in A and B and:
- bone marrow aspirate/biopsy for mycobacterial culture;
- mycobacterial blood culture (even if afebrile);
- abdominal ultrasound for intra-abdominal lymphadenopathy;
- radiography if osteitis is suspected;
- other systemic investigations as clinically indicated.

BCG confirmation: *M. bovis* BCG should be confirmed by culture and PCR or biochemical methods (required to differentiate from *Mycobacterium tuberculosis*)

- antimycobacterial drugs: for suspected or confirmed systemic disease:
  - isoniazid (INH)15–20 mg/kg/day;
  - rifampicin (RMP) 20 mg/kg/day;
  - pyrazinamide (PZA) 35 mg/kg/day (two months, or until tuberculosis excluded, as TB often co-exists; BCG is PZA-resistant);
  - ethambutol (EMB) 20–25 mg/kg/day;
  - ofloxacin (OFL)15 mg/kg/day or ciprofloxacin 30 mg/kg/day.

A. Local or regional BCG disease
- Treat medically:
  - Consider using the above five drugs until disseminated disease is excluded (if suspected).
  - For local/regional disease – INH, RMP, EMB (and PZA until TB excluded).
- Consider therapeutic aspiration if node fluctuant.
- Two–four weekly follow-up; if no improvement, or deterioration of adenitis after six weeks antituberculosis therapy, consider excision biopsy.
- If on antiretroviral therapy, ensure antiretroviral therapy is anti-tuberculosis-drug compatible.
- Refer to infectious disease service.
- Monitor for drug toxicity.
- Notify as vaccine adverse event to the Provincial Expanded Programme on Immunization (EPI) if fulfilling case definition.
- BCG-related IRIS lymphadenitis does not require anti-mycobacterial drugs.

B. Suspected or confirmed distant or disseminated BCG disease – Suspect in infants with Clinical WHO Stage 4 disease, especially if right axillary adenopathy and severe CD4 depletion (<25% in first year of life)
- Treat medically as above – *use five drugs including PZA until TB excluded.*
- Expedited initiation of antiretroviral therapy.
- Monitor for drug toxicity.
- Report as vaccine-related adverse event to EPI.

C. Local or regional disease not conforming to EPI criteria, local or regional BCG-IRIS with no suspected dissemination
- Observe, follow regularly for progression.
- Report as vaccine-related adverse event if progression to case definition.

12 HIV and infant feeding

Background

Breastmilk is the optimal nutrition for all newborn infants and for the first few months of life. Breastmilk contains all of the nutrition that the growing infant requires, as well as providing crucial protective immunological factors (Walker, 2010). Worldwide, there is a movement to promote and protect breastfeeding, particularly in developing countries, where the levels of breastfeeding are sub-optimal (Arabi et al, 2012).

Research shows that replacement feeding leads to diarrhoeal disease and malnutrition, which are major causes of morbidity and mortality in developing countries (WHO, 2000; Bahl et al, 2005).

Benefits of breastfeeding are particularly pertinent for the HIV -exposed/-infected infant. Some of the benefits of breastfeeding by HIV infected mothers include:

- Nutritional needs: breastmilk provides the perfect nutrients; this is particularly important in HIV infection.
- Breastmilk is easily digested and used by the body.
- Breastfed infants have fewer allergies.
- Breastmilk protects against infectious diseases, especially diarrhoea and pneumonia.
- Infants infected at birth progress to AIDS more slowly if breastfed.
- Birth spacing: breastfeeding delays a new pregnancy.
- Breastfeeding is economical.
- Breastfeeding protects a mother's health/decreases frequency of breast cancer.

Whilst the benefits of breastfeeding are significant, one important risk is the transmission of HIV-1 infection through breastmilk. Without any interventions, such as ART prophylaxis, the risk for six months of breast-feeding varies between 2% and 8%. The level of risk depends on various factors, which include:

- the stage of HIV disease in the mother;
- the length of the breastfeeding period;
- the presence of cracked nipples and mastitis;
- oral lesions/ulcers in the infant; and
- mixed feeding.

Considerable research has been carried out on breastfeeding and infant feeding by HIV infected mothers. Evidence shows that the risk of HIV transmission can be decreased by various measures.

Four general strategies have been proposed to reduce the risk of HIV transmission through breastfeeding:

1. Exclusive breastfeeding during the first 6 months:
   - Evidence from several studies has shown that exclusive breastfeeding for up to six months has a two to four fold decreased risk of HIV transmission.
2. Flash heating of expressed breastmilk (HTEBM):
   - Flash heating will inactivate "spiked" cell-free HIV-1 as detected by reverse transcriptase activity (Israel-Ballard et al, 2007).
3. Use of maternal HAART during breastfeeding (Mofenson, 2010):
   - Maternal prophylaxis with HAART (highly active antiretroviral therapy) aims to reduce the risk of transmission primarily by reducing the viral load in breastmilk.
   - Additionally transfer of antiretrovirals (ARVs) to the infant through breastmilk ingestion also occurs, which could provide some indirect ARV prophylaxis to the infant.
   - It is important to note that infants who become infected despite maternal HAART may have the virus with drug resistance mutations.
4. Use of infant ARV prophylaxis during breastfeeding (Coovadia et al, 2012):
   - The infant ARV prophylaxis strategy aims to protect the infant during the period of HIV exposure during breastfeeding.

Table 12.1 summarises some of the key studies on prevention of mother-to-child transmission (PMTCT) and breastfeeding, published recently:

Table 12.1 Summary of key studies on prevention of mother-to-child transmission (PMTCT) and breastfeeding

Study	ART Regimen	Reduction in transmission	Vertical Transmission Rate
HPTN 046	NVP to 6/12	50% at 6/12	0.7%
SWEN	NVP to 6/52	53% at 6/52	2.5%
PEPI Malawi	NVP to 14/52	69% @ 14/52	2.6%
	NVP to 6/12	70% @ 6/12	1.7%
BAN Malawi	Maternal HAART to 6/12	49.1% @ 6/12	2.9%

Based on the evidence from research studies and programmatic experience, both the World Health Organization (WHO) and the South African Department of Health have published updated guidelines around HIV and infant feeding.

The WHO followed strict principles for developing evidence-based guidelines on infant feeding that would lead to the best outcome of HIV-free survival. This process culminated in the development of new WHO HIV and infant feeding guidelines (2010).

The South African government adopted these guidelines as an approach to infant feeding that maximizes child survival, and not only the avoidance of HIV transmission.

The South African government also takes cognizance that infant feeding recommendations for HIV-infected women should not be implemented in isolation but within the umbrella of the Infant and Young Child Feeding Policy of the country (NDoH, 2005). The following principles of safe infant feeding for the whole population should also be considered:

- Trained health care personnel should provide high quality, unambiguous, and unbiased information about risks of HIV transmission through breastfeeding, ART prophylaxis to reduce this risk, and risks of replacement feeding.
- Counselling on infant feeding must commence after the first post-test counselling session in pregnancy.
- Infant feeding should be discussed with women at every antenatal visit.
- Mixed feeding during the first six months of life should be strongly discouraged as it increases the risk of childhood infections.
- Mass mobilization and communication on infant feeding and HIV should be done through mass media, including distribution of informal information in communities.

In development of the guidelines, cognizance was taken of programmatic evidence of the dangers of mixed messages, inadequate counselling and inappropriate feeding choices. This information led to the WHO recommending to countries that they consider their own conditions and decide which feeding option is likely to give the majority of HIV-exposed children the biggest chance of HIV-free survival and then principally support this one intervention, namely breastfeeding with ARV prophylaxis or formula feeding.

The new South African Infant Feeding Guidelines for HIV-infected women

South Africa has taken the decision, based on its current profile of infant mortality (Doherty et al, 2011), to follow the WHO guidelines to counsel and support HIV-infected mothers to breastfeed their infants exclusively in the first six months, and thereafter continued breastfeeding with complementary foods until 12 months of age. During the 12 months of breastfeeding, infants should receive nevirapine prophylaxis. Breastfeeding before 12 months should only be stopped if a nutritionally adequate and safe diet without breastmilk can be provided.

Table 12.2 NVP Infant Dosing Guide

Drug	Birth Weight	Dose	Quantity
NVP syrup (10 mg/ml)	Birth to 6 weeks <2.5kg birth weight*	2 mg/kg/d for 14 days then 4 mg/kg/d	(10 mg/ml)
	Birth to 6 weeks >2.5kg birth weight	15 mg/d	1.5 ml
	For all:		
	6 weeks to 6 months	20 mg/d	2 ml
	6 months to 9 months	30 mg/d	3 ml
	9 months to end BF	40 mg/d	4 ml

* For very low birth weight infants, consult local hospital guidelines as national guidelines are not yet finalised.

What if the mother is on lifelong ART treatment?

If the mother is on ART treatment she can still breastfeed her infant. However, the infant will only receive nevirapine for six weeks. It is unnecessary for him/her to have additional prophylaxis since the breastmilk HIV viral load in a mother receiving ART treatment is likely to be very low.

Is it still important for mothers to breastfeed exclusively in the first six months if their infants are receiving nevirapine prophylaxis?

Yes, there is considerable evidence showing that not only does exclusive breastfeeding reduce the risk of HIV transmission but also that it has other health benefits for the infant. It is therefore important that mothers are supported to practice exclusive breastfeeding in the first six months.

What should happen when mothers decide to stop breastfeeding?

They should stop gradually within one month and the infants who should have been receiving nevirapine prophylaxis must continue prophylaxis for one week after breastfeeding is fully stopped.

What should infants be fed when mothers stop breastfeeding?

Infants should be provided with safe and adequate replacement feeds to enable normal growth and development.

Alternatives to breastfeeding include:
For infants less than six months of age:
- commercial infant formula milk as long as safe home conditions are available; or
- expressed, heat-treated breastmilk.

Note that clinical evidence suggests that home-modified animal milk is not recommended as a replacement food in the first six months of life.
For children over six months of age:
- commercial infant formula milk as long as safe home conditions are available; or
- animal milk (boiled for infants under 12 months), as part of a diet providing adequate micronutrient intake.

Despite best efforts, there may be situations where the mother cannot breastfeed or makes the choice not to breastfeed. In such situations, the options for feeding the infant are:
- heat treated breastmilk (Israel-Ballard et al, 2007); or
- replacement formulas.

Conditions needed to formula feed safely

Mothers known to be HIV-infected should only give commercial infant formula milk as a replacement feed to their HIV-uninfected infants or infants who are of unknown HIV status, when the following specific conditions are met:

- safe water and sanitation are assured at the household level and in the community;
- the mother, or other caregiver can reliably provide sufficient infant formula milk to support normal growth and development of the infant;
- the mother or caregiver can prepare it cleanly and frequently enough so that it is safe and carries a low risk of diarrhoea and malnutrition;
- the mother or caregiver can, in the first six months, exclusively give infant formula milk;
- the family is supportive of this practice;
- the mother or caregiver can access health care that offers comprehensive child health services.

Note: infants who are started on formula feeding from birth should receive six weeks of daily nevirapine prophylaxis.

When should heat-treated, expressed breastmilk be used?

HIV-infected mothers may consider expressing and heat-treating breastmilk as *an interim feeding strategy*:

- in special circumstances such as when the infant is born with low birth weight or is otherwise ill in the neonatal period and unable to breast-feed; **or**
- when the mother is unwell and temporarily unable to breastfeed or has a temporary breast health problem such as mastitis; **or**
- to assist mothers to stop breastfeeding; **or**
- if antiretroviral drugs (for mother or baby) are temporarily not available.

How to heat-treat expressed breastmilk

- Express between 50-120ml milk into a clean 450ml glass jar.
- Place jar of milk in a 1-litre aluminium pot with sufficient water to cover the level of breastmilk (about two fingers above). Lid should be off during the heating process.
- Place the pot on a heat source and allow the water to boil. When the water is boiling rapidly take the jar of milk out of the water, place the lid on and allow to cool down before feeding to the baby.

What should happen in terms of cessation of breastfeeding for HIV-infected infants?

Mothers are strongly encouraged to continue exclusive breastfeeding if their infant tests positive when the routine PCR test is done at six weeks and then continue breastfeeding as per the recommendations for the general population, that is up to two years or beyond.

Important things to bear in mind for mothers who have chosen to avoid all breastfeeding

- Formula feeding mothers require support at every well child/routine visit to facilitate and support exclusive formula feeding.
- Formula milk preparation should be demonstrated at the first post-natal visit and as needed thereafter.
- Health care personnel should provide clear guidance regarding the volume and frequency of feeding needed at each age.
- They should also discuss the dangers associated with bottle-feeding and if they are used, how bottles should be cared for.
- Cup-feeding should be discussed and demonstrated as a recommended alternative to bottle-feeding.
- Home support for avoiding breastfeeding should also be considered so that the mother has a supporter outside the health facility to help her avoid all breastfeeding.

Contra-indications to breastfeeding

There are relative and absolute contraindications to breastfeeding, both in the mother and in the infant.

In the mother:
- anti-TB treatment;
- cavitating TB;
- breast cancer;
- psychosis; and
- antithyroid drugs.

In the infant:
- galactosaemia; and
- phenylketonuria.

References and further reading

Arabi, M., Frongillo, E.A., Avula, R., Mangasaryan, N. 2012. Infant and Young Child Feeding in Developing Countries. *Child Development* 83(1): 32–45.

Bahl, R., Frost, C., Kirkwood, B.R., Edmond, K., Martines, J., Bhandari, N., Arthur, P. 2005. Infant feeding patterns and risks of death and hospitalization in the first half of infancy: multicentre cohort study. *Bulletin of the WHO* 83: 418–425.

Bedri, A., Gudetta, B., Isehak, A., et al. 2008. Extended-dose nevirapine to 6 weeks of age for infants to prevent HIV transmission via breastfeeding in Ethiopia, India, and Uganda: an analysis of three randomised controlled trials. *The Lancet* 372(9635):300–313.

Chasela, C.S., Hudgens, M.G., Jaimeson, D.J., et al. 2010. Maternal or infant antiretroviral drugs to reduce HIV-1 transmission. *N Engl J Med* 362: 2271–2281

Coovadia, H.M., Brown, E.R., Fowler, M.G., et al. 2012. Efficacy and safety of an extended nevirapine regimen in infant children of breastfeeding mothers with HIV-1 infection for prevention of postnatal HIV-1 transmission (HPTN 046): a randomised, double-blind, placebo-controlled trial. *The Lancet* 379: 221–228.

Doherty, T., Sanders, D., Goga, A., Jackson, D. 2011. Implications of the new WHO guidelines on HIV and infant feeding for child survival in South Africa. *Bulletin of the WHO* 89: 62–67.

Israel-Ballard, K., Donovan, R., Chantry, C., Coutsoudis, A., Sheppard, H., Sibeko, L. & Abrams, B. 2007. Viral safety of flash-heated breast milk: A method to reduce mother-to-child transmission of HIV in resource-poor countries. *J AIDS* 45: 318–323.

Kumwenda, N.I., Hoover, D.R., Mofenson, L.M., Thigpen, M.C., Kafulafula, G., Qing, L., Mipando, L., Nkanaunena, K., Mebrahtu, T., Bulteys, M., Fowler, M.G., Taha, T.E. 2008. Extended antiretroviral prophylaxis to reduce breast-milk HIV-1 transmission. *N Engl J Med* 359: 119–129

Mofenson, L.M., 2010. Protecting the next generation – eliminating perinatal HIV-1 infection. *N Engl J Med* 362(24):2316–2318.

National Department of Health, South Africa. 2005. *Report – Infant and Young Child Feeding Policy.*

South Africa DoH. 2011. *PMTCT guidelines.* South African guidelines website reference http://www.info.gov.za/view/DownloadFileAction?id=77877

Walker, A. 2010. Breast Milk as the Gold Standard for Protective Nutrients. *J Pediatr* 156: S3–7.

WHO. 2000. Collaborative Study Team on the Role of Breastfeeding on the Prevention of Infant Mortality. Effect of breastfeeding on infant and child mortality due to infectious diseases in less developed countries: a pooled analysis. *The Lancet* 355: 451–455.

WHO. 2010. *HIV and infant feeding. Guidelines on Principles and recommendations for infant feeding in the context of HIV and a summary of evidence*. UNAIDS, UNICEF and World Health Organization.

WHO. 2010. *Antiretroviral drugs for treating pregnant women and preventing HIV infection in infants*. World Health Organization.

13 Expressed breastfeeding in hospital

Breastmilk is the ideal nutritional source for the newborn and special efforts should be made to promote breastfeeding for all infants. Women should be informed during pregnancy of its advantages. Successful breastfeeding depends largely on early initiation after birth. Breastfeeding forms an integral part of 'kangaroo mother care' (skin-to-skin nursing of the naked infant between the mother's breasts), the preferred method of care for preterm infants. Expression of breastmilk is indicated when immediate breastfeeding post-delivery is not possible because the baby is too ill, too premature to suckle, or requires transfer to another hospital. Frequent, thorough emptying of the breasts, either manually or with a breast pump, will stimulate prolactin release and lactogenesis.

Necrotizing enterocolitis (NEC) is associated with formula milk feeding in very low birth weight (VLBW) (≤1.5 kg) infants (4× higher risk) with maternal HIV infection being an additional risk factor. The importance of breastmilk feeding and the safety of pasteurized expressed breastmilk (PEBM) for premature infants must be explained to all HIV-1 positive mothers who deliver prematurely.

Pasteurized donor EBM is administered to VLBW infants if the mother is too sick to express breastmilk or has died.

HIV, CMV and hepatitis B can be transmitted through unpasteurized breastmilk. Because the practice of feeding expressed breastmilk (EBM) to very low birth weight (VLBW) (≤1.5 kg) infants has become the norm many bottles containing EBM are stored in refrigerators in neonatal wards. Unless stringent precautions are implemented these viruses can be transmitted to infants. The HIV status of every mother should therefore be confirmed before or on admission of her baby to a neonatal ward. Neonatal wards must have strict protocols to prevent the inadvertent administration of EBM from an HIV-positive mother to someone else's infant. A dedicated 'EBM Manager' must be identified for every shift in a neonatal ward to oversee the expressing, correct handling, labelling, pasteurization and issuing of the correct breastmilk to each baby. In large neonatal units permanent EBM Manager positions must be established.

Expressed breastmilk

- Every health care worker, including doctors, should be trained in lactation management *with special emphasis placed on the risk of HIV transmission through EBM.*
- The mother should be educated on all the aspects of sterility, hygiene, collection of milk, containers for collecting EBM, correct and accurate labelling of containers, storing of the milk, frozen milk and the technique of pasteurizing EBM. Written instructions and wall charts should also be provided.
- Expression by hand may not be as effective as an electric or manual breast pump, but is the method of choice where microbial contamination through breast pumps and breastmilk expression kits is possible.
- In State hospitals breast pumps are not permitted due to the risk of cross infection.
- Breastmilk may only be expressed manually.

Containers and labelling

- Use a sterile glass or polyethylene hard plastic container with a wide mouth because it is difficult to direct the streams of milk into a small opening. Plastic bags or non-sterile containers such as fruit juice bottles, etc. may not be used because of the risk of leakage/contamination. Containers must have airtight caps.
- A different sterile container should be used for each expressing session. Milk from different expressing sessions must not be mixed as this increases bacterial load and risk of infection.
- Should a sterile EBM container not be available, a suitable, thoroughly washed container and lid can be submerged in boiling water for 10 minutes.
- Used milk bottles should be thoroughly washed with soap and water (or in a specially designed dishwasher) and a brush should be used to remove all organic material. Autoclaving (120 °C for 15 minutes) of bottles is more reliable and preferable to chemical disinfection.
- The container of EBM must be labelled immediately with the baby's name and surname, hospital number, date and time of expression.
- The label must be placed high up on the container so that it is not immersed in water during thawing or if the EBM is pasteurized.

Handling expressed breastmilk to prevent contamination

- Stringent hand-washing procedures must be followed by anyone in contact with EBM or the equipment.
- Freshly expressed breastmilk may not remain out of the fridge beyond 1 hour, as this will increase the risk of bacterial growth. The container of EBM must not be left at the bedside/incubator.
- While being administered to the infant EBM should be kept at room temperature for no longer than four hours.
- The EBM Manager and the mother should check that the milk is correctly labelled (see details above) before the EBM Manager places the milk in the fridge/freezer.
- If not used within 24 hours, EBM must be frozen (between –12 and –18° C).
- Containers designated for freezing should only be 2/3 full as frozen milk expands.
- The EBM fridge must be locked and the key kept by the EBM Manager or nurse.
- Only the EBM Manager or nurse may remove milk from the fridge. No mother may take milk from the fridge herself.
- EBM from an HIV-positive woman or a woman who has refused to be tested for HIV may only be placed in the fridge or freezer after pasteurization.

Handling expressed breastmilk of HIV-positive mothers

- EBM of HIV-positive mothers must be pasteurized immediately after expressing preferably using the Flash Heating Method.
- The mothers must be educated and supervised on the method of pasteurization by the EBM Manager or Ward staff before doing it by themselves.
- Before the pasteurized expressed breastmilk (PEBM) is refrigerated, the EBM Manager must confirm correct labelling with the baby's name, surname, hospital number, date and time of expressing as well as date and time of pasteurization.
- A sticker with a different colour, to indicate that the milk has been pasteurized, must also be applied to the container.
- The label and sticker must be applied near the top of the container so that it remains intact even when the container is immersed in water during thawing.

- PEBM must be clearly marked and stored separately from other EBM. This can be in a separate fridge or on a separate shelf in the same fridge.
- Each mother must have a designated tray or container (such as a 2 L ice cream tub) for her own her containers of pasteurized milk in the refrigerator.
- Unpasteurized breastmilk from a known HIV-positive or untested mother may not be placed in the fridge or freezer.
- The milk must remain with the mother until it has been pasteurized.

Handling expressed breastmilk of mothers who refuse to be tested for HIV

- Breastmilk from these mothers must be assumed HIV-positive.
- Breastmilk from a mother with an unknown HIV status carries a high risk of HIV transmission if administered to the wrong baby.
- Nurses must be vigilant to identifying which mothers are untested and ensure that their EBM is pasteurized. Apart from expressing breastmilk, such a mother will breastfeed her baby as well and it can therefore be wrongly assumed that she is HIV-negative.
- EBM of all untested mothers must be pasteurized and correctly labelled before being placed in the fridge by the EBM Manager.
- The above only applies to women who refuse to be tested whose premature infants are fed their own mother's milk.
- Explain to the mother that her EBM is being pasteurized to destroy all virus in order to make the milk safe for her baby.
- The label on the container of EBM must indicate that the EBM has been pasteurized. This sticker should be a different colour to unpasteurized EBM.
- All mothers should be tested for HIV and Flash Heating should be used while results are pending.

Storage of expressed breastmilk

- Ideally all neonatal wards require a designated ward milk kitchen with a designated fridge/freezer for storage of EBM.
- This kitchen must be separate from the general ward kitchen, or at the very least the neonatal ward should have a separate area with a designated lockable fridge and an area for pasteurization..
- The dedicated fridge/freezer in the ward milk kitchen must have refrigeration and freezer space with a functional temperature gauge.

- An EBM Manager (or nurse appointed as EBM Manager for each shift) is responsible for the ward milk kitchen.
- Health care workers with infections such as infected skin lesions, upper respiratory tract infections, conjunctivitis, diarrhoea, etc, must not be allowed in the milk kitchen.
- No parents are allowed in the central or ward milk kitchen. Restrict access to staff only.

Administering expressed breastmilk

- At each feed two nurses must check the baby's name, the hospital number, and the date of collection on the container of milk before it is administered to the baby and sign the relevant nursing documentation in the infant's folder.
- The name of the nurse, signature, date, and time that the milk was checked must be noted in the infant's folder.
- Nurses should identify and administer stored breastmilk as for blood products.
- *A mother's EBM may never be given to any baby other than her own.*
- Discard milk if doubt exists regarding hygiene or identification of expressed milk.

Thawing of expressed breastmilk

- It is preferable that milk be thawed overnight in the fridge (4° C)
- If frozen milk needs to be used immediately the container of frozen milk can be placed in a container with luke warm, not hot, water but must remain upright. Ensure that the temperature of thawed milk does not exceed 37°C.
- The water should not cover more than half the bottle and the label should never be submerged.
- The label on the container of EBM must remain intact.
- Never thaw expressed milk from different mothers simultaneously in the same container of warm water as contamination or swapping may occur.

Techniques for pasteurizing expressed breastmilk

Commercial pasteurization (Holder Method)

- This system is used if large volumes of breastmilk are pasteurized such as in the case of a Breastmilk Bank usually found in a large hospital.
- The Holder Method necessitates that a special pasteurization bath be installed in the central milk kitchen. It must be operated according to specific instructions which are available from the existing Breastmilk Banks.

Flash Heating or Pretoria Pasteurization methods

- Both can be used in hospital or at home after discharge.
- Every hospital should have a designated area close to the ward milk kitchen where mothers can pasteurize their own EBM (Pasteurization station).
- Staff working with postnatal mothers and their babies must receive training on the institution's preferred pasteurization method.
- The trained staff members must demonstrate the preferred method to mothers who intend pasteurizing their breastmilk.
- A wall chart should be available for reference.
- Ensure that mothers use good hand expressing techniques.
- Emphasize meticulous hand-washing and hygiene of equipment and worktop surfaces.
- Mothers must be supervised when pasteurizing their breastmilk for the first time.
- Mothers must be provided with the appropriate sterile glass jars for expressing breastmilk.
- Plastic jars are *not* suitable for Pretoria or Flash pasteurizing.
- Jars must be labelled with the baby's name, surname, hospital number, date and time of expressing as well as date and time of pasteurization.
- A sticker with a different colour, to indicate that the milk has been pasteurized, must also be applied to the container.
- The label and sticker must be applied near the top of the container.
- Labels must be replaced if not legible after pasteurization.
- Initially, small volumes of colostrum tend to solidify but can be added to pasteurized milk from a verified HIV-negative donor and then repasteurized. The final volume should be 50ml.

FLASH PASTEURISATION METHOD

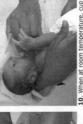

1. Equipment: Stove or flame, pot(±1L), glass jar, weight to stop jar toppling over, feeding cup.

2. Wash hands well with soap and hot water and dry with clean towel

3. Express 50 to 150ml breastmilk into sterile glass jar, cover jar.

4. Place pot with the jar of expressed breastmilk (EBM)on stove.

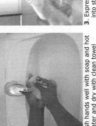

5. Place weight on jar of EBM to keep it stable.

6. Pour **tap** water into the pot to 2 fingers above level of EBM in jar.

7. a) **Switch stove on high.**
b) **Bring water in pot to rapid boil**
c) Switch stove off and......

8. **Immediately remove;**
a) Weight from jar,
b) Pot from stove and
c) **Jar of EBM from hot water.**

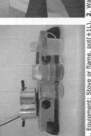

9. Cool EBM before feeding baby. Pasteurised EBM can be kept in the fridge for up to 24 hours

10. When at room temperature, cup feed pasteurised EBM to your baby.

11. Wash the jar, lid and cup in hot, soapy water. **12. To sterilise:** Place in pot, sub-merge in hot water and boil on stove for ± 10 minutes

- Once pasteurized, the cooled EBM can be used immediately or stored in the designated milk fridge for up to 24 hours.
- Pasteurized expressed breastmilk (PEBM) may also be frozen.
- After use, the jar should be washed and returned for routine sterilization in the central milk kitchen.
- In smaller hospitals, the jars should be returned to an area designated for cleaning and sterilization.
- It is preferable that mothers who are expressing at home pasteurize their EBM in the ward kitchen on return to the hospital, rather than at home.

Flash heating pasteurization – preferred method

Equipment:
- Pot with approximately 1 liter capacity;
- Sterilized glass jar with approximately 400 ml capacity e.g. empty glass peanut butter jar;
- A weight to hold down the jar of milk in the water, e.g. another jar with water;
- Electric/gas stove/hot plate;
- White insulation boards on which to place hot pot;
- Patient stickers;
- Permanent marker/stickers – 2 colours;
- Pen to write date on patient sticker.

Procedure:
- Express 50–150 ml breastmilk into the sterile glass jar.
- Place the lid on the jar.
- Place the jar with EBM into the pot and place on the stove.
- Place the weight on the jar.
- Pour approximately 450 ml tap water into the pot. Water level must be 2 fingers (2 cm) above the level of the expressed milk.
- Heat the water and milk together on a high heat setting, until the **water** is at a rolling boil.
- Immediately remove the pot from the stove and the EBM from the hot water and allow the breastmilk to cool at room temperature.

Pretoria Pasteurization method (secondary – use only if hot plate unavailable for Flash Heating)

Equipment:
- 1 × 1-litre pot (for Pretoria Pasteurization: Hart^R aluminium 1 litre pot);
- Sterilized glass jar of approximately 400 ml capacity;

- Kettle/Urn/Hydroboil;
- Measuring jug;
- A weight to hold down the jar of milk in the water;
- White insulation boards on which to place hot pot;
- Patient stickers;
- Permanent marker/stickers – 2 colours;
- Pen to write date on sticker;
- Wall clock.

Procedure:
- Express 50–150 ml breastmilk into the sterile glass jar.
- Place the closed jar in the aluminum pot.
- Put a weight on the jar to hold it down.
- Add freshly boiled water to the pot. Fill to 1 cm from the top.
- Leave the jar with EBM for 30 minutes in the hot water.
- Remove from hot water and cool before use.

Management of an infant unintentionally exposed to another woman's breastmilk

General information

- Post-exposure prophylaxis (PEP) must be administered as soon as possible to ensure maximal benefit (see below).
- All events should be clearly documented in the recipient baby's notes. This should include a clear description of the incident, 'donor' details, actions taken and all discussions with the parent/s.
- A Register should be kept for all inadvertent exposures in which the following must be documented:
  o name of the recipient infant;
  o name of the donor mother;
  o HIV status of both the infant's own mother and that of the donor mother and, if the infant is tested, of the infant;
  o date and time of the incident;
  o whether or not the milk was pasteurized.
- A Morbidity Form must be completed for each incident and this must be handed to Hospital Management and to the Quality Assurance Manager of the hospital.
- Copies of the Morbidity Form must be sent to the Hospital Superintendent and Nursing Services Managers, and should also be placed in the folder of the infant.

- The incident must be discussed at the monthly Morbidity Meeting.
- The reason for the exposure should be determined and action taken to avoid recurrence.

Immediate management

- Aspirate the milk via a nasogastric tube.
- Report the incident to the ward consultant and sister in charge.
- The ward doctor (or the 'on-call' doctor) must inform parents immediately and discuss the actions to be taken. Counselling is important.
- *After informed consent is obtained, test both mothers immediately for HIV and Hepatitis B (confirm that an RPR has been done in both mothers).*
- A rapid test can be used to screen for HIV. The Determine® Test is preferred. Many laboratories also have a rapid test for Hepatitis B surface antigen.
- Test results should be documented clearly in the recipient baby's notes and in the register in which inadvertent exposure is noted.
- If either the donor mother or recipient's mother refuses testing, obtain permission to screen her infant for HIV exposure using a rapid test.
- Positive rapid tests must be confirmed in the laboratory. An infant with a positive rapid test requires a HIV DNA PCR.
- Assure parents that confidentiality will be maintained.
- Do not introduce parents to one another.
- Decide whether post-exposure prophylaxis (PEP) is indicated.

Post-exposure prophylaxis (PEP) of the recipient baby

PEP is indicated if the donor mother is HIV-positive or her HIV status is unknown:

- Commence PEP as soon as possible, preferably within one hour of exposure.
- Complete the 28-day prophylactic course. If the recipient baby has a positive HIV DNA PCR test, review by a paediatric HIV clinician.

Three antiretrovirals are used in combination:
zidovudine (AZT):

term baby: (≥38weeks) 4.0 mg/kg orally every 12 hours for 28 days
preterm baby: (<38 weeks): 1.5 mg/kg orally every 12 hours for the first two weeks, *then* 2 mg/kg orally every six hours for two weeks

lamivudine (3TC):
>   <30 days of age: 2 mg/kg/dose orally every 12 hours for 28 days
>   >30 days of age: 4 mg/kg/dose orally every 12 hours for 28 days
- lopinavir/ritonavir (Kaletra®):
  300 mg/m²/dose orally 12 hourly for 28 days if older than 42 weeks post conception

To calculate the surface area of the baby: BSA = $(0.05 \times WT$ in kg)
- For infants below 42 weeks post conception (ie premature infants), give a single dose of nevirapine at 2 mg/kg in place of lopinavir/ritonavir
- Do baseline full blood count (FBC), alanine amino transferase (ALT) on the baby
- Complete the 28-day prophylactic course *unless* the recipient baby has a positive HIV DNA PCR test *in which case* the infant's treatment should be reviewed by a paediatric HIV clinician.

PEP if the donor mother is on antiretroviral therapy:
- Counsel the infant's parents/caregivers.
- Screen the recipient infant's mother for HIV.
- If the infant's mother or the infant has a positive rapid test, send baby's blood for HIV DNA PCR and hepatitis B serology.
- Do baseline FBC and ALT.
- Consult *urgently* with an HIV paediatrician to decide on the appropriate PEP for the recipient infant.

PEP if the recipient baby is HIV-infected:
The baby should be on antiretroviral therapy for its own health.

If the donor is HIV-negative:
Stop PEP immediately.

If the donor is positive or has unknown status and the recipient baby's mother is HIV-negative:
Provide PEP for 28 days as described above.

If an HIV-exposed recipient infant converts to a positive PCR:
Continue PEP and urgently consult with an HIV paediatrician.

Follow-up of exposed infants

- Continue in the ward if still hospitalized or at the infant follow-up clinic after discharge.
- Keep the parents informed.
- Obtain Hepatitis B results and act accordingly.
- If the 'donor' mother is Hepatitis B s antigen positive, give the exposed infant hyperimmune Hepatitis B immunoglobulin and the first Hepatitis B immunization immediately.
- Assess the 'donor' mother's infant at the same time. Also give hyperimmune Hepatitis B immunoglobulin and the first Hepatitis B immunization immediately.

Special investigations for infants on PEP

- At two weeks: do Hb. If unwell, do FBC and ALT.
- At four weeks: do Hb. If unwell, do FBC and ALT.
- Follow-up HIV testing: PCR at six weeks and if negative repeat at 12 weeks.
- Repeat ELISA test at six months to identify infants with late seroconversion.

Donor expressed breastmilk for the HIV-exposed VLBW infant

- Because of the increased risk of NEC, donor EBM (DEBM) is important for HIV-exposed VLBW infant when the mother is too ill to express or has died.
- Donor milk may be obtained from HIV-negative mothers in the neonatal ward or the community.
- Only DEBM of a mother with a recent (within the last month) written, confirmed negative blood HIV-1 result is accepted.
- HIV-1 tests are repeated every three months.
- *All donor milk is pasteurized (PDEBM) and thereafter tested for microorganisms.*
- DEBM may only be pasteurized in Level 3 and 2 hospitals under supervision of a paediatrician and the head of neonatal nursing.
- If DEBM is used at a small hospital (such as a Level 2 hospital) which does not have a commercial pasteurizer, the Flash Heating Method (use Pretoria Pasteurization method if hotplate unavailable) should be used to first pasteurize the milk before it is used.

- In these small hospitals donor milk is pasteurized in the ward milk kitchen.
- A senior registered nurse or EBM Manager who works in the neonatal ward of a smaller hospital is in charge of the pasteurization, consent forms and documentation of DEBM.
- All information on use of DEBM must be documented in the recipient baby's folder and a register must be kept in the milk kitchen.
- The authenticity of the DEBM must be checked against the donor's records and be given a donor and batch number before processing.
- Each jar of PDEBM must be clearly labelled with the donor number and date of pasteurization.
- The *recipient* parent/guardian must be given verbal and written information about PDEBM and sign consent for the administration of PDEBM.
- The recipient baby's details must include his/her name and folder number and feed number (if applicable).
- PDEBM can be defrosted; in a fridge overnight or left at room temperature but must be refrigerated while still cold (4°C), until it is to be used.
- The cold chain must be maintained when PDEBM is transported to the wards and what is not immediately used must be stored in the ward fridge (maintained at 4°C) for no longer that 24 hours.
- PDEBM that has been defrosted for longer than 24 hours must be discarded.

Distribution of PDEBM

- Written consent must be obtained from the mother, father or legal guardian of the baby before administration of PDEBM. If none of the above are available for consent, request permission from the hospital superintendent.
- All PDEBM must be labelled with the date pasteurized and the donor *number* rather than the donor name, before being issued.
- The designated staff must keep meticulous records of all DEBM received, whether pasteurized or unpasteurized, from other sources as well as DEBM from in-house donors. Once pasteurized, the records must include the date and the volume of PDEBM received from each donor, using their donor number and the recipient babies' names and folder numbers.
- Defrosted milk must be labelled with the date and time of when it was defrosted and the name and hospital number of the recipient baby.

- *Before PDEBM is administered, the EBM Manager (or nurse assigned as EBM Manager for that shift) and another nurse must check that the recipient baby's name and hospital number correspond with the donor number as indicated on the PDEBM container, and record accordingly.*
- PDEBM should be kept at room temperature for no longer than 4 hours while being administered to the infant.
- Frozen DEBM must remain frozen until it is defrosted for pasteurization.
- DEBM can be defrosted; in a fridge overnight or left at room temperature but must be refrigerated while still cold (4°C), until pasteurization.
- Once defrosted it must be pasteurized within 24 hours.
- DEBM that defrosts during transit or because of a faulty freezer cannot be refrozen but must be pasteurized within 24 hours.

Handling pasteurized donor-expressed breastmilk

- All PDEBM must be frozen unless used within 24 hours.
- PDEBM can be defrosted in a fridge overnight or left at room temperature but must be refrigerated while still cold (4°C), until used.
- Defrosted PDEBM must be refrigerated at between 0 and 4°C for up to 24 hours.
- When being administered e.g. via syringe driver, keep at room temperature for no longer than 4 hours.
- PDEBM that defrosts during transit or because of a faulty freezer cannot be refrozen but must be used within 24 hours.
- Alternatively it can be repasteurized, stored and used as PDEBM (described above).
- PDEBM cannot be pasteurized a third time.

Acknowledgements

Prof Brian Eley, Dr Helena Rabie, Dr Adri Bekker, Mrs Ellie Warrington, Dr Max Kroon and Mrs Elisna Lessing.

References and further reading

Arnold, L. D. W. 1999. *Recommendations for collection, storage and handling of a mother's milk for her own infant in the hospital setting.* 3rd edition. Denver: Human Milk Banking Association of North America.
Ayliffe, G. A. J. et al. eds. 1992. 'Preparation of infant feeds and the use of milk kitchens.' *Control of Hospital Infection.* 3rd edition. London: Chapman and Hall Medical.

Jeffery, B. S. and K. G. Mercer. 2000. 'Pretoria pasteurization: A potential method for the reduction of postnatal mother to child transmission of the human immunodeficiency virus.' *Journal of Tropical Pediatrics*; 46:219–223.

Kirsten, G.F., Goosen, L., Warrington, E., Kirsten, C.L., Rabie, H., Eley, B. et al. *Protocol for the use of expressed breastmilk in the Western Cape.*

Spicer, K. 2001. 'What every nurse needs to know about breast pumping. Instructing and supporting mothers of premature infants in the NICU'. *Neonatal Network*; 20:35–41.

UNICEF. 10 steps to successful breastfeeding. www.unicef.org

14 Nutrition

Without optimal antiretroviral therapy, disturbed growth and nutrition are inevitable in HIV-infected infants:

- Mean birth weight is lower in the infants of HIV-infected mothers than in the infants of uninfected mothers.
- Linear growth is reduced in HIV-exposed infants, whether infected or uninfected.
- Mean birth weight is lower in infants born to mothers with AIDS than to seropositive mothers without AIDS.
- Postnatal growth is compromised throughout childhood.
- Stunting and under-weight-for-age are common problems.
- Wasting syndrome (see textbox) is common.
- Preferential muscle wasting over fat wasting (i.e. lean body mass attrition) occurs.
- Depletion of somatic and visceral protein and of essential amino acids occurs.
- Multiple trace element, vitamin, and electrolyte deficiencies are frequent.

The aetiology and pathogenesis of growth failure and malnutrition are complex and vary in each child. The causes include:

- reduced dietary intake, owing to poverty and food shortages;
- oropharyngeal and oesophageal disease;
- anorexia and neurological complications;
- intestinal malabsorption and increased excretion of nutrients;
- abnormal energy, protein, and/or fat utilization;
- increased macronutrient and micronutrient requirements; and
- multiple micronutrient deficiencies, which occur frequently.

Deficiencies of nutrients essential for normal immunological function such as the vitamins A, B6, C, and E and the trace elements zinc, copper, iron, and selenium increase the risk of opportunistic infection (OI) in HIV-infected infants. This overview focuses on the practical aspects of the nutritional management of HIV-infected children in resource-poor settings.

Wasting syndrome is an AIDS-defining illness characterized by:
- persistent weight loss >10% of baseline; or
- downward crossing of at least two of the following percentiles on a weight-for-age chart (97th, 75th, 50th, 25th, 5th) in a child ≥1 year of age; or
- <5th percentile on a weight-for-age chart on two consecutive measurements, ≥30 days apart, *plus* chronic diarrhoea (i.e. at least two loose stools per day ≥30 days) or documented fever for ≥30 days, intermittent or constant.

Failure to thrive, unresponsive to dietary intervention and treating underlying causes such as tuberculosis is a WHO Stage III disorder.

Food security and nutrition

In sub-Saharan Africa, HIV infection and food insecurity have combined to have a devastating effect on the nutritional status of individuals, households and communities. The long-term consequences include social and economic collapse. Over the last few years countries in southern Africa have experienced significant food crises. In South Africa more than 14 million people, or about 35% of the population are vulnerable to food insecurity, many as a result of HIV/AIDS.

Figure 14.1 Bi-directional relationship between HIV/AIDS and food security (Source: Save the Children and Oxfam)

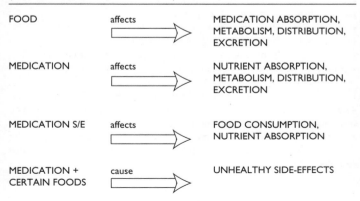

FOOD	affects →	MEDICATION ABSORPTION, METABOLISM, DISTRIBUTION, EXCRETION
MEDICATION	affects →	NUTRIENT ABSORPTION, METABOLISM, DISTRIBUTION, EXCRETION
MEDICATION S/E	affects →	FOOD CONSUMPTION, NUTRIENT ABSORPTION
MEDICATION + CERTAIN FOODS	cause →	UNHEALTHY SIDE-EFFECTS

Feeding during early infancy

(See also Chapter 12: HIV and infant feeding.) Breastfed infants with proven HIV infection should continue breastfeeding.

Treatment of HIV infection and opportunistic infections

The deleterious effect of HIV infection on linear growth correlates with the level of viraemia. Antiretroviral therapy will arrest and reverse stunted growth and nutritional deterioration in many HIV-infected children.

OIs are catabolic events that may aggravate the nutritional deterioration of HIV-infected children. All infective episodes should be treated vigorously. Parasitic infestation may facilitate the progression of HIV infection. Regular deworming at four to six month intervals with albendazole or mebendazole is recommended from the age of one year.

Nutritional effects of antiretroviral therapy

Combination antiretroviral therapy is associated with improvements in many growth parameters including weight-for-age, weight-for-height ratio, body mass index, arm muscle circumference, and to a lesser extent stature.

Shortly after the introduction of combination antiretroviral therapy, a clinical syndrome of fat redistribution and metabolic changes was described in adults. The lipodystrophy syndrome includes insulin resistance, dyslipidaemia, and lipodystrophy (truncal obesity, dorso-cervical fat pad, and extremity and facial wasting). Affected individuals demonstrate differing patterns of fat maldistribution. Prevalence of the lipodystrophy syndrome in children ranges from 1–43%. Although the protease inhibitors (PIs) have been implicated in the pathogenesis of lipodystrophy syndrome, fat maldistribution may occur with non-PI regimens. Lipoatrophy is caused by the nucleoside reverse transcriptase inhibitors (NRTIs), particularly stavudine.

Dyslipidaemias resulting in a proatherogenic lipid profile (elevated LDL, low HDL, hypercholesterolaemia, hypertriglyceridaemia) are strongly associated with PI administration. Dyslipidaemia may occur in the absence of clinically evident lipodystrophy. The prevalence of PI-induced dyslipidaemia ranges from 20% of children on a single PI to >90% of children on regimens containing two PIs.

Nutritional support

Many HIV-infected children unable to gain access to antiretroviral therapy rely on nutritional interventions to slow the progression of their disease. Wasting contributes to the morbidity and mortality of HIV infection. Even with antiretroviral therapy, nutritional support continues to be an important ancillary treatment.

Monitoring

During clinic visits parents should be asked about feeding problems, gastrointestinal symptoms, intercurrent infections, and features that suggest tuberculosis. Growth indices (weight-for-age, height-for-age, weight-for-height) should be plotted serially. Measurements of haemoglobin and red blood cell indices three to four monthly will help to establish treatable causes of anaemia.

Advice

Preventing infections in the home, safe food preparation, and measures to increase the nutritional value of meals should be discussed regularly.

Preparing food

Advise parents to take the following precautions when preparing food:
- Wash hands before preparing food.
- Clean bottles, teats, and other feeding utensils thoroughly before preparing milk and food.
- Use clean water to prepare milk.
- If a fridge is unavailable, prepare one feed at a time.
- Cover food to protect it from contamination by flies.
- Unless a fridge is available, buy fresh foods on the day of use.
- Cook meat, fish, and poultry thoroughly.
- Cook eggs until the yolks are hard.

Improving the nutritional value of meals

The nutritional value of meals can be improved by:
- adding 1–2 teaspoonfuls of vegetable oil, margarine, or peanut butter to the child's porridge, samp, rice, or potatoes;
- using wholewheat flour or brown bread instead of white bread;
- eating beans, peas, lentils, or soya products if meat is unaffordable;
- consuming fish, chicken, eggs, and meat when possible;

- choosing chicken and meat with less fat and bone;
- buying vegetables and fruit that are in season;
- providing more vegetables if fruit is expensive;
- not overcooking vegetables;
- cooking potatoes and sweet potatoes with the skins intact; and
- cultivating a food garden.

Dietary management

Nutritional requirements for HIV-infected children are largely based on theoretical considerations and could be different to those in uninfected children. Age-related macronutrient and micronutrient requirements have not been optimized. Recommended daily allowances (RDAs) applicable to uninfected children are used as guidelines. These may be obtained from standard paediatric textbooks. Children who fail to thrive or have overt malnutrition require additional support.

Unless data on energy expenditure is available to determine precise caloric objectives, 150% of the RDA for caloric and protein intake is a reasonable target for children with failure to thrive. An alternative method for calculating macronutrient requirements is to use the formula:

$$\frac{(\text{RDA for age} \times \text{ideal weight-for-height})}{(\text{actual weight})}.$$

Increased calories may be provided by adding cooking oil, glucose polymer, or medium-chain triglyceride preparations to feeds. Enteral supplementation through either a nasogastric or gastrostomy tube improves weight-for-age and weight-for-height, but does not increase height-for-age or lean body mass.

Total parenteral nutrition has not been extensively researched in children, but does improve growth in HIV-infected adults. Because these measures do not improve the survival of HIV-infected individuals significantly, and are technically challenging to implement, they are largely inappropriate in the management of HIV-infected children in Africa.

Regular vitamin A supplementation reduces morbidity and mortality in children with HIV infection. Oral supplementation should be administered every six months:

- children <6 months: 50 000 IU;
- children 6–12 months: 100 000 IU; and
- children >12 months: 200 000 IU.

If vitamin A preparations are not available, a multivitamin/trace element preparation which ensures a RDA for vitamin A of 3 000 to 5 000 IU should be prescribed regularly.

Food supplementation: In South Africa, the integrated nutrition programme coordinates an inter-sectoral approach to nutritional problems. Within its conceptual framework, vulnerable/at risk individuals, groups and communities are targeted for nutrition interventions. Growth faltering in childhood is defined as a growth curve that flattens or drops over two consecutive months, and is an indication for nutritional support. Age-appropriate products are supplied through 'PEM schemes', and include formula milk, infant cereal, energy drinks and other food supplements.

Acute severe malnutrition

Marasmus is more frequently encountered than kwashiorkor in paediatric HIV infection. Severe malnutrition, particularly kwashiorkor, should be managed according to standard clinical practice.

Pharmacological preparations

Megestrol acetate, a progesterone-like drug, acts as an appetite stimulant. Administered at a dosage of approximately 8 mg/kg/day to children with HIV infection and failure to thrive; it improves weight-for-age by increasing fat stores. It does not improve lean body mass, and weight gain is not sustained after discontinuation of the medication. Other agents that may improve appetite and body weight include glucocorticosteroids and cyproheptadine. Limited research in children has shown that growth hormone may improve body weight and lean body mass over short periods. These agents have limited application in sub-Saharan Africa.

Lipodystrophy syndrome

The replacement of a PI with either a non-nucleoside reverse transcriptase inhibitor (NNRTI) or abacavir does not reverse fat abnormalities despite improvements of metabolic derangements. In contrast, switching to NRTI-sparing regimens or changing certain NRTIs (e.g. replacing stavudine with abacavir or zidovudine) leads to improvement of lipoatrophy.

At present there is no consensus on the treatment of fat maldistribution in the absence of other metabolic abnormalities.

Dyslipidaemias

Lifestyle changes are recommended as the first intervention. These include dietary restriction of total fat to 25 to 35% of total caloric intake, and saturated fat to less than 7% of total calories, reduced dietary cholesterol, use of plant sterols, increased intake of soluble fibre, weight reduction when indicated and increased exercise.

There are no published reports on the use of lipid lowering agents in HIV-infected children with dyslipidaemia. The American Academy of Pediatrics recommends drug treatment for children older than 10 years if after six to 12 months of dietary modification, serum LDL cholesterol ≥4.9 mmol/L or ≥4.1 mmol/L with a family history of coronary artery disease or the presence of two other cardiac risk factors. Therapeutic options include bile acid sequestrants, HMG CoA reductase inhibitors and fibrates.

Another approach to managing dyslipidaemia is to switch from a PI to a PI-sparing regimen. This strategy ameliorates the observed lipid abnormalities.

References and further reading

Henderson, R. A., and J. M. Saavedra. 1995. 'Nutritional considerations and management of the child with human immunodeficiency virus infection.' *Nutrition*; 11:121–128.

Semba, R. D., and A. M. Tang. 1999. 'Micronutrients and the pathogenesis of human immunodeficiency virus infection.' *British Journal of Nutrition*; 81:181–189.

Miller, T.L. 2003. 'Nutritional aspects of HIV-infected children receiving highly active antiretroviral therapy.' *AIDS*; 17:S130–S140.

McComsey, G.A. and E. Leonard. 2004. 'Metabolic complications of HIV therapy in children.' *AIDS*; 18:1753–1768.

American Academy of Pediatrics. Committee on Nutrition. 1998. 'Cholesterol in childhood.' *Pediatrics*; 101:141–147.

Diarrhoea

Diarrhoeal disease is one of the most important complications of HIV infection. The majority of children with HIV infection will suffer from multiple episodes of diarrhoea in the first two years of life. These episodes are often severe, recurrent and prolonged, leading to malnutrition and increased mortality. Co-morbid conditions such as septicaemia and pneumonia often complicate the course and management.

The pathogenesis is multifold. Common stool pathogens are frequently detected and opportunistic infections (OI) are important in advanced disease. In addition, severe mucosal injury, malabsorption of sugars and fat, and bacterial overgrowth contribute to diarrhoea. A number of protease inhibitors, (e.g. nelfinavir, amprenavir, ritonavir and saquinavir) may also cause diarrhoea.

History and examination are key in evaluating diarrhoeal disease.

History

Important aspects to include in the history are:
- previous episodes of diarrhoea and hospital admissions;
- past drug history, including recent antibiotic use;
- history of exposure to infectious diseases;
- nutritional history;
- sanitation factors, (e.g. the source of the family's drinking water);
- social circumstances; and
- growth rate (which is charted on the 'Road to Health' booklet).

The symptom enquiry should cover:
- duration of symptoms;
- fever;
- vomiting;
- refusal of feeds;
- dysphagia;
- blood or mucus in the stool; and
- abdominal pain.

Examination

Children are initially evaluated for signs of dehydration and shock (see Appendix 15.1).

Nutritional evaluation includes:
- anthropometry and growth rate;
- subcutaneous fat and muscle mass;
- oedema;
- signs of anaemia;
- vitamin (e.g. vitamins A and D) and trace element (e.g. zinc) deficiencies.

In the general examination, look for:
- lymphadenopathy;
- thrush;
- dermatitis;
- signs of associated conditions such as pneumonia;
- hepatomegaly, splenomegaly, and abdominal distension (these are common); and
- anal fissures (occasional).

Examine the stool for blood and mucus.

Diagnostic approach

Initially, a conservative approach is appropriate. Episodes of diarrhoea will frequently resolve with standard supportive treatment. A more extensive evaluation is warranted for prolonged diarrhoea, advanced disease, or severe malnutrition.

General

Acid-base, serum electrolytes, albumin, and haematology should be assessed as part of the initial evaluation. Hypokalaemia is frequent. Other electrolyte abnormalities such as hypernatraemia, hyponatraemia, hypophosphataemia, and hypomagnesaemia occur. Blood cultures and a chest radiograph are performed where appropriate.

Lactose or sucrose intolerance frequently occurs, leading to a prolonged course of diarrhoea. Watery stools with a low pH (turns litmus paper red) and reducing substances in the stool suggest sugar malabsorption.

Osmotic diarrhoea occurs due to loss of brush border enzymes. The 'milk ladder' can assist in managing malabsorption. Specialized formulas are costly and need only be used until the malabsorption has resolved.

Table 15.1 The milk ladder

Villus with brush border enzymes	Diagnosis	Recommended formula
Lactase	Stool reducing substances: 5 drops stool + 5 drops water + Clinitest tablet: 1–2% positive	Lactose free formula: Soya based formula, other low lactose formula
Sucrase	As above: If negative add HCl: becomes positive with presence of sucrose.	Sucrose and lactose free milk
Maltase		Extensively hydrolysed formula

Stool

Stool specimens are examined for viruses (rotavirus, adenovirus), bacteria, and parasites. Yield is increased if adequate volumes of stool are submitted along with at least two specimens for bacterial culture. Specimens should reach the laboratory promptly. Alert the laboratory regarding the patient's immune status, and request appropriate tests for OIs.

The spectrum of organisms isolated is similar to those found in immuno-competent children in Africa: rotavirus is common; important bacterial pathogens are *Escherichia coli*, *Salmonella* spp., *Shigella*, *Campylobacter*, and *Yersinia* spp. Giardia frequently causes diarrhoea and reinfection is common.

Opportunistic infections

Cryptosporidium infection in immunocompetent children usually results in self limiting diarrhoea. Children with HIV, however, develop severe secretory diarrhoea leading to large water and electrolyte losses. Malabsorption with severe weight loss ensues and the mortality is high. The infection is often chronic with prolonged excretion of oocytes in the stools.

In addition to the intestine, the gall bladder, bile ducts and pancreas may be infected. Nitazoxanide for three days, has been registered by the FDA for immunocompetent children. A recent clinical trial however found that nitazoxinide is less effective in HIV-1-infected children. Anecdotal evidence suggests a higher dose and longer duration of therapy. Immune function should be restored using antiretroviral therapy. Poor absorption may mitigate beneficial effects. Protease inhibitors may also directly inhibit infection by the protozoan.

Prevention includes the boiling and subsequent cooling of drinking water. Ideally HIV-infected infants should not attend day-care centres where the risk of faeco-oral transmission is high. Guardians and other HIV-infected patients should avoid contact with faecal material. Hand washing is important.

Cytomegalovirus (CMV) is an important enteric pathogen. The colon is most frequently involved, followed by the oesophagus and small bowel. Diarrhoea and fever are the most frequent presenting symptoms. Serious complications include severe lower intestinal haemorrhage, perforation and colonic strictures. In addition the liver, bile ducts, and pancreas may be infected. Stool cultures are usually not helpful and the diagnosis relies on endoscopy (colonoscopy or gastroduodenoscopy) or surgical biospies for histopathology and viral culture. Patients may respond to ganciclovir. Severe CMV colitis may also be due to IRIS after introduction to antiretroviral therapy.

Colitis

Campylobacter jejuni, *Salmonella*, and *Shigella* should be sought in the stool. Test for *Clostridium difficile* toxin, if possible, in the stool of children who have been hospitalized or recently exposed to antibiotics. Adenovirus, herpes simplex, *Mycobacterium avium* complex (MAC), *Pneumocystis jirovecii*, *Cryptosporidium*, *Histoplasma*, and *Coccidioides* cause colitis in immunocompromised adults and are probably implicated in children. Severe colitis also occurs in the absence of identifiable pathogens.

Invasive investigations

Invasive procedures may be necessary in a child with persistent diarrhoea and negative stool cultures.

- Sigmoidoscopy is often valuable in children with unexplained persistent diarrhoea. Histology (electron microscopy) and culture of mucosal biopsies are useful to diagnose CMV, adenovirus, MAC, and other organisms not easily cultured in the stool. Non-specific colitis, resembling inflammatory bowel disease, may occur.

- Colonoscopy is indicated if sigmoidoscopy is inconclusive (colitis may be limited to the caecum and ascending colon). Colonoscopy is uncomfortable, and should be limited to patients with prolonged diarrhoea unresponsive to treatment.
- Oesophagogastroduodenoscopy is useful where no pathogen has been identified. Candida oesophagitis, bacterial overgrowth, and OIs may be diagnosed with upper gastrointestinal endoscopy, aspiration of duodenal fluid, and mucosal biopsy.

Treatment

- The same principles of resuscitation and rehydration apply to both HIV-infected and HIV-negative children. Children are initially evaluated for hypovolaemic shock. Shock is corrected with a rapid intravenous or intra-osseous infusion of resuscitation fluid (20–30 mL/kg). In the absence of shock and severe dehydration, oral or nasogastric rehydration therapy is effective. Oral rehydration is safe, easy to administer, and avoids the need for intravenous lines.
- Feeds are started as soon as shock and severe dehydration have been corrected. Routine interruption of feeds is not beneficial. As soon as the patient's appetite permits, additional energy intake is encouraged.
- In the presence of lactose intolerance, the following could be used: a lactose-free formula (e.g. soya formula), a low-lactose formula (e.g. Pellargon®), or fermented milk products (see textbox). Sucrose intolerance occasionally necessitates the introduction of sucrose-free feeds.

> Preparing fermented milk:
> Bring 500 mL milk to boiling point.
> Allow to cool to 38–46 °C (slightly warm to touch).
> Add 2 tablespoons Bulgarian yoghurt and stir.
> Keep warm for six to eight hours (wrap in a towel or keep in oven with pilot light on).

Bacterial overgrowth of the small bowel may lead to prolonged diarrhoea and malabsorption. The limited data available suggest that treatment with cholestyramine and antibiotics (such as gentamicin) may be effective in non-cryptosporidial diarrhoea. Specific treatments are available for a number of pathogens (see Table 15.2). Empiric treatment for suspected *C. difficile* infection should be instituted if the stool cultures are negative and *C. difficile* toxin cannot be determined in the stool.

Nutritional support is essential. Feeds should not be interrupted unless absolutely necessary. When possible the intake of additional feeds should be encouraged. Adequate energy and protein intake should be supplemented with vitamins. Zinc supplementation reduces the incidence and duration of diarrhoea in children at high risk for zinc deficiency and is beneficial when administered during an acute episode of diarrhoea. Regular vitamin A supplementation reduces the morbidity and mortality associated with diarrhoeal disease. Supplementation during an acute episode of diarrhoeal disease, however, does not confer the same benefit.

Antidiarrhoeal agents are not routinely used in the treatment of children and infants with diarrhoea. They are contraindicated for dysentery. Certain antidiarrhoeal drugs, (e.g. diphenoxylate) can lead to severe central nervous system depression in infants and young children and should be avoided. Loperamide can, however, give symptomatic relief with prolonged diarrhoeal disease unresponsive to treatment. Even though microsporidial diarrhoea is uncommon, a therapeutic trial of albendazole should be attempted in all children with refractory diarrhoea, especially where laboratory testing is not possible.

Infants and children with prolonged diarrhoeal disease should be considered for antiretroviral therapy. This will usually be delayed until resolution of the diarrhoea due to the unpredictable absorption of the drugs in patients with diarrhoea. If however the diarrhoea follows an unremitting course initiation of therapy should be discussed with practitioners experienced with antiretrovrial treatment.

Table 15.2 Drugs and dosages for organisms causing diarrhoea in HIV-infected children

Organism	Drug
Shigella	Nalidixic acid (12.5 mg/kg 6 hourly for 5 d.); 3rd-generation cephalosporin (e.g. cefotaxime, ceftriaxone)
Salmonella spp.	According to sensitivity; Mainly 3rd-generation cephalosporins
C. difficile	Metronidazole (5–7 mg/kg/dose 8 hourly, maximum 250 mg 6 hourly); vancomycin (10 mg/kg/dose 6 hourly, maximum 250 mg 6 hourly)

Giardia	Metronidazole (1–3 yr., 500 mg/d.; 3–7 yr., 600–800 mg/d.; 7–10 yr., 1 g/d. for 3 d.); Alternatively, 15 mg/kg/d. in divided doses for 5–7 d. Albendazole (over 2 yr. 400 mg daily for 5 d.)
Cryptosporidium	No effective treatment; May need prolonged therapy (up to 4 mo.) depending on response; Paromomycin 25–35 mg/kg/d. given 12 hourly (not currently available in SA); Azithromycin 5–12 mg/kg once daily;
Microsporidium	Albendazole only effective against the *encephalitozoon* species of *Microsporidium* (over 2 yr. 400 mg 12 hourly for 5 d.)
CMV	Ganciclovir (5 mg/kg 12 hourly for 14–21 d.), if available
Non-specific diarrhoea	Cholestyramine 1 g 6 hourly; Gentamicin 50 mg/kg per d. (maximum 360 mg/d.) 6 hourly po, but 1 h. apart from cholestyramine
Loperamide HCL	0.2 mg/kg/day
Zinc sulphate	10 mg elemental zinc daily

Appendix 15.1 Evaluation of hydration status in children

The evaluation of dehydration is imprecise and dependent on experience. Studies that have evaluated the validity of the clinical signs in acute diarrhoea have yielded inconsistent results. No single clinical sign provides an accurate assessment of hydration. The combination of signs improves the accuracy. Important signs include delayed capillary refill time, abnormal skin turgor, and an abnormal respiratory pattern (due to metabolic acidosis). The evaluation of capillary fill time is dependent on technique and ambient temperature. Skin turgor is influenced by the amount of subcutaneous fat: excess subcutaneous fat may disguise the presence of significant dehydration and if wasting is present skin turgor is reduced even in the absence of dehydration. Metabolic acidosis may be due to dehydration or bicarbonate loss. Consequently an acidotic breathing pattern does not necessarily indicate dehydration. Lethargy may be due to dehydration or associated disease. Consequently, the child who appears lethargic should receive urgent attention. Although parental history is inaccurate a history of decreased urine excretion (fewer than normal wet diapers/nappies) alerts the clinician to dehydration.

Table 15.3 Evaluation of hydration status in children

Degree of dehydration	Signs	Comments	Treatment
Severe	Two of the following signs: • Lethargic or unconscious • Sunken eyes • Not able to drink or drinking poorly • Skin pinch goes back very slowly	Urgent attention required (may indicate associated disease). Ask the care-giver what the child's eyes normally look like.	Intravenous resuscitation. Fluid: • Ringer's Lactate • Normal Saline Volume: • 20 mL/kg rapidly • give additional boluses of 10–20 mL/kg if circulation does not improve
Moderate (Some dehydration)	Two of the following signs: • Restless, irritable • Sunken eyes • Drinks eagerly, thirsty • Skin pinch goes back slowly	Consider other causes, e.g. meningitis. Children with wasting will appear more dehydrated than they are, obese children will have little reduction in skin turgor in the presence of dehydration.	Oral Rehydration 50–100 mL/kg over 4 hours (CDC guidelines) Maintenance Up to 2 years: 50–100 mL po after each loose stool. 2 years and more: 100–200 mL after each loose stool (IMCI)

Modified from WHO, IMCI and CDC Recommendations

Paediatric tuberculosis

HIV infection increases the risk of tuberculosis (TB). In the absence of antiretroviral therapy HIV-infected infants have a 24-fold higher risk to develop TB disease compared to HIV-uninfected infants in areas of high TB incidence. An increased incidence of congenital TB has also been noted.

Clinical features

Diagnosis of TB in children has always been challenging, but is now more complex because of overlap with other HIV-related lung diseases. Both over- and under-diagnosis are likely, depending on TB incidence and the health worker's experience.

Patient history

It is important to consider the following points when taking a history:
- TB can present at any age, even in neonates.
- Symptoms of pulmonary and extrapulmonary TB (EPTB) are more often acute in HIV-infected children.
- WHO criteria for the diagnosis of TB (cough >2 weeks, failure to thrive, and/or weight loss) are more common in HIV-infected children than in HIV-uninfected children with TB, but other HIV-related conditions can cause similar symptoms.
- Chronic fever is common in HIV-associated TB.
- *A history of contact with an adult TB source case is most important.* This is often the first hint of diagnosis. A history of a known contact is identified in up to 66% of cases.
- The drug susceptibility test results of the source case(s) are essential for the proper management of the childhood contacts.
- Previous antituberculosis treatment in the child or the adult source case is associated with a higher rate of drug resistance.

A history of any of the following may indicate the need for invasive investigations to establish a definite diagnosis:

- absence of an expected response to other treatments (e.g. antibiotics for two weeks);
- previous abnormal chest radiograph findings; or
- persistent lung disease.

Physical examination

- Generally, children present with primary pulmonary TB that is more symptomatic than that found in HIV-uninfected children.
- EPTB affects similar sites in both HIV-infected and uninfected children. Peripheral lymph node and central nervous system (CNS) involvement are quite common. Unusual sites, such as the middle ear (causing chronic otorrhoea) need special attention. The increased association of EPTB with HIV infection is not as clear as it is in adults. Note that HIV disease itself results in generalized lymphadenopathy and hepatosplenomegaly.
- There is an increased risk for TB in HIV-infected children without a BCG scar.

Special investigations
Tuberculin skin test

A Mantoux tuberculin skin test (TST) should be performed. The Mantoux TST consists of an intradermal injection of five tuberculin units (TU) of purified protein derivative (Japanese strain) or two TU of PPD RT23 (Danish strain). Induration is measured transversely in millimetres after 48 to 72 hours. A negative result does not exclude TB. For the HIV-infected child, induration >4 mm denotes a positive result. Repeating a negative TST after nutritional rehabilitation in a severely malnourished child may yield a positive TST. Positive TST results are reported in 40% to 55% of HIV-infected children with TB. Low CD4 counts and progressive HIV disease were associated with negative TST.

Interferon-gamma Release Assays (IGRAs)

IGRAs are specific T-cell-based assays developed to identify patients with TB infection. Two types of IGRAs are commercially available: the ELISA-based QuantiFERON-TB Gold In-tube assay (Cellestis Limited, Australia), and the ELISPOT-based T-Spot.*TB* assay (Oxford Immunotec, UK). These assays have the same sensitivity for identifying TB infection as TST, but they have an increased specificity to TST in high-burden areas of tuberculosis mainly because they are negative with BCG and most non-tuberculous mycobacteria. There currently is no evidence that the IGRAs have any advantage over TST in high tuberculosis burden areas.

Chest radiography

The typical reticulonodular (miliary) picture, with or without lymph-adenopathy, could indicate miliary TB, but lymphocytic interstitial pneu-monitis (LIP), which has become rarer with combination antiretroviral therapy (cART), could mimic it. A miliary picture in a child aged <1 year or on cART, or an evenly spread, fine, nodular pattern favours miliary TB. Clubbing, generalised lymphadenopathy and swollen parotids would favour LIP, but both can be present simultaneously. Culture-confirmed TB cases often have paratracheal lymphadenopathy, hilar lymph-adenopathy, and large airway compression. The increase in pleural and pericardial effusions observed in adult HIV/TB patients has not been seen in children. No radiological feature distinguishes TB from other HIV-associated lung conditions, and chest radiographs in HIV-infected and uninfected children with TB are similar.

Microscopy and culture

Microscopy of gastric aspirates or induced sputa for acid-fast bacilli has a low yield (5–10%) in children, and does not distinguish *Mycobacterium tuberculosis* from non-tuberculous mycobacteria.

Cultures from every available source (i.e. early morning gastric aspirate, induced sputum, nasopharyngeal aspirate, fine needle aspiration (FNA) of lymph nodes, bone marrow aspirate, bronchoalveolar lavage fluid, ear swabs, cerebrospinal fluid, pleural fluid) are important when TB is suspected. Histology and cultures for *M. tuberculosis* of lymph node (only if FNA unsuccessful), liver, lung, and trephine biopsies may be indicated for persistent or chronic lung disease. Susceptibility testing should be performed on *all* isolates. It is important to note that TB is not excluded until culture negativity at eight weeks. Follow-up cultures, while on treatment and after completion, are advisable if pathology remains. See Appendix 16.1: Procedure for obtaining sputum samples.

Supportive investigations

The elevated serum ESR, adenosine deaminase, lactate dehydrogenase, and globulins have limited benefit in the diagnosis of TB in HIV-infected children.

Therapeutic trial of antituberculosis treatment

Extreme care must be taken when instituting therapeutic trials, as poorly conducted trials may lead to drug resistance. Also, antituberculosis treatment can treat other conditions. Clinical and radiological response must, therefore, be monitored.

Treatment issues

Evaluate the following factors that will influence the choice of treatment:

- Is the child just infected with M. tuberculosis (TST positive without clinical or radiological evidence of tuberculous disease) or does the child have tuberculous disease? This distinction determines whether chemoprophylaxis or treatment is necessary.
- Is the child on antiretroviral therapy? If so, which antiretroviral drugs? Note that protease inhibitors and non-nucleoside reverse transcriptase inhibitors interact with rifampicin.
- Should both cART and antituberculosis treatment be introduced? (There may be immune reconstitution inflammatory reaction [discussed below] or overlapping side-effects if they are initiated simultaneously.)
- Is the drug-susceptibility test pattern from either the child's or the source case's *M. tuberculosis* isolate known?
- Did the child or source case receive any previous antituberculosis treatment? (Consider the risk of acquired drug resistance.)

Prophylaxis (isoniazid preventive treatment [IPT])

Post TB exposure prophylaxis is indicated in any child <5 years of age, or HIV-infected irrespective of age and cART (even if TST negative) when the child has had contact with an infectious adult source case (*after excluding disease*). Prophylaxis should be repeated with every contact with new TB source cases.

IPT for six months should be offered to all HIV-infected infants who initiate ART after three months of age once TB disease has been excluded and considered in all older HIV-infected children without TB disease.

Treatment regimens for prophylaxis [IPT] include:

- isoniazid 10 mg/kg daily (maximum 300 mg daily) for six to nine months; and
- isoniazid and rifampicin daily for three months, the latter only as directly observed therapy (not recommended by the South African National TB programme).

Treatment

- Rifampicin-based short course chemotherapy with directly observed treatment is indicated. If rifampicin is not included for the full duration, the minimum course is nine months. Regimens without rifampicin are not recommended, being significantly inferior.

- Most TB guidelines, including those of South Africa, recommend that treatment duration be the same for HIV-infected and uninfected TB patients. In our experience, treatment for nine to 12 months should be considered. Clinical, radiological, and, when indicated, microbiological evaluations must be performed at the end of treatment to confirm the response to treatment.

- Irregular adherence to therapy: If the patient misses more than two weeks (10 consecutive doses) of antituberculosis treatment early on, (i.e. irregular adherence to therapy), the entire treatment schedule should be recommenced.

- Corticosteroids are useful for TB meningitis (prednisone 2–4 mg/kg/day, with the higher dose for severe disease, [maximum 60 mg/day] for one month and taper), large airway compression due to enlarged mediastinal lymph nodes and pericardial TB (2 mg/kg/day).

- Treatment for multidrug-resistant MDR-TB, (i.e. resistance to isoniazid and rifampicin, with or without resistance to other drugs) should be individualized according to the drug susceptibility test results of the child or adult source case, or standardized based on the clustering in a community. An increased incidence of drug-resistant TB in HIV-infected patients has been reported. The first reports of childhood HIV/TB cases also showed a high incidence (20–30%) of drug resistance. These cases are best referred to an expert.

- Drug dosages for first-line antituberculosis treatment in children have recently been increased by the WHO and also SA NTP. New recommended dosages are: INH 10 mg/kg/day (range 10–15 mg/kg/day); rifampicin 15mg/kg/day (range 10–20 mg/kg/day); pyrazinamide 35 mg/kg/day (range 30–40 mg/kg/day) and ethambutol 20 mg/kg/day (range 15–25 mg/kg/day). See table for weight-band dosages. All HIV-infected children should receive pyridoxine (vit B6) supplementation and co-trimoxazole prophylaxis during TB treatment.

Antituberculosis treatment and antiretroviral therapy

(See Chapter 4: Interactions between HIV and tuberculosis.)

When to start

TB treatment takes precedence over antiretroviral therapy, but in general cART should be initiated within one to eight weeks after starting antituberculosis treatment. Infants below one year of age and critically ill children have the highest mortality for both TB and HIV. Therefore, antiretroviral therapy should be commenced one to two weeks after starting TB treatment or even sooner if there is advanced disease. Pulmonary TB is a WHO stage 3 event, but does not imply that antiretroviral therapy is immediately indicated. Rather evaluate the child. If stage 4 disease, extreme CD4 depletion or suspected MDR-TB, initiate antiretroviral therapy one to two weeks after starting TB treatment.

Overlapping drug side-effects

Side-effects from antituberculosis drugs occur slightly more often in HIV-infected patients. Most side-effects occur within two months of starting therapy. Hepatotoxicity, skin rash, nausea and vomiting, leukopenia, anaemia, and peripheral neuropathy could be due to either TB drugs or antiretroviral drugs. The severe cutaneous reactions seen in adults treated with thiacetazone also occur in children and it is therefore not used.

Immune reconstitution inflammatory syndrome (IRIS)

IRIS is the temporary exacerbation of symptoms, (e.g. fever) and signs, (e.g. lymph node enlargement, worsening chest radiograph appearance) which is called paradoxical TB-IRIS, and can occur when introducing cART and antituberculosis treatment. TB disease presenting acutely after a negative TB screen before commencing cART is called unmasking IRIS. It is ascribed to a hypersensitivity reaction to antigens released by non-viable bacilli and subsides spontaneously. Some cases are quite severe and treatment with steroids could be indicated. *This is not treatment failure.*

Prognosis for HIV-infected children with tuberculosis

In almost all adult and paediatric studies, TB mortality is higher among HIV-infected TB patients than in uninfected TB patients. Death is often due to other HIV-related infections or complications. Furthermore, the morbidity is also increased, as demonstrated in children with TB meningitis.

Recurrence of TB and failure to respond to antituberculosis treatment is often seen.

Possible causes for relapse and failure to respond include:

- incorrect diagnosis;
- poor compliance or incorrect treatment regimens;
- drug-resistant TB;
- progressive immune suppression;
- re-infection;
- impaired drug absorption (possibly HIV related); or
- duration of treatment too short (slow response).

Remember that a second or even a third episode of TB is possible.

Non-tuberculous mycobacteria

Non-tuberculous mycobacterial infection mainly involves the *M. avium* complex, an environmentally acquired mycobacterium. This causes peripheral lymphadenitis in young children. Disseminated disease is possible in children with advanced HIV-disease and markedly reduced CD4 counts. Clinical presentation can be indolent and slowly progressive. Fever, loss of weight, or failure to gain weight, abdominal pain, and severe anaemia are common. Diagnosis is by blood or tissue culture and DNA polymerase chain reaction probe. Median survival without treatment is about five to 10 months. Death is usually related to advanced HIV infection.

Treatment options include clarithromycin or azithromycin, along with ethambutol and/or rifampicin. The rescue treatment includes the newer generation fluoroquinolones (e.g. levofloxacin) and intravenous or intramuscular amikacin.

The World Health Organization strategy to control tuberculosis

The aim of the WHO strategy to control TB is to identify 70% of the infectious cases and to have a cure rate of 85%. Cornerstones of the strategy include:

- passive case finding;
- ensuring regular drug supplies;
- enhancing adherence; and
- standardizing the system of reporting.

Table 16.1 Weight band antituberculosis treatment for children <8 years of age (Acknowledgement: Paediatric Expert Review Committee for EDL)

Intensive phase:

Regimens 3A (without ethambutol) and 3B (with ethambutol):

Body weight kg	Intensive Phase (2 months) Treatment given 7 days a week		
	RHZ* 60,30,150	Additional isoniazid (5 mg/kg to make total isoniazid dose to 10-15 mg/kg) Isoniazid 100 mg tablet	Ethambutol 100 mg or 400 mg tablets
2–2.9 kg	½ tablet	–	50 mg (½ tablet if 100 mg ethambutol tablet) Alternatively, give ethionamide 62.5 mg (¼ of 250 mg tablet)
3–3.9 kg	1 tablet	¼ tablet	
4–5.9 kg	1 tablet	¼ tablet	100 mg
6–7.9 kg	1½ tablets	½ tablet	150 mg
8–11.9 kg	2 tablets	½ tablet	200 mg
12–14.9 kg	3 tablets	½ tablet	300 mg
15–19.9 kg	3½ tablets	½ tablet	300 mg
20–24.9 kg	4 tablets	1 tablet	400 mg
25–29.9 kg	5 tablets	1 tablet	500 mg
30–34.9 kg	6 tablets	1 tablet	600 mg

Continuation phase:
Regimens 3A and 3B: HR – using the combination of RH 60/30 plus additional isoniazid tablets or RH 60/60.

Body weight kg	Continuation phase (4 months) Treatment given 7 days a week			RH 60,60
	RH 60,30	Additional isoniazid (5 mg/kg to make total isoniazid dose to 10–15 mg/kg) Isoniazid 100 mg tablet		
2–2.9 kg	½ tablet	–		½ tablet
3–5.9 kg	1 tablet	¼ tablet		1 tablet
6–7.9 kg	1½ tablet	½ tablet	OR	1½ tablets
8–11.9 kg	2 tablets	½ tablet		2 tablets
12–14.9 kg	3 tablets	½ tablet		2½ tablets
15–19.9 kg	3½ tablets	½ tablet		3 tablets
20–24.9 kg	4 tablets	1 tablet		4 tablets
25–29.9 kg	5 tablets	1 tablet		5 tablets
30–35.9 kg	6 tablets	1 tablet		6 tablets

References and further reading

Coovadia, H. M. et al. 1998. 'Childhood human immunodefficiency virus and tuberculosis co-infection: Reconciling conflicting data'. *AIDS*, 12: 1185–1193.

Department of Health. 2009. *National Tuberculosis Management Guidelines*. Department of Health

Edmonds, A. et al. 2009. Anti-retroviral therapy reduces incident tuberculosis in HIV-infected children. *Int J Epidemiol*, 38:1612–21.

Jeena, P. M. et al. 2000. 'Lymph node biopsies in HIV-infected and non-infected children with persistent lung disease.' *International Journal of Tuberculosis and Lung Disease*, 4:139–146.

Madhi, S. A. et al. 2000. 'HIV-1 co-infection in children hospitalised with tuberculosis in South Africa'. *International Journal of Tuberculosis and Lung Disease*, 4:448–454.

Machingaidze S, et al. 2011. The Utility of an Interferon Gamma Release Assay for Diagnosis of Latent Tuberculosis Infection and Disease in Children: A Systematic Review and Meta-analysis. *Pediatr Infect Dis J*, 30:694–700.

Mandalakas, A.M. et al. 2011. Interferon-gamma release assays and childhood tuberculosis: systematic review and meta-analysis. *International Journal of Tuberculosis and Lung Disease*, 15:1018–32.

Schaaf, H. S. et al. 2000. 'Clinical insights into the interaction of childhood tuberculosis and HIV in the Western Cape.' *The Southern African Journal of HIV Medicine*, July; 1 (1): 33–35.

Schaaf, H.S. et al. 2007. Culture-confirmed childhood tuberculosis in Cape Town, South Africa: a review of 596 cases. *BMC Infect Dis*, 29;7:140.

Thomas, P. et al. and the New York City Paediatric Spectrum of Disease Consortium. 2000. 'Tuberculosis in human immunodeficiency virus-exposed children in New York City'. *Paediatric Infectious Diseases Journal*, 19: 700–706.

Walters, L.E. et al. 2008. Clinical presentation and outcome of tuberculosis in human immunodeficiency virus infected children on anti-retroviral therapy. *BMC Pediatrics*, 8(1):1 doi:10.1186/1471-2431-8-1. Article is available from: http://www.biomedcentral.com/1471-2431/8/1

Appendix 16.1 Procedure for obtaining sputum samples

This section reviews basic procedures for common methods of obtaining sputum in children: expectoration, gastric aspiration, and sputum induction.

Expectorated sputum

Background: All children who are able to produce a sputum specimen should have it sent for smear microscopy, and where available, myco-bacterial culture. Children who can produce a sputum specimen may be infectious, so, as with adults, they should be asked to do this outside, and not in enclosed spaces (such as toilets) unless there is a specially-equipped room for this purpose.

Procedure

- Give the patient confidence by explaining to him/her (and any family members) the reason for sputum collection.

- Instruct the patient to rinse his/her mouth with water before producing the specimen. This will help to remove food and any contaminating bacteria in the mouth.
- Instruct the patient to take two deep breaths, holding the breath for a few seconds after each inhalation and then exhaling slowly. Ask him/her to breathe in a third time and then forcefully blow the air out. Ask him/her to breathe in again and then cough. This should produce a specimen from deep in the lungs. Ask the patient to hold the sputum container close to the lips and to spit into it gently after a productive cough.
- If the sputum is insufficient, encourage the patient to cough again until a satisfactory specimen is obtained. Remember that many patients cannot produce sputum from deep in the respiratory track in a few minutes. Give him/her sufficient time to produce an expectoration which s/he feels is produced by a deep cough.
- If there is not expectoration, consider the container used and dispose of it in the appropriate manner.

(Adapted from World Health Organization. *Laboratory Services in Tuberculosis Control. Part II: Microscopy.* WHO, Geneva, 1998.)

Gastric aspirate

Note: Gastric aspirates are not generally an aerosol-generating procedure. As young children are also at low risk of transmitting infection, gastric aspirates can be considered low risk procedures for TB transmission, and can safely be performed at the child's bedside or in a routine procedure room.

Background

Children with TB may swallow mucus that contains *M. tuberculosis*. Gastric aspiration is a technique used to collect gastric contents in order to culture the *M. tuberculosis*, confirm the diagnosis of TB and determine susceptibility of the organism to antimicrobials. Smear microscopy can also be performed on gastric aspirates, but these specimens are rarely smear positive (except in very young infants) and can sometimes yield false-positive results (especially in HIV-infected children who are at risk of having nontuberculous mycobacteria). This procedure is most useful on young hospitalised children. It is most useful if the specimen can also be cultured for *M. tuberculosis* in the laboratory.

Gastric aspirates are used for collection of mycobacterial cultures in young children when sputa cannot be spontaneously expectorated nor induced using hypertonic saline. Even when three gastric aspirates are collected, only 25–50% of children with active TB will have a positive culture, so a negative gastric smear or culture *never* excludes TB in a child. Do not use tap water for this procedure, as it can sometimes contain nontuberculous mycobacteria.

Gastric aspirates are collected from young children suspected of having pulmonary tuberculosis. During sleep, the lung's mucociliary system beats mucus up into the throat. The mucus is swallowed and remains in the stomach until the stomach empties. Therefore, the highest yield specimens are obtained first thing in the morning.

Three gastric aspirates on consecutive mornings should be performed for each patient. This is the number that seems to maximize yield. Of note, the first gastric aspirate collection has the very highest yield and should be collected using the best possible technique.

Children not fasting for at least four hours (three hours for infants) prior to the procedure and children with a low platelet count or bleeding tendency should not undergo the procedure.

Equipment needed for gastric aspirates:
Helper (performing the test properly usually requires two people)
Gloves
Nasogastric tube (usually 10 French or larger)
5, 10, 20, or 30 cc syringe with appropriate connector for your tube
Litmus paper
Specimen cup and lab forms
Pen (to label specimens)
Sterile water or normal saline
Bicarbonate (8%) solution for bedside neutralization

Get everything ready before starting (the syringe needs to fit the NG tube).

How to do the procedure

- Do the procedure first thing in the morning when the child wakes up but is not active.
- Children should have fasted for at least four hours (infants for three hours) prior to the procedure.
- Find an assistant to help (this procedure requires two people).

- This procedure should be done on the ward at the child's bedside, or in a procedure room on the ward (if one is available).
- Prepare all equipment for the procedure.
- Position the child on his or her back or side and have the assistant help to hold the child.
- Measure the distance of the tube to stomach (from nose to stomach) to estimate distance that will be required to insert the tube.
- Attach a syringe (10–20 ml) to the nasogastric tube (size 10 French).
- Gently insert the nasogastric tube through the nose and advance it into the stomach.
- Withdraw (aspirate) gastric contents using the syringe attached to the nasogastric tube (2–5 mL).
- To check that the position is correct, use litmus paper: blue litmus turns red (acidic stomach contents). (You can also check by pushing some air from syringe into the stomach [e.g. 3–5 mL] and listening with a stethoscope over the stomach).
- If no fluid is aspirated, insert 5–10 mL of sterile water or normal saline (0.9% NaCl) and attempt to aspirate again:
  o If still unsuccessful, attempt this again.
  o Do not repeat more than three times (even if the nasogastric tube is in the incorrect position and normal saline inserted into the airways, the risk of adverse events is still very small).
  o Withdraw the gastric contents (ideally at least 5–10 mL).
- Transfer gastric fluid from syringe into a sterile container (sputum collection cup).
- Add an equal volume of sodium bicarbonate to the specimen (in order to neutralize the acidic gastric contents and so prevent destruction of tubercle bacilli).

After the procedure

- Wipe the specimen jar with alcohol/chlorhexidine to prevent cross-infection and label specimen cup.
- Fill out lab requisition forms.
- Transport the specimen (in a cool box) to the lab for processing as soon as possible (within four hours).
- If it will take more than four hours, place specimens in the fridge and store at 4–8 °C until transport.
- Give the child the usual feed after the procedure.

Induced sputa (IS) have a higher yield and are useful in outpatient settings as one IS is equivalent to three gastric washings. There is, however, an appreciable risk of nosocomial spread, so precautions must be taken.

References and further reading

WHO. *Guidance for national tuberculosis programs on the management of tuberculosis in children*. Geneva; 2006.

Zar, H.J., Hanslo, D., Apolles, P., Swingler, G., Hussey, G. 2005. 'Induced sputum versus gastric lavage for microbiological confirmation of pulmonary tuberculosis in infants and young children: a prospective study.' *The Lancet*, 365(9454):130–134.

Sexual abuse

Awareness of sexual offences against children has increased dramatically. Children who are sexually abused suffer great physical and/or emotional consequences. An addition to this ordeal is that sexual offenders may transmit HIV. According to the Criminal Law (sexual offences and related matters) Amendment Act of 2007, Chapter 5 (implemented from 2008), application for compulsory HIV testing of the alleged sex offender by the victim (>14 years of age) or interested person can be made where appropriate.

Definition

Child sexual abuse (CSA) is defined as using a child for sexual gratification. This can take different forms, e.g. voyeurism, fondling and fingering, and intercourse. Intercourse includes extra-genital, vaginal, anal, or oral penetration.

Presentation of child sexual abuse

The presentation of CSA may occur through:
- disclosure by the child or a third party;
- physical indicators, e.g. injury to the genitalia or anal area, sexually transmitted infections (STIs) etc.;
- psychosomatic indicators, e.g. secondary enuresis; or
- behavioural indicators.

The role of the doctor

Take a complete medical history (including immunization status), but do not obtain details about CSA from the child, unless the child discloses spontaneously. The social worker or investigating police officer has the responsibility to obtain details about the CSA event.

Undertake a full clinical examination of the child, including growth parameters, stage of sexual development, physical injuries, and systemic examination. Only after completing the general examination should the genital and anal area be examined. Explain every step to the child. Collect medico-legal evidence. A crime kit, supplied by the investigating police officer, should only be used if the child presents within 72 hours of the abuse.

Do further special investigations as clinically indicated, including:

- full blood count and clotting profile;
- skeletal radiographs and CT;
- syphilis, hepatitis B and HIV serology;
- smears and cultures for STIs; and
- pregnancy testing, if the female child is pubertal (Tanner stage 3 or more).

Notify the Director-General of Social Services or any designated officer when CSA is suspected. Do not confront the parent(s)/guardian, but explain the findings to them and inform them that a suspicion of child abuse is legally notifiable. Do not try to manage the problem on your own. Involve a social worker and other members of the CSA management team. Together with the social worker and/or police, ensure the safety of the child before discharge. Write detailed notes and draw sketches of the injuries. Complete the J88 form supplied by the police officer, if you are asked to do so. Treat current infections and other medical problems. Refer the child, as indicated, for surgical and mental health problems.

Prophylaxis

It is important to provide:

- post-exposure prophylaxis (PEP) for HIV if the child presents within 72 hours of the CSA (see below); and
- pregnancy prophylaxis, if indicated;
- guidelines for the prevention of HIV transmission (<14 years of age);
- counselling.

Counsel the child's parent/guardian about the potential risk of HIV transmission and offer antiretroviral therapy if the child presents within 72 hours of the abuse. The minimum antiretroviral therapy is zidovudine (AZT) and lamivudine (3TC), with or without a protease inhibitor.

Counsel the parent/guardian by explaining:

- what HIV/AIDS is;
- why hepatitis B and syphilis tests must be done;
- the importance of knowing the child's initial HIV, hepatitis B and syphilis status;
- the common side-effects of the drugs;

- the importance of compliance; and
- that the effectiveness of antiretroviral therapy in preventing post-sexual exposure is not known, but it does reduce transmission in other forms of exposure.

No PEP should be given to children presenting more than 72 hours after abuse, as antiretroviral therapy will have no impact on preventing HIV transmission.

HIV testing

Informed consent must be obtained from the child (>12 years of age – Children's Act 83 of 2005), parent or legal guardian before testing. Initial HIV testing should be performed to obtain the child's baseline HIV status. If immediate HIV testing is refused, revisit the issue at the one-week follow-up appointment.

Regimen for prophylaxis

AZT and lamivudine (3TC) forms the basis of PEP. The dosage for AZT depends on the body surface area (BSA): 180 to 240 mg/m^2 per dose 12 hourly for 28 days after 6 months of age. The dosage of lamivudine is 4 mg/kg/dose 12 hourly. Weight band dosing may be used.

To calculate the BSA:
- determine the weight and height/length of the child and use a BSA nomogram; or
- estimate by using the formula:

$$BSA = \sqrt{\frac{wt(kg) \times height(cm)}{3\,600}}$$

or use the weight-based chart.

Prescribe or give only enough AZT and 3TC to last until the one week follow-up appointment. If the patient has complied, prescribe AZT and 3TC for the remainder of the 28-day course. A third antiretroviral drug, (usually a protease inhibitor) should be added for severe trauma or if the perpetrator is also on antiretrovirals. Routine full blood count and liver enzyme tests for prophylactic antiretroviral therapy are not recommended. Relative contraindications to the use of AZT include significant renal or liver impairment.

Vertical transmission prevention studies have shown that two drugs are more effective than one (P1043). For this reason we usually recommend two antiretrovirals. Protease inhibitors increase the side effects and are often associated with poor adherence.

Follow-up testing

Follow-up is essential. After one week, meet to discuss the test results, identify new problems, treat, and continue prophylaxis to prevent HIV transmission.

All children negative for HIV at baseline, and in whom CSA was confirmed, should have subsequent HIV and syphilis testing at six weeks, three months and six months. Children who were initially HIV-infected, and those who become infected, should be referred to an appropriate health facility for long-term management.

Further information

ChildLine Toll-free 0800 0 55555

Setting up an HIV/AIDS clinic for children

HIV infection remains incurable but access to antiretroviral therapy can greatly prolong life. In the antiretroviral era it is increasingly clear that optimal health care delivery to children with HIV/AIDS requires efficient professionals working in a functional team. The paediatric HIV/AIDS clinic has become a venue of operations for multidisciplinary teams made up of nurses, counsellors, pharmacists and physicians. At most levels of care, a family orientated approach should be adopted. This makes provision of health care for families affected by the disease more accessible and efficient. The needs of children should not however be subverted by this approach.

The nature of an HIV clinic

The clinic serves as a multi-disciplinary platform where the team exercises its capacity to screen and triage patients, provide appropriate care and deliver successful antiretroviral therapy and overall health care. For optimal health care, patient flow into the clinic through screening procedures must be efficient and the clinic must be in the right place, both geographically and for appropriate referral systems. Antiretroviral therapy is a component of integrated, comprehensive primary health care (PHC) care for people with HIV/AIDS.

Comprehensive PHC is based within the district health system. Key components that should be maintained in a family service are: child-friendly and -centred care and attention to the psychosocial and economic needs of the family delivered as community-based care. These components are part of a chronic care module within the IMCI (Integrated Management of Childhood Illness) model. This form of integrated PHC necessarily requires strong elements of leadership and outreach.

Clinics must sustain high levels of performance over very long periods to deliver care to chronically ill patients and their families. Management must understand the psychological burden of this work. There must be agreement on the clinic's aims and goals, and how these are to be achieved. The diverse range of skills delivered by all members of the team should be recognized as necessary contributions to successful care. Optimal levels of knowledge and skills are required by the entire treatment team to sustain high levels of professional performance, patient and staff retention.

Children reaching adolescence present new challenges to treatment teams. Adolescents and young adults benefit from appropriate life skills training, manifest in improved adherence and more regular clinic attendance.

Families must be supported and encouraged to feel powerful enough to demand what is needed for themselves and their children and must be given an opportunity to exercise choice of services. Long-term adherence to antiretrovirals is most likely where families are self-motivated and supported to take on appropriate lifestyle options.

Clinics must be geared to deliver a comprehensive health care package. The clinic itself should aim to offer a 'one stop' service, with easy referral networks to resources it cannot provide.

At a recent conference for treatment teams, 23 teams from nine sub-Saharan African countries summarized the elements of an ideal clinic in the following table:

Table 18.1 Elements of an ideal clinic

ELEMENTS OF AN IDEAL CLINIC	
	Rationale
PHYSICAL ENVIRONMENT Child friendly Spacious, natural light, well ventilated Welcoming reception area Good signage, possibly with the use of colour Food (subsidized) available Appropriate and ergonomic furniture, storage A physical structure that facilitates flow	Child friendly: Recognize children's developmental need for mobility and exploration in play. Areas need to be safe and welcoming. Good signage improves patient flow and order. Adequate light and ventilation decrease error in care settings. Nourishment is an issue for health and well being.
PATIENT FLOW Triage by a trained nurse to ensure that patients are appropriately directed Appointments and records system streamlined by some pre-visit organization Continuity of care Access to transport, existing facilities, referral resources Identification and separation of adolescents or adults who are coughing and may transmit TB. Both should be wearing masks. Coughing children should also be separated	Adequate patient flow is a key quality indicator as is decreased patient waiting time. Children may be ill and require rapid care or a shortened clinic visit if rapidly directed to the practitioner they need to see. Seeing familiar practitioners each time improves patient satisfaction and retention in care and adherence.

CLEAR REFERRAL NETWORKS

Good linkage with PMTCT programmes to identify children requiring treatment

Clear links and transport between clinic and referral centres

Liaison between clinic and the community

Clinics should develop links with the referral hospital and with down-referral smaller clinics

Familiarity with individuals at all levels of care facilitates referral

Establishing district networks and regular meetings are helpful

Delayed referral and complicated or delayed transport can increase morbidity and mortality in paediatric populations.

STAFF ENVIRONMENT

Recognition for multidisciplinary team

Counsellors are vital

Whole staff needs to have been trained in communication with children and families

Staff rooms close but separate from clinic, safe space for active stress management

Tea and lunch breaks must be taken

The psychological burden of work with sick children can affect staff morale, illness and result in absenteeism. Care is complex and requires cooperating and smoothly functioning multidisciplinary teams. Improved work relationships increases quality of care and staff retention. Communication between management and clinical staff must be direct and supportive.

USE OF ANCILLARY STAFFING

Clerical administrative staff–data management

Nurse aide/community member trained to play with and care for children. Recognize and facilitate development related needs

Social services liaisons officer to facilitate grant applications

A patient-manager to guide clients through the clinic visit and ensure that information has been received and well understood

Use PWHA* to enhance service delivery. PWHA can do data management. Can improve patient retention and adherence with simple strategies through companioning, play and drawing. Experienced care-givers can field client questions, facilitate flow, provide community liaison.

*person with HIV/AIDS

The ideal clinic, collectively designed by the same group of health care workers, and represented in the schema in Figure 18.1, requires an architectural design that enhances interaction between team members and meets the needs of children and their families.

Figure 18.1 An ideal clinic structure

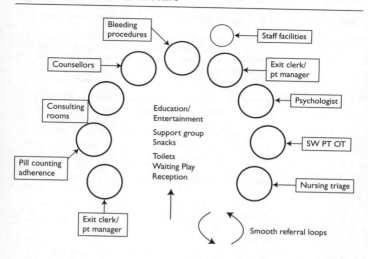

Supporting the quality of care

Care consistent with current professional knowledge must be delivered and has been defined as the degree to which health services delivered to individuals and populations increase the likelihood of desired health outcomes.

Quality improvement requires that clinics and treatment teams set targets and measure appropriate indicators of outcome and performance that can feed back on clinical and managerial operations. Table 18.2 lists the elements of quality health care and suggests some outcome indices to measure quality of care delivery.

Practical issues for paediatric services

Booking systems; defaulter tracing mechanisms, paper or computer-based records which readily provide medical history; adequate child-friendly space, equipment to run a paediatric service, pharmaceutical systems to ensure constant supplies of antiretrovirals and other necessary medication and laboratory services with reasonable turn-around times.

Table 18.2 Elements of quality health care in an HIV/AIDS clinic

Element of care	Features in an HIV Clinic	Outcome indicator
Safety	Following correct drug regimens Vigilance for adverse events and OIs Adverse event reporting Access to necessary levels of care	Adverse events Failure to gain access to hospital/ICU Prescription error rate Dispensing error rate
Effectiveness	Service based on scientific knowledge In-service training and CME for all staff Monitoring CD4 counts and viral loads Prompt responses to treatment failure and OIs Appropriate switching to palliative care Surveillance of outcomes Modification of care models in response to adverse outcome indicators	Rate of conversion to undetectable viral load Retention in care Adherence rate Hospital admission rate Bed use
Timeliness	Appropriate and prompt responses Reducing waits and harmful delays Management of clinic visits and medicine collection	Records of delays Clinic attendance rate Medicine collection rate
Equity	Equal care regardless of gender, ethnicity, geographic location, socioeconomic status Geographic location of service Support for transport costs Income generation projects Other social entrepreneurship	Frequency of outreach visits Attendance by gender Rate of uptake of grants Rate of uptake of income generation opportunity
Efficiency	Avoiding waste of equipment and supplies Workplace strategies that enhance teamwork Respect between professions	Staff satisfaction survey Rate of staff transfer out Stock surveys Time-and-motion studies

Lack of any requirement should not inhibit starting a service for children, as waiting for everything to be in place will exacerbate child morbidity and mortality.

Staff requirements

The appropriate staff:patient ratio has not yet been established for children.

The factors that influence health care worker requirements include task assignments, delivery models, other staff responsibilities, programme size, visit schedule and level of care provided.

Managing children may require longer consultations due to their more complex adherence requirement. In 2005 at the Tygerberg Hospital Family Clinic (THFC), the average time for a doctor to see an adult was 10 minutes and a child 20 minutes. Children visit more frequently for dosing adjustment as the child gains weight. Nurses or clinical officers with basic HIV knowledge can manage stable infants and children.

Access to management guidelines (i.e. WHO, national or regional) is essential. Training should accompany implementation. Basic paediatric knowledge of normal primary care of paediatric patients (IMCI Integrated Management Childhood Illness) is a prerequisite as common childhood illnesses occur frequently.

Allow for task shifting. New and innovative ways to address staff shortages must be developed. For example in Uganda, high school graduates receiving an intensive course in HIV management were successfully employed to lighten the load of more formally trained medical staff.

Community-based advocates are essential for tracking children requiring home-based support or lost to follow up.

Space

Safe and child-friendly spaces in the waiting area and consultation room, especially where adults also receive care, is helpful. The overwhelming adult epidemic causes children's needs to be ignored. Exposure to harmful organisms in the waiting room is a threat to children. Although effective care can be delivered in shared clinician space, sensitive issues should be discussed in private, particularly as children grow older. Personnel should have a high awareness for TB.

Apparatus

- *Infant and child scales for weight and weight percentile charts*
- *Tape measures and head circumference charts*
  Neurodevelopmental delay is common and under-recognised. Measuring head circumference and plotting on a percentile chart is an important component of the neurological assessment in children ≤3 years of age.
- *Stadiometer and length/height percentile charts*
  Regular measurement of height/length is not essential. However, for small infants <5 kg, length is essential to calculate body surface area, for antiretroviral dosages.
- *Appropriate specimen containers, needles and syringes*
  Use specimen containers requiring smaller blood volume. Equipment for gastric lavage or induced sputum for TB diagnosis is essential. TB specimens should be obtained in well ventilated areas, and HCWs should wear N95 disposable respirators.

Drug supply

Stable procurement, the correct transport, maintaining the 'cold chain' (for selected antiretrovirals, e.g. lopinavir/ritonavir solution) and correct storage conditions are essential. 'Room temperature' should not exceed 25 °C.

There should be Standard Operating Procedures for tracking and forecasting drug needs. Drugs close to expiry should be used first. Projected requirements for new enrolments and those already in care must be considered.

Laboratory support

Systems should be in place for managing the specimens and results. The 'turn around time' must be as short as possible. The clinic should develop a system of promptly reviewing and reacting to abnormal results.

Clinicians can often proceed with appropriate care and initiation of antiretroviral therapy in the absence of or while awaiting results.

Data capturing

Systems are needed for reporting and measuring outcomes. Data systems also assist in identifying problem areas and predicting future programme requirements. The most basic is a paper based register, although more than one type of register can be in use such as PMTCT, infant follow up, PCR and antiretroviral therapy. Clinics should have access to all the relevant documentation. Computer-based databases are helpful but depend on IT support and data capturing capacity. A useful strategy is to enter limited data immediately after seeing a patient.

The value of public-private partnership

It can be very difficult to strive for improvements in the quality of health care where material resources are severely constrained. Through developing their potential for social entrepreneurship healthcare workers in the public service can enhance the quality of health care they provide. Additional resources enable the development of ancillary projects that can provide income generation, support groups for children and care-givers, improved waiting area facilities, better equipment, transport funds, additional educational material and can even permit the employment of additional staff.

Non-governmental organizations, faith-based enterprises, large and small corporations, academic institutions, service organizations and individual donors are potential resources that can be engaged in partnership to improve conditions in financially constrained public service clinics. (See www.teampata.org and www.kidzpositive.org for examples and suggestions.)

While community participation in services is very helpful, constant attention needs to be placed on sustainability especially to avoid collapse of externally funded programmes.

References and further reading

PATA Conference Proceedings. 2005. The One to One Children's Fund. www.one2onekids.org

Crossing the Quality Chasm. 2001. Institute of Medicine. Washington, DC: National Academy Press.

WHO. 'Equipment for gastric lavage and induced sputum'. 2006. In *Guidance for national tuberculosis programs on the management of tuberculosis in children*. Geneva: World Health Organization.

PART 3

Approach to HIV infection in adults

19 Clinical assessment 189

20 Common emergencies 198

21 Evaluation of fever 213

22 Primary prophylaxis and immunization 219

23 Diet and nutrition 224

24 Adult tuberculosis 232

25 Sexually transmitted infections 262

26 Gynaecology 273

27 Contraception 280

28 Sexual assault 285

Clinical assessment

The initial assessment of an HIV-positive patient should be systematic and comprehensive. A clear management plan should emerge from this consultation, based on careful assessment, staging and evaluation of laboratory results. Adequate information is essential to the effective planning and provision of long-term care. Resistance to antiretroviral therapy and tuberculosis treatment is increasingly common, and infection with antibiotic resistant bacterial pathogens from healthcare facilities (nosocomial infection) is frequent. Clinicians need to obtain as much information as possible to assess resistance risks.

History

The history and examination can focus on the areas summarized in Table 19.1.

Table 19.1 History

HIV diagnosis	• Date of test • Reason for test • Response to diagnosis • Disclosure
Social background	• Relationships: sexual orientation, marriage, long-term partner, extra-marital or casual sexual relationships • Condom use and sexual practices • Support structures: people with whom the patient can discuss the diagnosis and who may be in a position to provide emotional support and participate in the patient's care • Home circumstances including number of people in the house, opportunities for privacy, electricity, running water • Children: age, state of health, HIV status • Other members of the family with HIV infection • History of tuberculosis (TB) within the household, including multi-drug resistant TB (MDRTB) • Deaths within the family, cause of death, coping strategies • Employment, other sources of income (family support, disability grant) • Awareness of diagnosis: by the partner, family, friends, colleagues in the workplace • Factors preventing full disclosure of HIV status

Medical background

HIV-related symptoms with prognostic significance:

- Hospital admissions (e.g. pneumonia)
- Constitutional symptoms: weight, including usual weight and duration of weight loss (should be quantified if possible)
- Drenching night sweats
- Fevers and chills
- Unusual fatigue of recent onset
- Cough, sputum production, pleuritic pain, haemoptysis
- Dyspnoea
- Herpes zoster, including number of episodes, extent, and dissemination
- Skin rashes, itchy and non-itchy
- Oral candidiasis
- Prolonged diarrhoea
- Dysphagia
- Headache
- Deterioration in cognitive function
- Gait problems

STIs:

- Condom use
- Penile or vaginal discharges, ulcers, dysuria
- Treatment received for STIs (usually syndromic)
- Syphilis serology
- Hepatitis B – infection or vaccination
- Number of separate episodes, completion of recommended treatment

Tuberculosis history:

- Including date/s of diagnosis, method of diagnosis (e.g. smear, culture, chest radiograph, clinical)
- Hospitalization
- Clinic attended
- Antituberculous therapy and TB treatment card
- Sputum smear results while on treatment
- Duration of treatment
- Treatment outcome (cured, completed, not completed)
- Number of episodes of tuberculosis
- Exposure to patients with multi-drug resistant or extreme-drug resistant TB (association with hospitalization)
- Persisting constitutional and respiratory symptoms on antituberculous therapy
- Culture and sensitivity results
- Molecular test results (resistance gene mutations), culture and drug susceptibility results

Laboratory and antiretroviral history:
- Initial CD4 count, subsequent CD4 count
- Antiretroviral history, including initiation date, previous regimens, duration on regimen, reasons for switching drugs, current regimen
- Viral load results, before initiation of antiretroviral therapy, and while on therapy
- Results of resistance testing (HIV genotyping results, *M. tuberculosis* drug susceptibility tests, and isolation of drug resistant bacterial pathogens

Evaluation for risks of drug-resistant infections:
- History of prior use of antiretroviral therapy, sexual contact with others taking antiretroviral therapy (consider testing for viral load and HIV resistance three months after starting anti-retroviral therapy)
- Exposure to patients with multi-drug resistant TB or patients who have died while taking treatment for TB, either at home or during hospitalisation (if TB symptoms present consider immediate molecular testing for resistance and mycobacterial culture with drug susceptibility testing)
- Hospitalization within the past six months (if presenting with severe sepsis start with broad-spectrum antibiotic cover determined by local sensitivity patterns and guidelines *after* taking blood cultures)

Other medical or surgical problems
Diabetes
Hypertension
Hyperlipidaemia
Angina, myocardial infarction or stroke

Psychiatric symptoms (See Chapter 36: Psychiatry)
Mood state
Prolonged low mood, unusual sleep patterns, social withdrawal, suicidal ideation, unusual anger
Unusually agitated behaviour
Auditory or visual hallucinations, feelings of persecution

Current medications and allergies (especially to co-trimoxazole and anti-convulsants)

Lifestyle:
Number of sexual partners
Smoking
Alcohol intake (potential drug interactions)
Recreational drug use
Diet
Exercise
Dietary supplements
Alternative medications and herbs (potential drug interactions)

Examination

Table 19.2 provides a summary of the examination.

Table 19.2 Examination

General impression	• Is the patient in good health, chronically unwell, acutely ill?
Mood state	• Attitude, behaviour, affect
Weight, height, body mass index (BMI) = $\frac{\text{Weight (kg)}}{\text{Height}^2 \text{ (m)}}$	
Temperature, blood pressure, heart rate	
Cutaneous signs with prognostic significance	• Herpes zoster scars • Seborrhoeic dermatitis • Onychomycosis • Itchy bump disease • Kaposi's sarcoma • Pallor
	Lymphadenopathy • Site, size, symmetry • Record normal findings • Use a 'stick-man' sketch showing the size and distribution of the nodes at each consultation • Symmetrical cervical, axillary, and epitrochlear nodes are normal in Stage 1 and 2 disease, but painful or tender nodes are always abnormal • Lymphadenopathy tends to regress with progressive immune suppression, and the development of new lymphadenopathy in a patient with advanced disease suggests TB, lymphoma, or Kaposi's sarcoma • See also Chapter 21: Evaluation of fever
	Oropharyngeal examination (See Chapter 39: Oral medicine) • Angular cheiitis • Candidiasis (pseudomembranous, erythematous, hyperplastic, median rhomboid glossitis) • Oral hairy leukoplakia • Aphthous ulceration • Kaposi's sarcoma of the palate • Gingivitis • Caries

Ear and nose
- Sinus tenderness
- Nasal discharge or post-nasal drip (and cough)
- Discharging ear
- Otitis externa
- Tympani – retracted, inflamed, or perforated

Chest
- Respiratory rate, recession
- Cyanosis and oxygen saturation (pulse oximetry) in room air
- Pleural effusion
- Signs of bronchial or parenchymal disease

Cardiovascular
- Pulse rate and blood pressure
- Pericardial syndrome (elevated venous pressure, oedema, rub, pulsus paradoxus)
- Murmurs – stigmata of infective endocarditis
- Cardiomyopathy

Abdomen
- Hepatomegaly and splenomegaly
- Ascites
- Adenopathy or masses
- Perianal inspection, rectal examination (if clinically indicated)
- Urine analysis (dipstick)

Genital
- Inguinal lymphadenopathy
- Examination of the penis or vagina and cervix (using a speculum) for ulcers or purulent discharge
- Cervical smear

Nervous system
- Tailor the extent of the examination to the patient's symptoms and degree of immune suppression (See Chapter 35: Neurology)

Screen for HIV encephalopathy
- Assessment of the appropriateness of behaviour and interaction
- HIV dementia score, or mini-mental state examination score
- Gait and tandem gait
- Smoothness of eye pursuit movements
- Anti-saccades
- Finger fine movements
- Dysdiadochokinesis
- Generalized hyperreflexia
- Frontal lobe signs

Screen for chronic meningitis
- Headache, altered mental status, meningism, and fever

Screen for focal CNS or spinal cord pathology
- Cranial nerve abnormalities
- Long tract signs
- Hemianopia and apraxias
- Paraparesis, sensory level, and bladder dysfunction

Screen for peripheral neuropathy
Numbness, dysthesias, reduced vibration sense and diminished ankle jerks

Fundoscopy
Microvasculopathy or retinitis
Papilloedema

Assessment

At the end of the consultation, assess the following:
- Does the patient have insight into the nature of HIV infection?
- Is the patient able and willing to use condoms?
- What social support structures are available to the patient?
- What current and previous opportunistic infections has the patient had?
- What are the current medical problems?
- Are there risk factors for atherosclerosis (age, gender, smoking, diabetes, hypertension)?
- What is the World Health Organization (WHO) Stage?
- Is prophylactic co-trimoxazole indicated?
- Could the patient have tuberculosis (TB)?
- How physically incapacitated is the patient? See Appendix 19.1: Karnofsky score.
- Is antiretroviral therapy indicated? What is the best antiretroviral option?

The *prognosis* for an individual patient can be determined using the WHO Staging System. The CD4 count and viral load add additional information (See Chapter 6: HIV transmission and natural history).

Follow-up visits

Further consultations can be more problem orientated, but do the following routinely:

- Inquire about condom use and sexual contacts.
- Inquire about symptoms of STIs.
- Ask about tuberculosis symptoms such as coughing, weight loss, or sweats.
- Recent hospitalization or contact with patients who may have MDR TB
- Make a non-judgemental assessment of adherence to antiretroviral therapy. (See Chapter 48: Adherence to antiretroviral therapy.)
- Discuss disclosure to partners, family, and friends.
- Weigh the patient and calculate the BMI.
- Examine the skin, mouth, and lymph nodes.

It is exceptionally useful to keep a front-page summary chart for each patient recording weight, BMI, any new clinical findings, WHO staging, with the CD4 count, viral load, full blood count, creatinine, alkaline phosphatase, alanine transaminase.

Initial investigations

Baseline investigations

Baseline investigations include the following:

- *CD4 count*: A count of <200 cells/µl implies significant immune suppression and is an indication for *Pneumocystis carinii* pneumonia (PCP) prophylaxis and initiation of antiretroviral therapy. Ideally, therapeutic decisions should not be based on a single reading. (See Chapter 5: Laboratory investigations.)
- *Full blood count and differential count*: TLC correlates fairly well with the CD4 count. A TLC of 1.25×10^9 cells/l is roughly equivalent to a CD4 count of 200 cells/µl. Haematological parameters should be monitored regularly when patients are taking antiretroviral therapy (especially the haemoglobin and absolute neutrophil count for patients taking zidovudine).
- *Syphilis serology*: Syphilis serology, (e.g. VDRL or RPR) should be done at baseline and repeated yearly in order to screen for latent syphilis. (See also Chapter 25: Sexually transmitted infections.)
- *Cervical smear*: HIV-positive women infected with human papilloma-virus (HPV) have an increased risk of cervical carcinoma. The initial Pap test should be repeated after six months and then annually.
- *Tuberculin skin test*: if isoniazid prophylaxis is being considered. (See Chapter 22: Primary prophylaxis and immunization.)

- *Sputum smears for tuberculosis*: Perform two sputum smears if the patient has a persistent cough or constitutional symptoms. (See Chapter 24: Adult tuberculosis, for a discussion of smear-negative tuberculosis.)

Second-line investigations

Subsequent investigations should be guided by the clinical setting:

- *Viral load* independently predicts the rate of progression of immuno-suppression and is the most meaningful way of determining a patient's response to antiretroviral therapy. The test is expensive and should only be done if antiretroviral therapy is about to be initiated, or is currently being taken (See Chapter 5: Laboratory investigations.)
- *Chest radiograph* is of value if the patient has fever, weight loss, or respiratory symptoms. Patients with significant immune suppression (WHO stage 2–4) should have a baseline radiograph before starting antiretroviral therapy, as tuberculosis is common during immune reconstitution.
- *Liver enzymes and bilirubin* should be checked if the patient has hepatomegaly or signs of a disseminated illness. They are also necessary if there is a history of liver disease, or if the patient is taking certain antiretroviral drugs, (e.g. when initiating nevirapine).
- *Hepatitis B and C serology* should be done as part of a work-up for transaminitis, but should only be checked routinely if resources permit. Negative Hepatitis B surface antibody and core IgG antibody tests are indications for vaccination. Hepatitis serology should be checked before antiretroviral therapy is initiated.
- *Electrolytes, urea, and creatinine* should be measured in acutely ill patients, or if the urine analysis or blood pressure is abnormal.
- *Fasting or random glucose* should be checked if there is glucose present on urine dipstick.
- *Lipid studies* should be checked if there are risk factors for athero-sclerosis or if the patient is taking a protease inhibitor.

Appendix 19.1 Karnofsky score

Able to carry on normal activity; requires no special care	100	Normal; no complaints of disease
	90	Able to carry on normal activity; minor symptoms or signs of disease
	80	Able to carry on normal activity with some effort; some symptoms or signs of disease
Unable to work; able to live at home and care for most of personal needs; requires a varying amount of assistance	70	Cares for self; unable to do normal activity or to do active work
	60	Requires occassional assistance but is able to care for most of own needs
	50	Requires considerable assistance and frequent medical care
Unable to care for self; requires equivalent of institutional or hospital care; disease may be progressing rapidly	40	Disabled; requires special care and assistance
	30	Severely disabled; hospitalization indicated although death not imminent
	20	Very sick; hospitalization necessary; active supportive treatment necessary
	10	Moribund, fatal processes progressing rapidly
	0	Dead

Common emergencies

The purpose of this chapter is to provide a quick reference for the diagnosis and management of common HIV-associated emergencies. Refer to chapters on specific topics for more detailed information.

Respiratory distress

Useful clinical features:
- shortness of breath;
- productive cough and colour of sputum;
- pleuritic chest pain;
- fever and chills;
- duration of symptoms;
- weight loss and drenching night sweats;
- use of antiretrovirals, most recent CD4 count;
- respiratory rate, heart rate, temperature;
- blood pressure, capillary filling time, oxygen saturation in room air;
- use of accessory muscles, cyanosis, mental state;
- chest auscultation for breath sounds, wheezes or crepitations.

Possible diagnoses

HIV-associated:
- community-acquired pneumonia;
- overwhelming sepsis;
- *Pneumocystis jirovecii* pneumonia;
- lactic acidosis;
- tuberculosis.

Other:
- status asthmaticus;
- infective exacerbation of chronic obstructive pulmonary disease;
- pulmonary oedema;
- pulmonary embolus;
- pneumothorax.

Essential special investigations
- chest radiograph;
- urine dipstick;
- arterial blood gases in room air.

Note: Abrupt onset of hypoxaemia and tachycardia in the presence of a normal (or unchanged) chest radiograph and normal white cell count suggests pulmonary embolism. Normal plasma D-dimers make the diagnosis unlikely but can be raised in conditions other than thromboembolism. If this diagnosis is being considered anticoagulate with heparin and arrange spiral CT scan of the pulmonary arteries.

Community-acquired pneumonia

Clinical features:
- symptoms for few days;
- purulent sputum;
- pleuritic chest pain;
- localized crackles, bronchial breathing;
- areas of dense air-space opacification on chest radiograph.

Clinical features suggesting the need for admission:
- severe pneumonia (see below);
- physical frailty, comorbidity including immune suppression;
- multilobar pneumonia;
- cyanosis, oxygen saturations <92%;
- poor socioeconomic status.

Clinical features suggesting severe pneumonia:
- altered mental status (acute confusional state);
- urea >7 mmol/L;
- respiratory rate >30 breaths per minute;
- hypotension – systolic blood pressure <90 mmHg, diastolic blood pressure <60 mmHg;
- physical frailty, or age >65 years.

Treatment:
- Outpatient treatment – oral amoxicillin-clavulanate 375 mg three times daily with amoxicillin 500 mg – 1 000 mg 3 times daily, with erythromycin 500 mg four times daily.

- Inpatient treatment – intravenous amoxicillin-clavulanate 1.2 g eight hourly *or* cefuroxime 1.5 g eight hourly *or* ceftriaxone 2.0 g daily *and* erythromycin 1.0 g eight hourly. Add gentamycin 5–6 mg/kg daily for severe pneumonia.
- *NB: Never use a fluoroquinolone* for the treatment of pneumonia in HIV-infected patients as these drugs are active against *Mycobacterium tuberculosis* including multidrug resistant organisms, and may cause false negative culture results.

Other supportive measures:
- oxygen by face mask to maintain oxygen saturation above 92%;
- intravenous fluids;
- if not improving or critically ill consider adding treatment for *Pneumocystis jirovecii* pneumonia and tuberculosis;
- consider admission to intensive care unit if oxygen saturations in 40% oxygen face mask are <92%, or mean arterial pressure <65 mmHg.

Severe sepsis

Clinical features:
- temperature >38 °C or <35 °C or hypothermia;
- heart rate >90 beats/min;
- respiratory rate >20 breaths/min (or PCO_2 <3.5 kPa);
- white cell count >11 or <4 × 10^9/L or >10% band forms on smear (left shift);
- hypotension (mean arterial pressure <65 mmHg), oliguria (<0.5 mL/kg/hr, delayed capillary filling time);
- hypoxaemia when breathing room air;
- altered mental status (acute confusional state/delirium);
- thrombocytopenia, prolonged prothrombin time and partial thromboplastin time, increased fibrin degradation products (i.e. coagulopathy);
- possibly signs of focal sepsis (e.g. pneumonia, urosepsis, peritonism).

Treatment:
Rapid, goal-orientated resuscitation is life-saving and the following should be achieved within 90 minutes from the time of presentation:
- Take blood culture and urine culture, immediately give intravenous ceftriaxone 2.0 g and gentamicin 5-6 mg/kg loading dose (continue if renal function and urine output normal).
- Check arterial blood gases, full blood count, differential, urea, creatinine, electrolytes, glucose.

- Insert urinary catheter and central venous line.
- Give intravenous crystalloids (e.g. Ringer's lactate or 0.9% saline) until central venous pressure 12–15 cm water, then start dobutamine 250 mg – 500 mg in 200 mL saline at 5–50 mL/hour to maintain mean arterial pressure >70 mmHg; add adrenalin infusion 4–8 ampoules in 200 mL saline at 5–50 mL/hour if necessary.
- Maintain central venous oxygen saturations at >70% (obtain the blood sample from the central venous catheter).
- Packed cell transfusion to maintain haemoglobin above 8 g/dL.
- Admit to intensive care unit if possible or stabilize and refer to regional level facility after initial resuscitation and antibiotic therapy.
- Consider continuous positive airway pressure or mechanical ventilation.
- Discuss case with a senior colleague.

Pneumocystis pneumonia

Clinical features:
- severe shortness of breath, inability to take a deep breath;
- non-productive cough;
- diffuse (bilateral) interstitial opacification and/or 'ground-glass' (alveolar) opacification on chest radiograph.

Treatment:
- co-trimoxazole 480 mg tablets – <60 kg four tablets three times daily; >60 kg four tablets four times daily;
- add prednisone if oxygen saturations are <90% in room air – not on TB treatment initially 40 mg 12 hourly, on TB treatment initially 60 mg 12 hourly;
- oxygen by facemask to maintain oxygen saturation above 92%.

Hyperlactaemia and lactic acidosis

Hyperlactaemia due to mitochondrial toxicity induced by nucleoside reverse transcriptase inhibitors (NRTIs) can cause substantial morbidity and mortality. Stavudine used in Regimen 1 is the commonest cause of hyperlactaemia. Didanosine (used in Regimen 2) has also been associated with severe hyperlactaemia.

Conditions such as sepsis and dehydration can unmask previously subclinical hyperlactaemia.

The following are risk factors for hyperlactaemia:
- female gender;
- BMI >28;

- weight >75 kg;
- weight gain >5 kg over three months;
- weight loss >5% body weight over three months.

Clinical features
- Asymptomatic hyperlactaemia is common, occurring in up to 25% of patients, and is *not* an indication to change the antiretroviral regimen.
- Clinical features of hyperlactaemia are a spectrum, ranging from subtle symptoms with hyperlactaemia to severe metabolic acidosis with cardiorespiratory failure.

Common symptoms include:
- nausea and vomiting;
- weight loss;
- abdominal pain;
- fatigue and dyspnoea.

Associated symptoms include:
- peripheral neuropathy;
- myalgia;
- peripheral oedema;
- lipodystrophy.

Response to symptoms

Any patient on NTRI-containing antiretroviral therapy should have point-of-care lactate checked on uncuffed venous blood (not capillary blood):
- Normal: <2.5 mmol/L
- Moderate elevation: 2.5–5 mmol/L
- Severe elevation, potentially life-threatening: 5–10 mmol/L
- Life-threatening elevation: >10 mmol/L

An elevated lactate level should be confirmed later the same day before antiretroviral management decisions are made.

Management of the hyperlactaemia patient in resource-limited settings

Once the diagnosis of hyperlactaemia has been confirmed clinicians in resource-limited settings need to consider:
- Is there a precipitating/alternative cause for the hyperlactaemia?
- Is it appropriate and safe to immediately substitute another NRTI for stavudine, or should antiretroviral therapy be suspended?

- Should Kaletra® be prescribed to cover the NNRTI tail?
- Should the patient be referred to a regional or tertiary level institution?
- If antiretroviral therapy was interrupted – can the patient subsequently take modified Regimen 1 (zidovudine/abacavir/tenofovir substituted for stavudine) or should an NNRTI-sparing regimen be prescribed? (Usually Kaletra® with efavirenz).

Step 1: Evaluation for precipitating causes of hyperlactaemia

Common causes of hyperlactaemia include:

Dehydration

Clinical features:
- diarrhoea, vomiting, reduced fluid intake, uncontrolled diabetes mellitus with polyuria;
- tachycardia;
- reduced urine output <1 mL per hour;
- concentrated urine: SG >1030 on dipstick;
- reduced skin turgor;
- postural drop in blood systolic pressure >10 mmHg;
- jugular venous pulsation not visible with patient lying flat;
- hypotension.

Management:
- intravenous saline at 250 mL/hr–1 000 mL/hr;
- check urea, creatinine, sodium, potassium;
- treat the underlying cause (e.g. vomiting, diabetes).

Severe sepsis

See above.

Cardiac failure

Clinical features:
- dyspnoea on exertion, orthopnoea, paroxysmal nocturnal dyspnoea;
- elevated jugular venous pressure at 45°;
- pedal and sacral oedema.

Management:
- restrict fluids to <1 500 mL daily;
- low salt diet;

- furosemide 40–120 mg IV eight hourly via short-line (plugged intravenous cannula);
- oxygen by face mask;
- thiamine 100 mg IV/PO daily;
- evaluation for cause of cardiac failure and selection of long term management plan.

Severe anaemia (see Chapter 30: Haematology)

Step 2: Evaluation for immediate substitution of another NRTI for stavudine or antiretroviral discontinuation

It is reasonable to make an immediate substitution for neuropathy or lipoatrophy but if symptomatic hyperlactaemia or decompensated lactic acidosis caused by an NRTI is suspected antiretroviral therapy *should always be discontinued*.

If antiretroviral therapy is interrupted for hyperlactaemia the patient should always be treated with vitamin B co tablets (four tablets twice daily) and thiamine 100 mg daily in order to provide mitochondrial co-factors.

Step 3: Should Kaletra® be prescribed to cover the NNRTI tail?

If antiretroviral therapy is discontinued and the regimen included an NNRTI prescribe Kaletra® 4 capsules 12 hourly (if taking efavirenz) or Kaletra® 3 capsules 12 hourly (if taking nevirapine) for seven to 14 days (to cover the NNRTI 'tail') unless:
- The patient is vomiting all medication.
- The patient is jaundiced or has bilirubin present on urine dipstick.
- The liver is enlarged (possible steatohepatitis).

Step 4: Assessment for transfer to a regional/tertiary facility

The main reasons for transfer are:
- To measure the patient's pH/bicarbonate (this will determine if the patient can subsequently be treated with zidovudine, or must be treated with abacavir or tenofovir or a NRTI-sparing regimen).
- Intensive care management for cardiorespiratory collapse.

If blood gases, pH and bicarbonate cannot be measured immediately refer if:
- lactate is >10 mmol/L; *or*
- *danger signs present*

- respiratory rate >20;
- heart rate >90;
- patient is too fatigued to walk >20 meters on the flat;
- dehydration, sepsis and heart failure have been excluded or treated for >24 hours.

If blood gases, pH and bicarbonate can be measured immediately refer if:
- lactate is >10 mmol/L; *or*
- bicarbonate is <15.

At the regional hospital consider the following treatment:
- If hypotensive, oliguric or hypoxic admit to an intensive care unit and manage using severe sepsis strategies (see above), give vitamin B support (see next point) and consider intravenous infusion of 4.2% sodium bicarbonate 200 mL hourly until pH >7.1.
- If intensive care is not needed give intravenous fluids at 100–200 mL/hour; intravenous or oral thiamine 100 mg daily and vitamin B3 (riboflavin) 50 mg daily (in vitamin B co tablets); and treat all inpatients empirically for sepsis with a third generation cephalosporin, e.g. ceftriaxone 2.0 g daily.

Step 5: Reintroduction of antiretroviral therapy

Once antiretroviral therapy has been discontinued the lactate should be monitored every three to seven days until <5 and then every 14 days until <2.5 mmol/L for >2 months.

Note: intercurrent illness can cause decompensated lactic acidosis even if NRTI therapy has been discontinued as mitochondrial recovery can take months. Suspect hyperlactaemia in any patient who has been exposed to antiretroviral therapy in the past six months. Refer if the lactate is >10 mmol/L or if danger signs are present.

Either: Modified Regimen 1 (with zidovudine or tenofovir or abacavir substituted for stavudine) can be prescribed if the patient is clinically well and the lactate has been <2.5 mmol/L for >2 months.

If zidovudine is prescribed remember to check the full blood count at baseline, one month and every six months.

Or: An NRTI-sparing regimen should be prescribed if the lactate was >10 mmol/L or bicarbonate was <15 mmol/L. Didanosine (ddI) should never be prescribed. Consideration can also be given to prescribing NRTI therapy associated with less mitochondrial toxicity, e.g. abacavir, tenofovir and lamivudine/emtricitabine if the patient has private funds, or these medications can be obtained through the state sector. This should be discussed with an HIV specialist.

Note: All antiretroviral-related adverse drug events should be reported to the Provincial Pharmacovigilance Committee using the Adverse Drug Reaction form.

Diarrhoea and dehydration

Possible diagnoses

HIV-associated:
- advanced HIV infection with coccidian parasite infestation or entero-pathy;
- due to antiretrovirals (e.g. didanosine and lopinavir/ritonavir);
- lactic acidosis (unusual);
- cytomegalovirus colitis (rare).

Other:
- gastroenteritis due to viruses, bacteria or bacterial toxins, protozoa;
- dysentery;
- cholera;
- malabsorption and inflammatory bowel disease (rare).

Diagnosis and treatment

Acute onset diarrhoea:
- Measure blood pressure lying and standing (if patient not too ill): postural drop of >10 mmHg indication for intravenous fluids.
- Exclude peritonism.
- Check urea, creatinine, electrolytes, blood gases, lactate (if on anti-retroviral therapy).
- Check stool for blood, mucous and white cells – if any are present give ceftriaxone 2.0 g IV/IM daily and metronidazole 400 mg eight hourly.
- Replace fluid and electrolyte losses.
- Treat nausea with metoclopramide or cyclizine and give loperamide two tablets six hourly.

Chronic HIV-associated diarrhoea:
- Measure blood pressure lying and standing (if patient not too ill): postural drop of >10 mmHg is an indication for fluid replacement.

- Exclude peritonism.
- Check urea, creatinine, electrolytes, blood gases, lactate (if on anti-retroviral therapy).
- Replace fluid and electrolyte losses.
- Treat nausea and give loperamide or codeine or morphine oral solution six hourly to control diarrhoea.
- Treat empirically for giardiasis and isosporiasis with metronidazole 400 mg eight hourly for five days and cotrimoxazole 480 mg tablets four tablets 12 hourly for 2–4 weeks followed by two tablets daily.

If not on antiretroviral therapy:
- Refer to an antiretroviral programme.

If on antiretroviral therapy:
- Exclude lactic acidosis (see above).
- Consider switching antiretrovirals if diarrhoea clearly related to drugs (get expert advice).

Severe headache
Possible diagnoses

HIV-associated:
- meningitis (bacterial, tuberculous, cryptococcal and viral);
- raised intracranial pressure (due to space-occupying lesion or menin-gitis).

Other:
- migraine;
- sub-arachnoid haemorrhage;
- hypertensive encephalopathy.

Severe headache associated with fever or vomiting suggests meningitis and the clinician needs to consider lumbar puncture (See Chapter 35: Neurology). Tension headache and migraine can also be associated with vomiting, and infections such as malaria and influenza can also cause headache. Meningism (neck stiffness), fever and altered mental status are other essential clinical clues to the diagnosis of meningitis – however all features are not always present.

CT scan of the brain should be performed before lumbar puncture if the patient has:

- papilloedema (if you need to dilate the pupils document this in the notes!);
- focal neurological signs;
- a decreased level of consciousness.

Do not do the lumbar puncture if the scan suggests raised intracranial pressure (mid-line shift or occlusion of the third or fourth ventricle). Treat the patient with ceftriaxone 2 g daily and seek expert advice.

See Chapter 35: Neurology for interpretation of CSF results.

Altered mental status and agitated or aggressive behaviour

Sub-clinical HIV dementia is common and can make patients more vulnerable to delirium or psychosis. It is essential to diagnose potentially treatable conditions including:

- Metabolic: Renal/liver failure; electrolyte abnormalities (Na, K, Ca); abnormal glucose;
- Oxygen: Hypoxaemia;
- Vascular: Stroke, hypotension, hypertensive encephalopathy, sub-arachnoid bleed;
- Endocrine: Abnormal thyroid hormones; (abnormal cortisol level – rare)
- Seizures: Post-ictal state;
- Trauma: Concussion; subdural or extradural bleed;
- Uraemia: Renal failure;
- Psychiatric: Primary psychiatric disorder including depression
- Infections: Pulmonary, urinary, cellulitis, meningitis, sinusitis, cholecystitis;
- Drugs: Alcohol withdrawal, recreational, prescription medications (e.g. antituberculous therapy) non-adherence to psychiatric treatment
- Dementia: Previously diagnosed.

Patients with psychosis tend to have auditory hallucinations and to remain orientated, although they can also have superimposed delirium (for example from substance abuse used to 'self-medicate' psychosis). Agitation and disturbed behaviour can be very troublesome. Delirium needs to be diagnosed and treated and the behavioural disturbance then needs to be treated with the lowest possible dose of neuroleptic.

Depression is very common, and the diagnosis is often missed. Tearfulness, diminished interaction with family and nursing staff, lethargy and appetite changes are clues to the diagnosis. It is important to ask directly for suicidal ideation: 'Are you feeling so sad that you keep thinking you do not want to carry on living?' Treatment with tricyclic antidepressants or serotonin reuptake inhibitors is effective, but initial doses need to be low to prevent side effects.

Sedation of aggressive and agitated patients in accordance with the Mental Health Care Act (MHCA)

- Offer sedation to patient: if accepted document this in notes. Consider offering oral sedation if appropriate.
- Attempt to de-escalate the situation by reassuring the patient and allowing personal space and privacy.
- If sedation is refused, sedate patient *after* gathering sufficient information to complete one MHCA 04 form, two MHCA 05 forms and one MHCA 07 form. Ensure these forms are completed as soon as possible.
- If parenteral sedation needs to be given and the patient is unable to cooperate: call six assistants:
  o five security guards – one for each limb and one for head/shoulders;
  o one doctor/nurse to assist with administering sedation;
- Give the following medications:
  o lorazepam 4–12 mg IVI / IMI;
  o haloperidol 10–20 mg IVI / IMI.
- Ensure that the resuscitation trolley is close at hand, and place the patient in the recovery position to prevent aspiration. Respiratory depression from the combination of neuroleptic drugs and benzodiazepines is very rare.
- *Repeat the doses* of haloperidol and lorazepam at 15–30 minute intervals until the patient is fully sedated. Remember that agitated patients may rapidly metabolize medications due to enzyme induction from recreational drugs, and will have high levels of sympathetic nervous system activation. In order to counteract these effects higher doses of sedating medications may be needed.
- Ensure that patient is fully sedated so that restraints are unnecessary.
- If the patient was violent at the time of presentation prescribe Clopixol Acuphase 50–150 mg IMI stat, which has an effect for up to 72 hours.
- Prescribe maintenance sedation with haloperidol (5–15 mg) and lorazepan (2–8 mg) to be given 3–6 hourly in order to ensure that the patient is sufficiently sedated so that the functioning of the ward is not disrupted.

Figure 20.1 Flow chart for the management of aggressive or agitated patients

STEP 1:

Patient with disordered mentation:
Aggressive   Disruptive and irrational
Destructive   Hallucinating
Running away from home   Agitated

STEP 2:

Obtain history of disordered thinking and behaviour from patient's escorts
Observe the patient's appearance and behaviour and document unusual features
Assess for features suggesting delirium:
Disorientation and incoherent speech; fluctuating level of attention or
consciousness; history of recent alcohol abuse, or drug abuse; history of
recent seizures or head trauma
RR >20, HR >90, Temp >38 C or <35 C, O_2 saturation <94% in room air
WCC <3.5 or >12, Ur >8, glucose >12 or <3, abnormal Na, K, or Ca
Abnormal cardiorespiratory or abdominal examination
Abnormal urine dipstick
Meningism or abnormal CSF analysis
Focal CNS signs
Asterixis.

STEP 3:

Sedate if patient's behaviour is dangerous or disruptive
Offer sedation to the patient – if this is accepted document this in the notes
If sedation is refused, or if patient does not have sufficient insight to give
consent, sedate patient *after* gathering sufficient information to complete the
following forms – one *MHCA 04*, two *MHCA 05* (signed by two healthcare
workers), and one *MHCA 07*.
Note that sedation may need to be given before the physical examination
and work-up for delirium is complete

STEP 4:

Delirious:
Diagnose underlying condition
Start appropriate treatment for both
the medical condition and the
behavioural disturbance

Not delirious:
Admit with a working
psychiatric diagnosis
Ensure that appropriate
medication is prescribed

- Vital signs should be monitored 2 – 6 hourly depending on the patient's level of sedation.
- Sedation should not be stopped until the ward doctor has reassessed the patient.
- Hydration and nutritional status should be regularly assessed and fluids and feeds provided accordingly. Prescribe thiamine 100 mg daily IV or PO.

Abdominal pain

Possible diagnoses

- lactic acidosis (if on antiretroviral therapy);
- pancreatitis (can be caused by antiretroviral therapy);
- hepatitis;
- perforation (often due to intra-abdominal tuberculosis).

Diagnosis and treatment:
- See above for lactic acidosis.
- Check bilirubin, liver enzymes, plasma glucose and INR if there is a tender hepatomegaly.
- If pancreatitis is suspected check serum amylase and lipase and treat with intravenous fluids, intramuscular morphine, nasogastric drainage and regular clinical review. If hypotension or respiratory distress develops admit to an intensive care unit.
- Request a surgical opinion.

Providing fluids, feeds and medications to HIV patients

Many patients will be very ill and unable to eat or take oral medications. The following may need to be used:
- Intravenous fluids and medications: ensure that the patient has a running intravenous line and that the fluids have been ordered on the communication chart. It is preferable (and cost effective) to prescribe once daily or twice daily intravenous medication (e.g. ceftriaxone 2.0 g IV daily).
- Nasogastric feeds and medications: especially important for comatose patients (e.g. stroke or meningitis). Remember that TB therapy cannot be given IV and therefore must be given by NG tube if the patient cannot swallow. Nasogatric feeds (e.g. Ensure) should be prescribed.

- Subcutaneous fluids (hypodermoclysis): this technique is especially appropriate for frail patients (e.g. advanced HIV) who are dehydrated but not shocked. An IV cannula is inserted under the skin of the anterior abdominal wall and connected to an IV line. Up to 4 L can be given daily: the fluid is rapidly absorbed into the lymphatic system and enters the circulation. Morphine and haloperidol can be added to the fluid for patients receiving palliative care. Other medications can be given IM or by NG tube.

Use of analgesics and local anaesthetic

Many patients experience severe pain. Take note of the following points:
- Lignocaine should be injected (maximum 20 mL 1% solution) before arterial puncture, lumber puncture, central line insertion, intercostal drain insertion, or percutaneous biopsy.
- Premedication with morphine should be given before elective procedures.
- Appropriate initial analgesia for meningitis is morphine injections and ibuprofen with paracetamol, all given regularly.
- Pleuritic or pericardial pain responds to ibuprofen with paracetamol/ codeine.
- Analgesia for intercostal drains should include morphine for the first 48 hours.
- Chronic pain should be treated according to WHO guidelines with paracetamol, ibuprofen, codeine or morphine (refer to the front pages of the *SAMF*).
- Oral morphine can be given as a solution (10 mg in 5 mL), or as 10 mg or 30 mg morphine sulphate tablets. Titrate up the morphine dose until pain is controlled. Note that morphine prescribed appropriately for pain is not addictive.
- Use adjuvant agents as appropriate (e.g. amitriptyline for neuropathy).
- Diclofenac or naproxen can be used for patients not responding to ibuprofen.

Evaluation of fever

Fever is a common presentation in the HIV-infected patient. The likelihood that fever is due to severe opportunistic diseases increases as the immune system progressively declines. Therefore the differential diagnosis expands as the CD4 count drops. However, several opportunistic infections (e.g. coccidian parasites causing diarrhoea, mucocutaneous herpes simplex and candida infections) typically do not cause fever. It is important to remember that HIV-infected patients are at increased risk of developing many infectious diseases prevalent in the community (e.g. influenza, dysentery, or malaria). HIV itself can cause prolonged fever, but this is uncommon and is a diagnosis of exclusion. Non-infectious causes of fever should be considered: important causes include malignancies (lymphoma and Kaposi's sarcoma), Castleman's disease, venous thromboembolism, and drug fever. Finally, fever is often a feature of the immune reconstitution inflammatory syndrome (see Chapter 50: Immune reconstitution inflammatory syndrome).

The acute presentation

Two key issues with acute presentations are to distinguish benign viral causes from bacterial infections, and to remember that although most opportunistic infections follow a sub-acute to chronic course, they can present acutely and mimic acute bacterial infections.

The following features suggest a benign viral cause for fever:
- coryzal symptoms (rhinitis, sneezing, pharyngitis without exudate);
- tracheobronchitis;
- diffuse myalgia and arthralgia;
- normal white cell count; and
- normal C-reactive protein (CRP).

The following features suggest bacterial infection:
- rigors;
- tachypnoea or tachycardia;
- focal pain (pleuritic, renal angle, dysuria, sinus tenderness, headache with neck stiffness, joint or muscle);

- purulent secretions (sputum, nasal discharge, dysentery, vaginal discharge);
- neutrophils in body fluids (urine, cerebrospinal fluid, stool, joint or pleural aspirate);
- elevated white cell count or left shift; and
- elevated CRP.

If no clear focus is found and a bacterial infection is suspected, useful tests include:
- chest radiograph;
- blood culture;
- urine culture;
- lumbar puncture (only if the patient has either a headache, meningism or altered mental status); and
- stool culture (only if the patient has diarrhoea).

Obtaining clinically appropriate specimens for culture is essential. Antibiotics should be used prudently, balancing the possibility of bacterial infection with the risk of inducing antibiotic resistance. Hospitalized patients should initially receive parenteral therapy.

Severe sepsis carries a high mortality, necessitating admission (preferably in a high care or intensive care unit). Features of severe sepsis include:
- an altered mental status;
- hypotension (mean arterial pressure <70 mmHg);
- elevated serum lactate; and
- organ failure (e.g. adult respiratory distress syndrome, disseminated intravasular coagulopathy, renal failure, ileus).

The sub-acute or chronic presentation

Tuberculosis is by far the commonest cause of a febrile sub-acute or chronic illness in southern Africa.

The following HIV-related infections can also present with fever and constitutional symptoms of insidious onset:
- disseminated fungal infections (cryptococcosis, histoplasmosis);
- *Pneumocystis jirovecii* pneumonia (PCP);
- *Mycobacterium avium* complex (MAC);
- acute hepatitis B;
- cytomegalovirus;

- nocardiosis; and
- bacillary angiomatosis.

Often OIs causing the sub-acute or chronic presentation will meet the criteria for fever of unknown origin (FUO). In HIV-infected patients, FUO can be diagnosed when:

- the temperature is >38 °C for >4 weeks during several out-patient visits, or for >3 in-patient days; and
- standard bacterial cultures are negative for at least two days; and
- diagnosis remains uncertain after three days of appropriate investigation.

Patients with fever and deteriorating functional status should be admitted for more rapid evaluation. Undiagnosed tuberculosis is often fatal and initially attention should be focused on excluding this infection, with spontaneous or induced sputum specimens for acid-fast bacilli (AFB) and/or nucleic acid amplification tests. A CD4 count above 200 cells/µL makes other opportunistic infections less likely. Peripheral tuberculous lymphadenopathy (tuberculous nodes are usually >2 cm in diameter) is also common. The diagnosis can be made most conveniently using wide-needle lymph node aspiration. If an induced sputum examination and lymph node aspiration are unhelpful, perform the following investigations:

- chest radiograph;
- abdominal and pericardial ultrasound scan;
- CRP (a normal CRP virtually excludes tuberculosis);
- mycobacterial urine culture and blood culture in a mycobacterial bottle (which is also suitable for the identification of bacteria and fungi); and
- serum cryptococcal antigen latex agglutination test.

Pleural and peritoneal effusions should be aspirated to exclude bacterial infection. Treat for TB if there are:

- suggestive features on chest radiograph;
- hilar, mediastinal, or intra-abdominal lymphadenopathy;
- pericardial effusion with constitutional symptoms; or
- pleural or ascitic lymphocytic exudates.

Even in the absence of these features a trial of antituberculous therapy should be considered in patients with FUO, provided their CRP is elevated. *Ideally at least two clinically relevant specimens should be sent for mycobacterial culture before starting antituberculous therapy.* Clinicians embarking on empiric antituberculous therapy should evaluate response. Fever typically responds within 10 days. The following features are helpful in documenting a response to treatment at two and eight weeks:

- weight gain;
- resolution of the presenting symptoms;
- rising haemoglobin;
- falling CRP levels; and
- patient performance of tasks improves (e.g. ability to work).

If there is deterioration or failure to respond to empiric antituberculous therapy the patient should be referred for further work up.

Immune reconstitution is an important cause of FUO within the first three months of antiretroviral therapy; importantly the fever can persist even when the underlying opportunistic infection is effectively treated (See Chapter 50: Immune reconstitution inflammatory syndrome). Patients starting antiretroviral therapy may develop FUO or may still not be thriving after six weeks of treatment. This may be because improving immune function unmasks previously occult OIs. The patient may develop pulmonary infiltrates, pleural and pericardial effusions, bone marrow or liver infiltrates, or lymphadenopathy. MAC is the commonest cause of immune reconstitution syndrome in the developed world, but in sub-Saharan Africa steps should be taken to exclude TB. Lymphoma is an important non-infectious cause of FUO. Disseminated visceral Kaposi's sarcoma, drug fever and deep vein thrombosis are less common but should be considered, as should infective endocarditis, autoimmune disease and thyroiditis. Drug fever may be associated with maculopapular rash and eosinophilia, and is most often caused by co-trimoxazole, abacavir, nevirapine or efavirenz, antituberculous drugs, β-lactam antibiotics and anticonvulsants. However many drugs can be implicated. Fever will resolve within 48 hours of withdrawing the drug. Abacavir hypersensitivty reaction causes fever and rash, seldom eosinophilia, and re-challenge can be life-threatening. Fever due to deep vein thrombosis should be suspected in immobile patients, and can be ruled out with a negative D-dimer test and negative doppler ultrasound scan of the leg veins. If the initial investigations are negative, or the patient does not respond to antituberculous therapy, or tuberculosis is thought unlikely, further investigation should be considered, guided by clinical findings. The following radiological procedures may be helpful to select the best diagnostic procedure in patients with FUO:

- CT scan of the mediastinum and hilar regions and a high-resolution CT scan of the lung parenchyma;
- abdominal CT scan;
- CT scan of the head and sinuses (uncontrasted and contrasted); and
- Gallium scan.

The following procedures may isolate the causative organism:
- lumbar puncture (only if the patient has either a headache, meningism or altered mental status);
- bone marrow biopsy (especially if neutropenia and/or thrombocytopenia are present);
- liver biopsy (if ultrasound or liver function tests are abnormal);
- lymph node biopsy (Trucut or excision, visceral nodes can be biopsied under CT scan guidance);
- skin biopsy (if nodular lesions are present); and
- lung biopsy (if there are pulmonary infiltrates).

Biopsy material should be divided equally into tissue for culture (placed into normal saline) and for histology (placed into formalin). Ask the laboratories to test for mycobacteria and fungi, and, in selected cases, stains for CMV and bacillary angiomatosis. Discussing diagnostic work-up of FUO with experienced colleagues is a rewarding exercise.

References and further reading

Chieng, D.C. et al. 1999. 'Utility of fine-needle aspiration in the diagnosis of salivary gland lesions in patients infected with human immunodeficiency virus'. *Diagnostic Cytopathology*, 21(4):260–264.

Ellison, E. et al. 1998. 'Fine needle Aspiration (FNA) in HIV+ patients: results from a series of 655 aspirates'. *Cytopathology*, 9(4):222–229.

Gamborini, E. et al. 2000. 'Fine-needle aspiration diagnosis of Kaposi's sarcoma in a developing country'. *Diagnostic Cytopathology*, 23(5):322–325.

Grossl, N.A. et al. 1997. 'Utility of fine needle aspiration in HIV-positive patients with corresponding CD4 counts. Four years' experience in a large inner city hospital.' *Acta Cytologica*, 41(3):811–816.

Hot, A. et al. 2007. 'Fever of unknown origin in HIV/AIDS patients.' *Infectious Disease Clinics North America*, 21:1013–1032

Hudson, C. et al. 2000. 'Diagnosing HIV-associated tuberculosis: Reducing costs and diagnostic delay'. *International Journal of Tuberculosis and Lung Disease*, 4 (3): 240–245.

Mayo, J. et al. 1997. 'Fever of unknown origin in the HIV-infected patient: New scenario for an old problem'. *Scandinavian Journal of Infectious Diseases*, 29: 327–336.

Nayak, S. et al. 2003. Fine-needle aspiration cytology in lymphadenopathy of HIV-positive patients.' *Diagnostic Cytopathology*, 29(3):146–148 .

Prego, V. et al. 1990. 'Comparative yield of blood culture for fungi and mycobacteria, liver biopsy and bone marrow biopsy in the diagnosis of fever of undetermined origin in human immunodeficiency virus-infected patients.' *Archives of Internal Medicine*, 150: 333–336.

Shenoy, R. et al. 2002. 'Fine needle aspiration diagnosis in HIV-related lymphadenopathy on Mangalore, India. *Acta Cytologica*, 46(1): 35–39.

Wilson, M. 1996. 'General principles of specimen collection and transport'. *Clinical Infectious Diseases*, 22: 766–767.

Primary prophylaxis and immunization

Most of the morbidity and mortality in HIV-infected patients results from opportunistic infections (OIs). Primary prophylaxis or immunisation can prevent many of these infections from occurring. Secondary prophylaxis refers to maintenance therapy to prevent recurrences following initial intensive therapy for many major OIs (see notes on specific infections).

Co-trimoxazole

Co-trimoxazole provides protection against *Pneumocystis jirovecii* (formerly *P. carinii*) pneumonia, toxoplasmosis, many bacterial infections, diarrhoea caused by *Isospora belli* or *Cyclospora* spp, and malaria. The standard dose is 960 mg daily (two single-strength tablets containing trimethoprim 80 mg/sulfamethoxazole 400 mg) but lower doses (480 mg daily or 960 mg three times a week) are probably as effective and cause fewer side-effects. The prophylactic use of co-trimoxazole has been shown to markedly reduce mortality and hospitalization. The current WHO guidelines recommend commencing co-trimoxazole prophylaxis in early HIV disease (WHO stages 2, 3 and 4 or a CD4 <350), following a study in Côte d'Ivoire. However, the morbidity seen in early disease was far higher and there was less antimicrobial resistance among the common bacterial organisms than occur in southern Africa. A South African cohort study failed to show benefit in early disease. The South African guidelines for initiating co-trimoxazole prophylaxis in HIV-infected adults therefore recommend initiating co-trimoxazole with more advanced HIV disease:

CD4 count <200 cells/µl
or
WHO Stage 3 or 4 disease.

The most common side-effect is a maculopapular rash. Because alternative prophylaxis (see below) prevents fewer infections than co-trimoxazole, try to treat through the rash or interrupt treatment and then desensitise (see Appendix 22.1). Only attempt this if there are no mucous membrane lesions (as in Stevens-Johnson syndrome, which is life-threatening), no blistering, and no features of systemic involvement (e.g. fever, hepatitis). Neutropenia may also occur. An alternative regimen is dapsone

100 mg daily, but this does not protect against bacterial infection and provides only limited protection against toxoplasmosis. Co-trimoxazole prophylaxis can be stopped in patients on antiretroviral therapy, once the CD4 count is greater than 200 cells/μl for more than three months.

Preventing tuberculosis

The most effective way to protect HIV-infected patients in a population is to achieve a high cure rate for all patients with smear-positive tuberculosis (TB). Randomized controlled trials have shown that preventive therapy reduces the risk of active TB by about 60% in HIV-infected patients with a tuberculin skin test reaction of ≥5 mm. Meta-analyses have failed to show a significant benefit in patients with a negative test. The WHO recommends giving preventive therapy to all HIV-infected patients in countries with high TB burdens if tuberculin skin testing cannot be done. Other high-risk categories of patients will probably also benefit from preventive therapy, irrespective of the tuberculin skin test status. TB preventive therapy is indicated for:

- individuals with TB contacts;
- health care workers;
- underground miners; and
- patients with a tuberculin skin test of ≥ 5 mm.

It is essential to exclude active TB prior to the start of TB preventive therapy. Screening for active TB in this setting is best achieved using symptom screening (any one of: active cough of any duration, weight loss, fever, night sweats), which has been shown to have high negative predictive value. It is not necessary to do routine chest radiographs or sputum examination in patients without TB symptoms.

Isoniazid (INH) at a dose of 300 mg daily, given for six months, is the best-studied regimen in HIV infection. However, the duration of benefit is relatively short-lived (about a year). A recent Botswana study has shown that 36 months' INH was much more effective than 6 months' INH. The Botswana study also confirmed that INH only benefits patients with positive tuberculin skin tests. There was evidence of harm with 36 months' INH in patients with negative tuberculin skin tests, who should therefore not receive prolonged INH. Pyridoxine 25–50 mg daily should always be prescribed to prevent INH-induced peripheral neuropathy. INH is potentially hepatotoxic, and patients starting prophylaxis should be informed of the low possibility (<1%) of drug-induced hepatitis. Patients should be instructed to stop treatment immediately if they develop nausea, vomiting, right upper-quadrant pain, yellow eyes, or dark urine. It is important that patients are seen monthly by a health care professional while on preventive therapy to detect adverse effects and to assess adherence.

Fungal infections

Fluconazole primary prophylaxis is controversial. Studies have shown reduction in the incidence of candida and cryptococcal infections, but no survival benefit. Prolonged fluconazole prophylaxis can select for azole-resistant candida species, which are difficult to treat.

Patients with CD4 counts <100 should have serum cryptococcal antigen tests done and be treated pre-emptively with fluconazole.

TB preventive therapy should be administered by HIV clinics rather than TB clinics in order to reduce the risk of exposure to TB. Antiretroviral therapy reduces the incidence of TB by about 80%, but incidence remains higher than in the general population even once CD4 counts rise to normal levels. It is unclear whether preventive therapy provides additional benefit.

Malaria prophylaxis

Malaria is more common in HIV infection, and more severe. Therefore antimalarial chemoprophylaxis should be used when travelling to malarial areas and for selected patients (e.g. pregnant women) in endemic areas. Doxycycline and mefloquine can be safely co-administered with antiretroviral therapy. Co-trimoxazole provides some protection against malaria, but is not recommended for travellers.

Immunization

Responses to immunization are poor if the CD4 count is <200 cells/μl. The immunological response is determined by the nadir CD4 count, so responses remain lower than HIV-uninfected people even if the CD4 count increases on antiretroviral therapy. Live-attenuated vaccines are absolutely contraindicated with symptomatic HIV disease or if the CD4 count is <200 cells/μl. Immunization causes a transient increase in the viral load. This does not cause harm, but viral load measurements should not be done for about four weeks after vaccination.

Pneumococcal vaccine

The polyvalent Pneumovax® currently available has been shown to be ineffective in a large Ugandan study of patients not on antiretroviral therapy. The risk of pneumonia was actually higher in patients receiving this vaccine and it is, therefore, not recommended. One of the new conjugate vaccines was evaluated in Malawian adults and adolescents who recovered from serious pneumococcal infection. The conjugate vaccine was safe and reduced the incidence of infection due to the strains covered by the vaccine. Therefore the conjugate pneumococcal vaccine should be offered to patients at high risk of pneumococcal disease (e.g. previous pneumococcal infection, chronic lung disease, splenectomy).

Hepatitis B

Vaccination should be considered for all who are non-immune. However, vaccine responses are poor if CD4 counts are <200, so vaccination should be deferred until CD4 count has risen to >200 on ART.

Influenza vaccine

This is recommended annually.

Vaccination for travellers

Patients with HIV disease can safely be given inactivated vaccines including hepatitis A and B. The yellow fever vaccine is contraindicated in patients with symptomatic HIV infection (WHO Stage 3 or 4 disease), or if the CD4 count is <200 cells/µl.

References and further reading

Badri, M. et al. 2001. 'Initiating co-trimoxazole prophylaxis in adult HIV-infected patients in Africa: an evaluation of the provisional WHO/UNAIDS recommendations.' *AIDS*, 15:1143–1148.

Centers for Disease Control and Prevention. 2009. Guidelines for Prevention and treatment of Opportunistic Infections in HIV-Infected Adults and Adolescents. *MMWR*, 58.

French, N. et al. 2000. '23-valent pneumococcal polysaccharide vaccine in HIV-1-infected Ugandan adults: Double-blind, randomized and placebo controlled trial'. *The Lancet*, 355 (9221): 2106–2111.

French, N. et al. 2010. A trial of a 7-valent pneumococcal conjugate vaccine in HIV-infected adults. *N Engl J Med*, 362(9):812–822.

Samandari T, et al. 2011. '6-month versus 36-month isoniazid preventive treatment for tuberculosis in adults with HIV infection in Botswana: a randomised, double-blind, placebo-controlled trial.' *The Lancet*, 377(9777):1588–1598.

Appendix 22.1

Co-trimoxazole desensitisation is safe and effective in about two thirds of cases using the regimen in the table. Desensitisation should be done under antihistamine cover, started one day before. After the initial dose of co-trimoxazole the patient should be observed for several hours.

(Use co-trimoxazole suspension 240 mg/5 mL)

DAY 1	1.25 mL daily
DAY 2	1.25 mL 12 hourly
DAY 3	1.25 mL 8 hourly
DAY 4	2.5 mL 12 hourly
DAY 5	2.5 mL 8 hourly
DAY 6	1 tablet (480 mg) daily

23 Diet and nutrition

Malnutrition is a common complication of HIV infection and, when accompanied by fever or unexplained diarrhoea, is the AIDS defining diagnosis in nearly 20% of patients. Malnutrition further exacerbates the immune suppression caused by HIV. Thus, malnutrition both contributes to HIV disease progression and is a result of HIV.

It takes two major forms:

- *Starvation* is a deprivation of food leading to weight loss. This is further divided into the macronutrient status, which reflects the total mass of the body, and the micronutrient status, which reflects the efficiency of the body's cellular functioning. Micronutrient deficiency may exist without macronutrient deficiency, while macronutrient deficiency almost always has associated micronutrient deficiencies. Feeding is usually sufficient to reverse starvation.
- *Cachexia* is a disproportionate depletion of lean body mass (LBM), owing to specific metabolic changes. The metabolic changes provide energy and the substrate needed to fuel the body's response to illness or injury. This leads to protein and, especially, skeletal muscle loss in the long term. Feeding is not sufficient to reverse the effects of cachexia.

Timely nutritional interventions are particularly important in patients with low body mass indices.

The body compartments can be divided into fat and lean tissue (fat-free mass). Lean body mass (LBM) may be further divided into skeletal and non-skeletal. The LBM is in turn divided into an extracellular component (connective tissues and extracellular component) and an intracellular component - the body cell mass.

Depletion of body cell mass has been correlated with shortened survival, increased risk of opportunistic infections, and poorer quality of life in AIDS patients, independent of the level of immune depletion, i.e. CD4 cell count.

Malnutrition and weight loss

- Unintentional weight loss is a diagnostic criterion in the classification of HIV infection.

- Several factors contribute to malnutrition and weight loss in HIV disease (see Figure 23.1). These factors are not mutually exclusive.
- Rapid episodic weight loss accompanies opportunistic infections, while slower progressive weight loss may occur in advanced HIV disease.
- Malnutrition is associated with immune suppression and even mild weight loss (5%) is predictive of increased morbidity and mortality.
- A low body mass index (BMI) predicts mortality, even in patients starting ART.
- The loss of muscle or LBM has been identified as a strong predictor of death. However, no simple method exists for the assessment of LBM in practice.

Food and medication interactions

Figure 23.1 The interaction between diet and medication

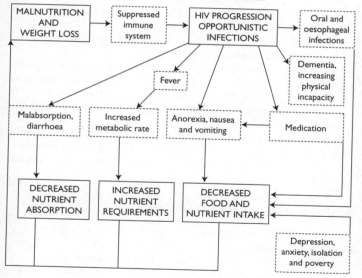

Guidelines for nutritional assessment

- *Body weight*. This should be measured at every clinic visit.
- *Weight loss*. This is measured by comparing the current body weight with an available baseline value, or with the highest value recorded during preceding assessments:
  - <10% unintentional weight loss indicates World Health Organization (WHO) Clinical Stage 2 HIV infection.
  - ≥10% unintentional weight loss indicates WHO Clinical Stage 3 HIV infection.
- *Calculating the BMI* is a measure of height compared to weight. It allows health workers to determine the nutritional status of a patient at a single point in time. This eliminates reliance on weight change over an interval, where a reliable previous weight is seldom available.
  - The BMI = weight (kg) / height (m) ^{2}
  - If the BMI is < 20 it indicates that the patient is underweight.
  - If the BMI is between 21–25 it indicates that the patient's weight is normal.
  - If the BMI is 26–29 the patient is considered overweight.
  - If the BMI is more than 30 the patient is obese.
- *Calculating height*. If a stadiometer is unavailable to measure height the arm span method could be used to approximate height, i.e. with upper extremities (including hands) fully extended and parallel, measure the distance between the tip of one middle finger to mid-sternum and multiply this by a factor of two.
- *Body composition*. Measurements to determine LBM are currently impractical. This requires trained nutritionists and the use of special-ized and costly equipment, such as skinfold callipers or a bodystat machine.

Malnutrition and HIV/AIDS

HIV infection affects nutrition through increases in resting energy expenditure, reductions in food intake, nutrient malabsorption, and complex metabolic alterations that culminate in the weight loss and wasting common in AIDS. The effect of HIV on nutrition begins early in the course of the disease, even before an individual may be aware that he or she is infected with the virus.

The following symptoms and illnesses commonly caused by HIV infection have nutritional consequences that can lead to malnutrition.

Anorexia

Anorexia, or loss of appetite, may occur with the onset of infection and when fever is present, or as a side effect of medications. It leads to general weight loss and is common when individuals are depressed or living in socially and emotionally unfavourable environments.

Diarrhoea

Diarrhoea is very common in HIV infection and has many causes. Diarrhoea may cause dehydration. Chronic diarrhoea often results in wasting. (See Chapter 38: Gastroenterology and hepatology.)

Fever

Fever is very common in HIV infection (see Chapter 22: Primary prophylaxis and immunization). The body's energy expenditure increases with fever, causing increased energy requirements.

Nausea and frequent vomiting

Nausea and vomiting can result from the drugs used to treat HIV/AIDS or from opportunistic infections. Nausea often causes reduced appetite and voluntary restriction of food, and vomiting lowers the amount of nutrients available to the body.

Oral thrush

This can result in difficulty eating foods, loss of appetite, reduced food intake, and malabsorption, leading to weight loss.

Anaemia

Iron deficiency from poor dietary intake and/or absorption of iron commonly causes anaemia.

Macronutrient requirements

Energy requirements

The HIV-infected person has additional energy needs because of:
- untreated HIV infection and opportunistic infections;

- nutrient malabsorption; and
- altered metabolism.

The various phases of the infection are marked by an increase in metabolism, increased energy needs, and nutrient depletion. These effects of infection often occur synergistically and result in weight loss and wasting. In the absence of symptoms (WHO stage 1), HIV-infected persons should increase energy intake by 10% over the level of energy intake recommended for healthy non HIV-infected persons of the same age, sex, and physical activity level. In the presence of symptoms (WHO stage 2 and above), HIV-infected persons should increase energy intake by 20% to 30% over the level of energy intake recommended for healthy non-HIV-infected persons of the same age, sex, and physical activity level. These recommendations are for HIV-infected persons, including those taking HIV-related medications such as antiretrovirals.

Protein requirements

HIV-infected people do not require more protein than the level recommended for healthy non-HIV-infected people of the same age, sex, and physical activity level. At the onset of opportunistic infections, the body loses nitrogen, which suggests a need for increased protein intake if opportunistic infections remain untreated. Studies have not demonstrated, however, that improved clinical outcomes occur from increased protein intake among HIV-infected individuals. Further research is needed on the optimal protein requirements of HIV-infected persons during the course of HIV disease. HIV-infected people often have pre-existing protein-energy malnutrition. Protein-energy malnutrition (PEM) results from inadequate intake or poor utilization of food and energy, not a deficiency of one nutrient and not usually simply a lack of dietary protein.

Fat requirements

There is no evidence that fat requirements are different because of HIV infection. However, certain antiretrovirals or certain infection symptoms such as diarrhoea may require changes in the timing or quantity of fat intake in some cases.

Micronutrient requirements

It is not recommend that micronutrients are supplemented beyond the level of recommended micronutrients for healthy non-HIV-infected persons of the same age, sex, and physical activity level. However, micronutrient deficiencies are common in HIV due to nutrient malabsorption and altered metabolism. Deficiencies of vitamins and minerals such as vitamins A, B-complex, C, E, selenium, and zinc, which are needed by the immune system to fight infection, are common. Deficiencies of antioxidant vitamins and minerals contribute to oxidative stress, a condition that may accelerate cell death and increase the rate of HIV replication. Good nutrition is best achieved by consuming a diverse diet with foods rich in micronutrients, especially vitamins A, B6, B12, and selenium, iron and zinc. A multivitamin supplement with added minerals, which contains no more than two times the Recommended Daily Allowance (RDA) for each nutrient, should be given to patients with malnutrition or poor food intake. For patients receiving isoniazid therapy, 25–50 mg pyridoxine (Vit B6) is advised to prevent peripheral neuropathy.

Key nutritional messages for people living with HIV/AIDS

- Eat a variety of foods.
- Make starchy foods the basis of each meal.
- Eat plenty of fruit and vegetables.
- Meat and dairy products may be eaten daily.
- Eat dried beans, peas, lentils and soya regularly.
- Include sugars, fats, and oils, especially after periods of weight loss.
- Use salt sparingly.
- Be as active as you can.
- Drink lots of clean, safe water.
- Do not drink alcohol.

With chronic vomiting, diarrhoea, and night sweats, dehydration is a serious concern. Fluid lost during each bout of diarrhoea or with each vomitus should be replaced with the easily prepared and affordable oral rehydration solution.

Table 23.1 Practical guidelines to cope with symptoms of HIV/AIDS

Symptom	Dietary advice
Loss of appetite	Drink high-energy drinks, e.g. milk, maas, mageu
	Eat small, frequent meals
	Avoid alcohol
	Exercise, e.g. walk before meals
	Eat with others and not alone
	Eat when you feel hungry
	Avoid drinking liquids with meals as these will fill you
Nausea and vomiting	Eat small, frequent meals
	Eat cold foods or foods at room temperature
	Avoid lying down after eating
	Eat plain foods
	Avoid rich, fatty foods
	Avoid foods with a strong smell and taste
Sore mouth and throat	Eat soft, moist foods, e.g. mashed potato, minced meat, pasta
	Use margarine or gravy to moisten cooked food
	Avoid sticky and rough foods e.g. peanut butter, potato chips and raw vegetables
	Avoid citrus fruits, pineapple, tomato, and spicy foods
	Eat cold foods or foods at room temperature
Diarrhoea	Eat small, frequent meals
	Drink isotonic fluids, e.g. oral rehydration solution
	Decrease/avoid milk and dairy products
	Decrease high-fat foods
	Include foods high in soluble fibre, e.g. bananas, oats porridge
	Avoid caffeine, e.g. coffee, cola drinks

Oral rehydration solution
- Use 1 litre clean, safe water.
- Add 8 level teaspoons sugar.
- Add half a teaspoon salt.
- Mix well.
- Store in a clean and covered container.
- Keep the solution in a cool place.
- Make a fresh solution every day.

References and further reading

Castetbon, K. et al. 2001. 'Prognostic value of cross-sectional anthropometric indices on short-term risk of mortality in Human Immunodeficiency Virus-infected adults in Abidjan, Cote d'Ivoire'. *American Journal of Epidemiology*; 154 (1): 75–84.

Kennedy, R.D. 2001. *The South African national guidelines on nutrition for people living with HIV/AIDS.* Pretoria: Department of Health.

Piwoz, E.G. and E.A. Preble. 2000. *A Review of the literature and recommendations for nutritional care and support in sub-Saharan Africa.* SARA project. Washington: USAID.

World Health Organization (WHO). 2003. *Nutrient requirements for people living with HIV/AIDS: Report of a technical consultation 13–15 May 2003.* Geneva, Switzerland: WHO, 2003.

Bonnard, P. 2002. *HIV/AIDS Mitigation: Using What We Already Know* (Technical Note 5). Washington D.C.: Food and Nutrition Technical Assistance Project (FANTA), Academy for Educational Development (AED).

Castleman, T., Seumo-Fosso, E., and Cogill, B. 2004. *Food and Nutrition Implications of Antiretroviral Therapy in Resource Limited Settings* (Technical Note 7). 2nd ed. Washington, D.C.: Food and Nutrition Technical Assistance Project (FANTA), Academy for Educational Development (AED).

24 Adult tuberculosis

Tuberculosis (TB) is the most common opportunistic infection in HIV-infected adults and the leading cause of death in South Africa. See Chapter 4: Interactions between HIV and tuberculosis for a discussion of TB epidemiology and pathophysiology. The HIV epidemic has complicated the diagnosis of TB, and the rising incidence of drug-resistance has compromised treatment outcomes. TB diagnosis relies on sputum microscopy for acid-fast bacilli (AFB), radiology and clinician judgement which are imprecise and labour-intensive, and on costly nucleic acid amplification tests and culture. These strategies are problematic in resource-limited settings. Delayed diagnosis is common. Clinical benefits from antituberculous therapy take several weeks to become apparent and TB mortality is highest in the first eight weeks of therapy.

Clinicians need to maintain a high level of concern for TB especially in patients living with HIV. Broadly, symptoms are due either to the presence of a focal TB disease process or to cytokine-mediated constitutional symptoms. Pulmonary and extrapulmonary disease can occur simultaneously.

Constitutional symptoms are present in most cases of TB and include:

- loss of weight;
- drenching sweats occurring on most nights for more than two weeks;
- feverishness, fatigue, and subjective muscle weakness (aesthenia).

Pulmonary symptoms include:

- cough for more than two weeks (with or without sputum production);
- pleuritic-type chest pain;
- dyspnoea (can occur with extensive pulmonary TB, massive pleural effusion, or tuberculous pericardial effusion, but other causes should be excluded, see Chapter 20: Common emergencies);
- haemoptysis (rare, as lung cavitation does not usually occur in HIV-infected patients).

Cough or fever of any duration, or night-sweats for three of the past four weeks is a sensitive (>90%) screening test for TB. Absence of current cough, fever, weight loss or night sweats is a good symptoms screen to rule out TB (negative predictive value >97%) as is a normal C-reactive protein (CRP) (negative predictive value >95%). However, asymptomatic sputum culture-positive PTB is increasingly being described in the literature.

Extrapulmonary symptoms include:

- asymmetrical enlargement of cervical, axillary or inguinal lymph nodes;
- abdominal distension or discomfort (due to tuberculous ascites, hepatic congestion from pericardial effusion, or massive intra-abdominal lymphadonopathy);
- headache with neck stiffness or altered mental status (due to tuberculous meningitis – refer for urgent lumber puncture – see Chapter 35: Neurology);
- pain and deformity of the spinal column, with or without paraplegia, or para-spinal mass extending into the iliac fossa and anterior thigh (due to TB of the vertebral column, extradural abscess and cord compression, or psoas abscess – refer for an urgent ultrasound scan and MRI scan);
- pain and swelling in one joint (due to tuberculous arthritis – refer for an orthopaedic opinion).

Renal tuberculosis is not a significant clinical entity in HIV-infected patients, although M. tuberculosis is frequently isolated from the urine.

Laboratory diagnosis of tuberculosis

Sputum examination for acid-fact bacilli (AFB) is likely to remain the first-line test for pulmonary TB in resource-limited settings in the medium term. However new molecular tests for *Mycobacterium tuberculosis* DNA, including gene mutations associated with drug resistance, are entering routine clinical care. High costs (for example the Xpert TB/RIF assay), imperfect sensitivity, and need for stringent laboratory conditions (for example the Genotype MDRTB assay) may limit widespread rollout. Urine testing for *M. tuberculosis* antigens such as lipoarabinomannan (LAM) will probably be most useful in patients with advanced HIV.

At present none of the mycobacterial-based assays can be used to rule out TB and mycobacterial culture is currently the most sensitive reference standard. Automated liquid culture platforms are widely used in South Africa but are expensive. Promising new low-cost assays such as the Microscopic Observation Drug Susceptibility test (MODS) and the Nitrate Reductase Assay (NRA) perform culture and phenotypic drug susceptibility testing directly from clinical specimens, but further development is required before these tests can be used in routine clinical care. The quality and number of clinical specimens submitted to the laboratory for culture remains of prime importance. Clinicians need to be aware of the limitations of the tests used in their laboratory and should discuss specific issues with a microbiologist.

Interferon-gamma release assays (IGRAs) detect lymphocytes that specifically react against *M. tuberculosis* antigens have no role in the diagnosis of active tuberculosis. Similarly, there is no role for antibody tests (serology) to diagnose active TB and the WHO has taken the unprecedented step of recommending that these tests be banned.

Diagnosis of smear-positive pulmonary tuberculosis

Any patient with tuberculous symptoms and a productive cough should have two (HIV-confirmed patient) or three (HIV-suspect or negative patient) sputum specimens sent for AFB staining using either the Ziehl-Neelsen, fluorescent auramine, or rhodamine stains.

2007 WHO guidelines suggest that pulmonary TB can be diagnosed if:
- one acid fast bacillus (AFB) is seen in at least one sputum sample (in countries with a well-functioning external quality assurance system).

This departure from previous guidelines ensures that the diagnosis of pulmonary TB is not missed in patients with paucibacillary disease.

Patients with a non-productive cough should have sputum induction with ultrasonic nebuliser and hypertonic saline. TB suspects who are too debilitated to cough can have a string test to detect AFB in swallowed respiratory secretions (see Appendix 21.1 in Chapter 21: Evaluation of fever).

It is essential that clinical staff have a good working relationship with the local laboratory to ensure rapid turn-around time for sputum specimens. Local initiatives should be encouraged to ensure rapid delivery of results (within 48 to 72 hours) by making effective use of human resources, and internet, cellphone or computer technology.

Smear-negative tuberculosis

About 60% of HIV-infected TB patients will have negative sputum smears. Implementation of the Gene Xpert (GXP) TB-RIF assay algorithm as a first-line investigation (Appendix 24.1) will likely improve detection of pulmonary tuberculosis, with up to 70% of smear-negative tuberculosis patients testing GXP-positive in research settings.

Smear-negative or GXP-negative tuberculosis

Response to antibiotic therapy is no longer a component in the diagnosis of smear-negative pulmonary TB, as patients may have both TB and pulmonary bacterial co-infection. A pragmatic response is to treat with a course of antibiotics, and to review the patient's overall condition after one and two weeks (if an outpatient) or in three to five days (if an inpatient) (See Chapter 32: Pulmonology). A patient with a bacterial respiratory infection would be expected to have shown substantially recovery over this period, and to have negative sputum smears, but remains a TB suspect until all symptoms have resolved at follow-up visits. Persisting symptoms suggests smear-negative pulmonary TB.

The WHO recommends that smear-negative pulmonary TB can be diagnosed when the following criteria are met:

- at least two sputum specimens negative for AFB; and
- radiographical abnormalities are consistent with active tuberculosis; and
- there is laboratory confirmation of HIV infection; or
- strong clinical evidence of HIV infection; and
- decision by a clinician to treat with a full course of antituberculosis chemotherapy.

Using a chest radiograph to diagnose smear-negative or GXP-negative tuberculosis

A chest radiograph is an essential investigation in all TB suspects with negative sputum smears.

Radiographic findings that suggest active HIV-associated TB are:

- asymmetrical air-space opacification;
- scattered 'soft' pulmonary nodules (which need to be distinguished from 'hard' calcified granuloma);
- miliary or micronodular infiltrates;
- cavitation (which may be subtle);

- pleural effusion;
- mediastinal or hilar adenopathy (see Appendix 24.2);
- increased cardiothoracic ratio (suggesting pericardial effusion);
- normal radiograph.

Note that pleural and pericardial TB, and mediastinal tuberculous adenopathy are classified as extrapulmonary TB by the WHO.

Several conditions have clinical and/or radiological similarities with smear-negative pulmonary TB. If unsure it is important to obtain a second opinion. Common conditions include:

- community acquired pneumonia with or without parapneumonic effusion;
- chronic bronchitis (that may be secondarily infected – look for bronchial wall thickening);
- bronchiectasis (with or without secondary infection – look for dilated bronchi and fibrocystic changes);
- lung abscess (look for an air-fluid level in the lung parenchyma);
- chronic bacterial sinusitis with post-nasal drip (ask about nasal congestion, purulent nasal discharge, and facial pain when bending forward);
- allergic rhinitis with post nasal drip (ask about seasonal sneezing, itchy nose, and nasal congestion, look inside the nose for oedematous mucosa over the turbinates);
- asthma (ask about wheezing and cough at night, or with exercise, relieved by salbutamol inhaler);
- cardiac failure (ask about orthopnoea and ankle swelling, look for pulmonary oedema on the chest radiograph);
- lung cancer;
- pneumoconiosis (ask about work under ground on the mines or living in a traditional hut with smoke exposure);
- sarcoidosis (look for skin plaques and check for uveitis).

HIV-associated conditions can also mimic smear-negative pulmonary TB, including:

- *Pneumocystis* pneumonia (look for symmetrical fine reticulonodular infiltrates and 'ground-glass' air space opacification – note that this infection can cause pulmonary cysts);
- pulmonary Kaposi's sarcoma (look for Kaposi's plaques in the skin and oropharygeal mucosa, but note that absence of these lesions does not rule out pulmonary Kaposi's sarcoma);

- pulmonary fungal infections including cryptococcus and histo-plasmosis;
- lymphoma;
- pulmonary nocardiosis (can be diagnosed on sputum culture).

> All patients diagnosed with smear-negative pulmonary tuberculosis should have at least one sputum specimen sent for liquid media culture. A negative culture does not rule out TB, but a positive culture confirms the diagnosis and conversion from culture-positive to culture-negative on follow-up cultures suggests that the patient is responding to treatment.

Response to a pleural effusion

TB pleural effusion can be diagnosed clinically in adults younger than 45 years if:

- *the aspirated fluid is not purulent and is clinically an exudate (straw-coloured fluid that forms a clot on standing.)*

In adults older than 45 years, or if the pleural fluid is not clearly an exudate, the following tests should be sent:

- blood and fluid total protein (a ratio of >0.5 suggests an exudate);
- cytology (neutrophils predominance suggests parapneumonic effusion, lymphocyte predominance [ratio lymphocyte count / neutrophil count ≥0.45] suggests TB, atypical cells suggest malignancy);
- elevated adenosine deaminase assay (ADA) suggests TB or (rarely) haematological malignancy, but a normal result does not rule out TB (especially in immune compromised patients).

Pleural biopsy should be considered for all atypical or non-resolving pleural effusions.

> Pleural (and ascitic) fluid inoculated under aseptic conditions into a mycobacterial blood culture bottle has a good culture yield for *M. tuberculosis*.

Extrapulmonary tuberculosis

The 2006 WHO guidelines recommend the extrapulmonary TB can be diagnosed if:

- one specimen from an extrapulmonary site is culture-positive for M. tuberculosis or smear-positive for AFB; *or*
- there is histological or strong clinical evidence consistent with active extrapulmonary tuberculosis; *and*
- there is laboratory confirmation of HIV infection; *or*
- strong clinical evidence of HIV infection; *and*
- decision by a clinician to treat with a full course of antituberculosis chemotherapy.

Common extrapulmonary manifestations of TB involve serous cavities or lymph nodes.

Serositis:
- pleural exudate;
- pericardial effusion with constitutional symptoms;
- ascitic exudate.

Lymphadenopathy:
- enlarged cervical, axillary and inguinal nodes;
- mediastinal or hilar lymphadenopathy;
- intra-abdominal lymphadenopathy or splenic hypoechoic lesions on ultrasound scan.

'Strong clinical evidence' usually means demonstrating at least one of these abnormalities. TB meningitis is considered in Chapter 35: Neurology.

> At least one TB culture should be sent for liquid media culture from all patients diagnosed with extrapulmonary TB. Induced sputum, biopsy material and pus and fluid aspirates have a good yield.

Response to a normal chest radiograph

If the chest radiograph is normal there are four possible options:
- biopsy asymmetrically enlarged peripheral lymph nodes (See Appendix 21.1 in Chapter 21: Evaluation of fever);

- if the patient is coughing send a sputum TB culture, review the patient two, four to six weeks later with a repeat chest radiograph. (Note that this only an option is the patient is ambulant, has good social support and easy access to medical care if deterioration occurs);
- refer the patient for abdominal and pericardial ultrasound scan, looking for pericardial effusion, intra-abdominal lymph nodes, hypoechoic splenic lesions, ascites;
- refer the patient for evaluation for fever of unknown origin (see Chapter 21: Evaluation of fever).

Response to ascites

Typically an ascitic exudate is diagnosed by demonstrating that the difference (gradient) between blood and ascitic albumin is <11 g/L. This rule becomes difficult to apply in debilitated HIV-infected patients who often have very low serum albumin. It is helpful to clinically rule out causes of ascitic transudate such as cardiac failure, portal hypertension and nephrotic syndrome. Demonstrating lymphocytes in the asctic fluid makes a diagnosis of TB more likely, as does an elevated ADA.

Treatment of tuberculosis

Antituberculous drugs are used for their bactericidal and bacteriostatic properties and also to prevent resistance. Isoniazid and rifampicin are the most powerful bactericidal drugs, with the widest spectrum of activity, and rifampicin has the most potent sterilising capabilities. Pyrazinamide is bactericidal against TB bacilli in an acidic environment in macrophanges, and streptomycin is bactericidal against rapidly multiplying bacilli. Some

Table 24.1 Essential antituberculous drugs (adapted from WHO 2003 treatment guidelines)

Essential drug (abbreviation)	Recommended dosage (dose range) in mg/kg Daily	Three times weekly
Isoniazid (H)	5 (4–6)	10 (8–12)
Rifampicin (R)	10 (8–12)	10 (8–12)
Pyrazinamide (Z)	25 (20–30)	35 (30–40)
Streptomycin (S)	15 (12–18)	15 (12–18)
Ethambutol (E)	15 (15-20)	30 (20-35)

sub-populations (strains) of TB bacilli remain dormant for long periods of time, and are metabolically active for only brief periods. This phenomenon necessitates prolonged treatment, and explains about half of cases of TB relapse (the other half are due to re-infection).

TB treatment consists of two phases: an initial phase lasting two months involving the greatest number of drugs (isoniazid, rifampicin, pyrazinamide and ethambutol) and a continuation phase, lasting in most cases for four months and involving fewer drugs (usually only isoniazid and rifampicin). During the intensive initial phase there is rapid killing of tubercle bacilli, with infectious patients rapidly losing their infectivity, usually within approximately two weeks. The sterilising effect of the continuation phase drugs eliminates remaining bacilli and prevents subsequent relapses. Combination pills such as Rimstar, Rimactazid, Rifafour-E275 and Rifinah are strongly recommended. An example of dosing combination pills is given below:

Initial phase:
Rifampicin 150 mg/isoniazid 75 mg/pyrazinamide 400 mg/ethambutol 275 mg combination tablet:
- weight 30–37 kg – 2 tablets;
- weight 38–54 kg – 3 tablets;
- weight 55–70 kg – 4 tablets;
- weight 71 kg and over – 5 tablets.

Continuation phase:
- rifampicin 150 mg/isoniazid 100 mg – patients weighing less than 50 kg: 3 tablets (450 mg rifampicin and 300 mg isoniazid);
- rifampicin 300 mg / isoniazid 150 mg – patients weighing 50 kg or greater: 2 tablets (600 mg rifampicin and 300 mg isoniazid).

Re-treatment cases include all TB patients who have been treated for more than one month previously and are currently smear or culture positive. Such patients have a higher likelihood of drug resistance. Re-treatment patients should receive an initial phase of three months involving treatment with five drugs (isoniazid, rifampicin, pyrazinamide, ethambutol and streptomycin), one month with four drugs (isoniazid, rifampicin, pyrazinamide, ethambutol) and a continuation phase of five months with three drugs (isoniazid, rifampicin, ethambutol). MDR-TB cases are most at risk of failure in the re-treatment regimen, despite full adherence. There is very little evidence to support the inclusion of streptomycin in the retreatment regimen, and drug susceptibility testing for all retreatment cases may be a more effective strategy.

Most forms of extrapulmonary TB can be treated with the regimens mentioned above for between six to nine months. For patients with TB meningitis, six months of therapy with continuous rifampicin has been shown to be as effective as the traditional nine to 12 regimens. Lastly, adjunctive steroids may be useful in pericardial and meningeal tuberculosis (see Chapter 29: Cardiology and Chapter 35: Neurology).

Antituberculous therapy and antiretroviral therapy

Rifampicin-based antituberculous therapy can be given with nucleoside / nucleotide and non-nucleotide reverse transcriptase inhibitor-based ART, and antiretroviral therapy should not be interrupted. However rifampicin interacts with protease inhibitors and dose modification is required (see Chapter 49: Drug-drug interactions).

Antiretroviral therapy (ART) in patients newly diagnosed with TB should be started within two weeks provided the treatment for tuberculosis is being tolerated, social support is in place and adequate antiretroviral training has been given. Patients with a CD4 count >50 cells/μL have the option of starting ART after the first eight weeks of treatment for TB to reduce the risk of mild immune reconstitution disease (See Chapter 50: Immune reconstitution inflammatory syndrome).

Efavirenz is preferable to nevirapine when ART is initiated in tuberculosis patients. Tuberculosis patients who start nevirapine are at increased risk of virological failure as liver enzyme induction caused by rifampicin may cause sub-therapeutic nevirapine levels when given during the first two weeks at a dose of 200 mg daily (if nevirapine is the best option consider initiating treatment at 200 mg twice dialy).

Side-effects of main antituberculous agents

Isoniazid (H) adverse effects:
– peripheral neuropathy;
– hepatitis (rare);
– generalised skin rash (rare);
– fever;
– joint pains.

Note: Isoniazid inhibits the metabolism of epileptic drugs such as phenytoin and carbamazepine. Dosages of these drugs may need to be reduced for the duration of treatment.

Rifampicin (R) adverse effects:
– gastro-intestinal: nausea, anorexia, mild abdominal pain;
– cutaneous reactions: mild flushing and itchiness of the skin;
– hepatitis (uncommon unless concurrent history of liver disease or alcoholism);
– colours urine, sweat and tears orange/pink.

Note: Rifampicin is an enzyme inducer. Be careful of drug interactions between rifampicin and drugs such as the oral contraceptive pill, warfarin, oral diabetic drugs, digoxin, anti-epileptics. Doses of contraceptive should be increased in patients receiving rifampicin, or other methods of contraception should be used.

Ethambutol (E) adverse effects:
– progressive loss of vision due to retrobulbar neuritis (colour vision affected first);
– skin rash;
– joint pains;
– peripheral neuropathy.

Note: Patients should be told to notify a health professional of any changes in vision. Visual disturbance should lead to the immediate discontinuation of ethambutol.

Pyrazinamide (Z) adverse effects:
– hepatotoxicity;
– arthralgia;
– skin rash on sun exposed areas.

Note: Patients with liver disease should not receive pyrazinamide.

Streptomycin (S) adverse events:
– cutaneous hypersensitivity, rash and fever;
– vestibular toxicity causing dizziness, vertigo, unsteadiness, vomiting;
– deafness;
– anaphylaxis;
– renal impairment.

Note: Avoid streptomycin in patients with pre-existing renal disease or patients >65 years. Streptomycin is contra-indicated in pregnancy and in young children.

Use of antituberculous drugs in specific categories of patients

TB in renal failure

Streptomycin and ethambutol are excreted by the kidney. These drugs may be given in reduced doses where facilities enable the close monitoring of renal function.

Liver failure

Isoniazid, rifampicin and pyrazinamide are all associated with hepatitis and rifampicin can also cause cholestasis. Pyrazinamide is possibly the most hepatotoxic drug and patients with established chronic liver disease should not receive the drug. Isoniazid plus rifampicin plus one or two non-hepatotoxic drugs such as streptomycin and ethambutol may be used for a total treatment duration of eight months instead (2SHRE/6HR). Alternative regimens include 9RE or 2SHE/10HE.

Pregnancy and breastfeeding

Most antituberculous drugs are safe in pregnancy with the exception of streptomycin which is ototoxic to the foetus and therefore contra-indicated in pregnancy. All antituberculous drugs are compatible with breastfeeding.

Management of antituberculous therapy with hepatitis or jaundice

Antituberculous therapy can cause clinically significant hepatitis (ALT >5x normal) at any time. The initial response to jaundice or hepatitis is to stop all antituberculous drugs and to review the results of a full liver panel. Elevated bilirubin with predominant elevation of the cannalicular enzymes (ALP and GGT) and ALT <3x normal suggests drug-induced cholestasis, hepatic infiltration, or biliary obstruction. Under these circumstances it is usually safe to continue antituberculous therapy, with close monitoring of the lever enzymes, bilirubin and INR. Ultrasound-scan of the liver may show dilated ducts, focal lesions or lymph nodes in the porta hepatis; if the scan is normal a liver biopsy may be helpful. Antituberculous therapy should always be discontinued if the ALT is ≥5x normal. If the patient is very ill, and MDR-TB is unlikely, ethambutol, streptomycin and ofloxacin have a low risk of hepotoxicity and can be prescribed. The ALT and bilirubin should be check at least twice weekly. When the bilirubin and ALT are <2x normal isoniazid and rifampicin can be reintroduced, either singly or together, with close follow up monitoring for seven to 14 days. In mild cases it is reasonable to reintroduce isoniazid, rifampicin, ethambutol and pyrazinamide together with close monitoring.

Treatment monitoring and adherence

Response to treatment should be monitored by sputum smear examination. This should be performed at the end of the second month and at six months of treatment. Persistent sputum positivity at the end of two months of treatment indicates one of the following: poor patient adherence, heavy initial bacillary load or drug resistant TB non responsive to first-line drugs. Sputum positivity at two months should lead to four months of treatment with initial phase antituberculous therapy, after which the smears are repeated and the continuation phase of treatment with two drugs is started. Drug susceptibility testing (DST) should be performed if the smear still remains positive at two to three months of antituberculous therapy. Negative patient smears at two months, followed by positive smears at six months are termed treatment failures and such patients should be retreated for TB under specialist supervision. All re-treatment and treatment failure patients should have a specimen sent for resistance mutation testing, culture and DST.

Patient adherence should be encouraged using a patient-centred approach, using directly observed therapy (DOT) for the initial phase of treatment in at least smear-positive cases and also in continuation phase regimens that include rifampicin. DOT is required to ensure patient treatment adherence and ensures healthcare accountability for their patients' adherence to antituberculous therapy.

Treatment monitoring for smear-negative and extrapulmonary TB

In these cases the efficacy of treatment is harder to determine as it is not possible to determine smear conversion. The WHO recommends clinical monitoring. Monitoring should focus on objective clinical status, and detection of complications (such as constrictive pericarditis or hydrocephalus). Objective improvement can be demonstrated by showing improving weight and haemoglobin, falling CRP, resolution of TB symptoms and improvement of functional status (e.g. using the Karnofsky score).

Multidrug resistant tuberculosis

The incidence of multidrug resistant TB (MDR-TB) is rising in southern Africa. Transmission of MDR-TB occurs both in the community and in healthcare settings. As with drug-sensitive TB the challenge is rapid identification of MDR-TB and early initiation of effective treatment.

Multidrug resistance is defined as:
- *resistance to at least rifampicin and isoniazid (the two most potent antituberculous drugs).*

Extreme drug resistance is defined as:
- resistance to rifampicin and isoniazid; *and*
- resistance to any flouroquinolone; *and*
- resistance to any one of three injectable second line drugs: capreomycin, kanamycin and amikacin.

Extensively drug-resistant TB (XDR-TB) has emerged as a serious threat to public health, especially but not solely in countries with high HIV prevalence. A notable outbreak of XDR-TB was reported in Tugela Ferry, KwaZulu-Natal Province, South Africa. 23% of 221 cases of MDR-TB were found to have XDR-TB. The emergence of XDR-TB raises concerns of TB epidemics with severely restricted treatment options that could jeopardise the progress already made in global TB control. Strengthening the coverage and quality of basic TB control is the most important measure to prevent MDR-TB and provides the means to deploy treatment strategies for drug resistant TB.

Traditionally, MDR-TB should be suspected in:
- retreatment patients who remain sputum smear positive after three months of intensive therapy;
- retreatment failure and defaulter cases;
- close contacts of MDR tuberculosis cases;
- chronic cases of tuberculosis.

However, HIV patients often have smear-negative disease and untreated MDR-TB can be fatal over a period of weeks. Increasing transmission of MDR-TB in the community means that most patients with resistant infection will not fall into recognized at risk categories. Therefore clinicians need to have a high index of suspicion for possible MDR-TB in TB patients who are 'failing to thrive' on antituberculous therapy ('TB non-responders'). The possibilities are:

- non-adherence to antituberculous therapy (with a drug-sensitive infection);
- malabsorption of antituberculous drugs;
- immune reconstitution disease (within three months of initiating anti-retroviral therapy);
- disease process other than TB, including other HIV-related conditions (e.g. lymphoma);
- MDR-TB.

Laboratory diagnosis of MDR-TB

Drug resistance can be suspected but not proven clinically – laboratory diagnosis is essential. The reference standard is phenotypic resistance testing in liquid or on solid culture media, demonstrating growth of *M. tuberculosis* in the presence of standardized concentrations of antitubercular antibiotics. Resistance testing can be technically challenging (for example to pyrazinamide and ethambutol) and testing for resistance to some second line drugs has not been standardized. Reference laboratory facilities are needed and a final result takes weeks. Molecular testing has the potential to transform the field but current technologies have significant limitations. The Xpert TB/RIF assay only detects resistance mutations to rifampicin, and is only positive only in about two thirds of smear-negative specimens. The Genotype MDR-TB assay tests for resistance mutations to both isoniazid and rifampicin but can only be used on smear-positive clinical specimens or positive liquid culture media samples. Standardized tests for resistance mutations to other drugs are not yet available.

Treatment of MDR-TB

Treatment for MDR-TB should only be given in specialized government-funded centres. Patients diagnosed with rifampicin-resistant mutations on Xpert TB/RIF should be treated for MDR-TB, with the option of adding isoniazid (to cover for possible rifampicin mono-resistance) and rifampicin (if the rifampicin result is thought to be false-positive [i.e. low pre-test probability]). Prior TB treatment, death of a close contact from TB, and recent hospitalization increase the probability of MDR-TB. Ineffective drugs can be stopped when DST results are available. MDR-TB cases should have monthly cultures and DST.

The WHO advocates the following guidelines be used when designing a MDR-TB patient treatment regimen:

- The regimen should be based on the patient's previous drug history.
- Prevalence of resistance to first-line and second-line drugs, as well as drugs and regimens commonly used locally should be taken into consideration.
- *At least* four drugs with either certain or almost certain efficacy should be included, based on drug sensitivity testing or the drug history of the patient.
- Drugs are administered at least six days per week.
- Note that, wherever possible, pyrazinamide, and fluoroquinolones should be given once per day as this may be more efficacious.
- When selecting a flouroquinolone the order of preference is moxifloxacin > levofloxacin > ofloxacin.
- Ethambutol is no longer used to treat MDR-TB as the background prevalence of resistance is high and routine sensitivity testing has poor reproducibility.
- An injectable agent (aminoglycoside or capreomcin) is used for a minimum of six months or at least four months after culture conversion, whichever is longer.
- Treatment is for a *minimum* of 18 months.
- Each dose is given as directly observed therapy (DOT), throughout treatment.
- DST, where available and reliable, should be used to guide therapy.
- Early MDR-TB detection and prompt initiation of treatment are important determinants of successful therapy.
- Weight-based standardized treatment of MDR-TB is shown in Table 24.2 and Table 24.3.

Table 24.2 Intensive Phase: Standardised Regimen for Adult MDR-TB Treatment

Patient weight	Drug	Dosage
<33kg	Kanamycin	15–20 mg/kg
	Ethionamide	15–20 mg/kg
	Pyrazinamide	30–40 mg/kg
	Moxifloxacin	400 mg (children: 7.5 to 10 mg/kg)
	Terizidone	15–20 mg/kg

33–50 kg	Kanamycin	500–750 mg
	Ethionamide	500 mg
	Pyrazinamide	1 000–1 750mg
	Moxifloxacin	400 mg
	Terizidone	750 mg
51–70 kg	Kanamycin	1 000 mg
	Ethionamide	750 mg
	Pyrazinamide	1 750–2 000 mg
	Moxifloxacin	400 mg
	Terizidone	750 mg
>70 kg	Kanamycin	1000 mg
	Ethionamide	750–1 000 mg
	Pyrazinamide	2 000–2 500 mg
	Moxifloxacin	400 mg
	Terizidone	750–1 000 mg

Table 24.3 Continuation phase: at least 18 months after TB culture conversion (treatment taken at least six times per week)

Patient weight	Drug	Dosage
<33kg	Ethionamide	15–20 mg/kg
	Pyrazinamide	30–40 mg/kg
	Moxifloxacin	400 mg (children 7.5–10 mg/kg)
	Terizidone	15–20 mg/kg
33–50 kg	Ethionamide	500 mg
	Pyrazinamide	1 000–1 750 mg
	Moxifloxacin	400 mg
	Terizidone	750 mg
51–70 kg	Ethionamide	750 mg
	Pyrazinamide	1 750–2 000 mg
	Moxifloxacin	400 mg
	Terizidone	750 mg
>70 kg	Ethionamide	750–1 000 mg
	Pyrazinamide	2 000–2 500 mg
	Moxifloxacin	400 mg
	Terizidone	750–1 000 mg

Antiretroviral therapy should be initiated as soon as MDR-TB is diagnosed irrespective of CD4 count. Note that the antacid in buffered didanosine preparation (seldom used in modern treatment regimens) prevents the absorption of flouroquinolones which should be given at least two hours later. Resection of affected lung is an important treatment modality for patients who are not responding to therapy and have localised disease.

Infection control

M. tuberculosis is transmitted by patients with pulmonary TB during coughing and sneezing. Aerosolized respiratory droplets evaporate to form droplet nuclei 1-2 μm in size than can remain suspended in a closed environment for several days. The droplet nuclei are inhaled into the lungs of other people in the room. Infection control depends on three essential components:

- control of respiratory secretions by coughing / sneezing into cupped hands (that are frequently washed), or tissues; and use of surgical masks to cover the mouth and nose of open TB cases;
- environmental control with good ventilation, and abundant sunlight (ultraviolet light (UVB) rapidly destroys *M. tuberculosis*);
- use of N95 masks by healthcare workers and family in prolonged contact with infectious TB cases.

If an MDR-TB patient is to be managed at home the patient should have his or her own bedroom that is well ventilated, should spend as much time as possible outside in the sunshine, and until culture negative should eat alone and wear a surgical mask when mingling with family members. Young children and family members with HIV infection, diabetes, or alcoholism should live elsewhere if possible. All family members should be tested regularly for HIV infection.

In healthcare facilities coughing patients in clinics should be rapidly triaged out of the general queue and should be asked to give sputum samples for AFB testing in a well-ventilated space. Sputum induction should be used if needed.

Isoniazid preventative therapy

HIV-positive adults with a positive tuberculin skin test (TST) are at increased risk of TB and isoniazid preventative therapy (IPT) given for at least six months reduces this risk. The incidence of tuberculosis begins to increase again as soon as IPT is discontinued. Giving long-term IPT is a reasonable strategy in highly adherent patients with a positive skin test and may also have a mortality benefit. Importantly, patients with a negative TST do not benefit from IPT and may be at increased risk of death if IPT is given for long periods.

IPT cannot be given to patients with active TB as this may cause isoniazid resistance. Patients should be screened for TB symptoms before IPT is considered – those with any symptom (cough, fever, sweats, weight loss) should have a chest radiograph and sputum smears/culture. A small group of patients without symptoms have sputum culture-positive TB and may inadvertently receive isoniazid monotherapy. Ideally, patients should be repeated screened for TB symptoms and have a screening chest radiograph before IPT is considered.

For the TST 0.1 mL of purified protein derivative (PPD) from M. tuberculosis is injected intracutaneously (into the skin) of the anterior forearm, avoiding structures such as veins or tendons. An intradermal bleb must be clearly visualized. The patient should return 48-72 hours later, and the transverse diameter of the inflammatory induration should be measured after delineating the edges with a ball-point pen. A positive test is ≥5 mm in diameter. Strongly positive tests may blister and ulcerate but will heal without scarring. IGRA is used to detect an immune response against M. tuberculosis in well-resourced settings, and it is assumed (but not proven) that IGRA positive patients will also benefit from IPT. Logistic factors that need to be considered in implementing a tuberculin skin testing service are shown in the box below.

Logistic considerations when establishing a tuberculin skin test service

- Institutional will to establish an HIV Wellness / IPT service.
- Allocation of TST/IPT staff and clinic space.
- Patient counselling on need for TST after HIV test and TB screening.
- Batching patients to maximize efficiency – fast-tracking / triage.
- In-service training.
- Quality control / supervision of placement technique.
- Return to have TST read at 48–72 hours – patient time and transport costs.
- Supply chain management of disposable items:
  o tuberculin vials – disposed 8 hours after opening;
  o refrigerator or cold bag – unbroken cold chain;
  o disposable syringes with 27 gauge needle;
  o sharps container and safe disposal of medical waste;
  o supervisor to regularly evaluate stocks and appropriately order stock.

Patients without TB symptoms and with a positive TST can be offered isoniazid 300 mg daily with pyridoxine 25-50 mg daily. The importance of good adherence should be emphasized. Hepatitis is a rare side-effect of isoniazid and patients should be advised to stop immediately treatment and present for clinical review if nausea, right upper quadrant pain or yellow discolouration of the eyes occurs.

IPT requires significant resources and more effective programmes such as initiation of ART at CD4 count of <350 cells/μL should take priority. Patients who are starting ART should wait at least three months before being screened for IPT to allow subclinical TB to become apparent and to increase the chances of a positive TST after immune reconstitution.

Holistic care of TB patients

All TB patients should be notified at the time of diagnosis and transferred to their local TB treatment centre using standardised forms. TB is a stigmatizing diagnosis. Healthcare workers should make the time to listen to the concerns of the patient and family and give practical responses to questions dealing with the likelihood of cure and risk of transmission to other family members. All HIV-infected patients should receive ongoing cotrimoxazole prophylaxis with two single tablets strength daily. TB patients qualify for a disability grant and should also receive food parcels for the duration of treatment. Young children who have been in contact with a smear-positive family member should be assessed for active disease or for prophylaxis.

Healthcare workers often need to provide end-of-life care to TB patients (see Chapter 56: Palliative care). Open discussion of the issues combined with effective control of symptoms is central to care. Morphine is an exceptionally effective drug for the control of dyspnoea, cough and pain (combined with paracetamol and non-steroidal anti-inflammatory drugs).

References and further reading

Boehme, C.C., Nicol, M.P., Nabeta, P., et al. 2011. Feasibility, diagnostic accuracy, and effectiveness of decentralised use of the Xpert MTB/RIF test for diagnosis of tuberculosis and multidrug resistance: a multicentre implementation study. *The Lancet*, 377:1495-505.

Donald, P.R., McIlleron, H. 2009. 'Antituberculous drugs'. In *Tuberculosis: A Comprehensive Clinical Reference.* Schaaf, H.S., Zumla, A. (Eds.). Elsevier Inc.

Getahun, H., Kittikraisak, W., Heilig, C.M., Corbett, E.L., Ayles, H., Cain, K.P., Grant, A.D., Churchyard, G.J., Kimerling, M., Shah, S., Lawn, S.D., Wood, R., Maartens, G., Granich, R., Date, A.A., Varma, J.K. 2011. Development of a standardized screening rule for tuberculosis in people living with HIV in resource-constrained settings: individual participant data meta-analysis of observational studies. *PLoS Med,* 18;8(1):e1000391.

Lawn, S., Churchyard, G. Epidemiology of HIV-associated tuberculosis. 2009. *Curr Opin HIV AIDS,* 4: 325–333.

Mendelson, M. 2007. Diagnosing tuberculosis in HIV-infected patients: challenges and future prospects. *British Medical Bulletin,* 81 and 82: 149–165

Republic of South Africa. Department of Health. 2009. *South African National Tuberculosis Management Guidelines.* http://familymedicine.ukzn.ac.za/Libraries/Guidelines_Protocols/TB_Guidelines_2009.sflb.ashx

South African Department of Health. 2011. MDRTB policy and treatment guidelines. http://www.info.gov.za/view/DownloadFileAction?id=165278

South African Department of Health. 2011. Policy framework for the management of MDRTB in South Africa. http://www.doh.gov.za/docs/policy/2011/policy_TB.pdf

TB Online http://www.tbonline.info/ (*information for activists, patients, health workers & researchers working to end TB*) http://www.tbonline.info/media/uploads/documents/guidelines_prog_management_mdr_2011.pdf

WHO. 2004. *TB/HIV: A Clinical Manual.* 2nd ed. Stop TB WHO.

WHO. 2007. *Improving the diagnosis and treatment of smear-negative pulmonary and extrapulmonary tuberculosis among adults and adolescents. Recommendations for HIV-prevalent and resource-constrained settings.* Stop TB WHO.

WHO. 2011. *Guidelines for the Programmatic Management of Drug-Resistant Tuberculosis: 2011 update.*

WHO. 2012. *The Global Plan to Stop TB 2011 to 2015.* Stop TB WHO. http://www.stoptb.org/global/plan/

Wilson, D., Howell, V., Toppozini, C., Dong, K., Clark, M., Hurtado, R. 2011. Against all odds: diagnosing tuberculosis in South Africa. *J Infect Dis*, 204 Suppl 4:S1102-9.

Wood R, Middelkoop K, Myer L, Grant AD, Whitelaw A, Lawn SD, Kaplan G, Huebner R, McIntyre J, Bekker LG. 2007. Undiagnosed tuberculosis in a community with high HIV prevalence: implications for tuberculosis control. *Am J Respir Crit Care Med*, 175:87-93.

Appendix 24.1

Algorithm for the implementation of the Gene Xpert TB/RIF (GXP) assay in tuberculosis suspects

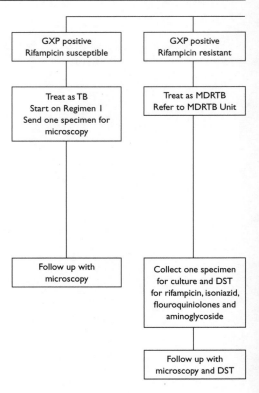

ALGORITHM FOR
(TB and DR-TB contacts, non-contact symptomatic
Collect one sputum specimen

GXP positive Rifampicin susceptible	GXP positive Rifampicin resistant
Treat as TB Start on Regimen I Send one specimen for microscopy	Treat as MDRTB Refer to MDRTB Unit
Follow up with microscopy	Collect one specimen for culture and DST for rifampicin, isoniazid, flouroquiniolones and aminoglycoside
	Follow up with microscopy and DST

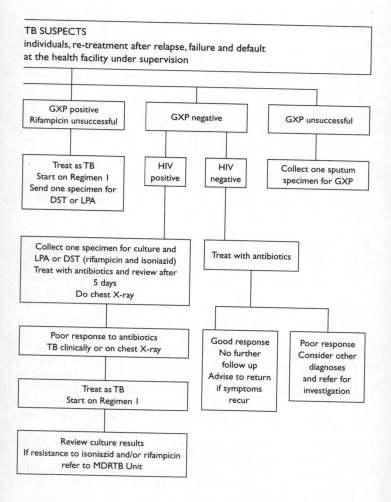

TB SUSPECTS
individuals, re-treatment after relapse, failure and default
at the health facility under supervision

GXP positive
Rifampicin unsuccessful

GXP negative

GXP unsuccessful

Treat as TB
Start on Regimen 1
Send one specimen for
DST or LPA

HIV
positive

HIV
negative

Collect one sputum
specimen for GXP

Collect one specimen for culture and
LPA or DST (rifampicin and isoniazid)
Treat with antibiotics and review after
5 days
Do chest X-ray

Treat with antibiotics

Poor response to antibiotics
TB clinically or on chest X-ray

Good response
No further
follow up
Advise to return
if symptoms
recur

Poor response
Consider other
diagnoses
and refer for
investigation

Treat as TB
Start on Regimen 1

Review culture results
If resistance to isoniazid and/or rifampicin
refer to MDRTB Unit

Appendix 24.2 Radiological signs of mediastinal and hilar adenopathy

Look for mediastinal and hilar adenopathy in both the frontal and lateral chest radiographs.

On the frontal film:

- The width of the superior mediastinum above the aortic arch in a young patient is not usually wider than the vertebrae – but it does widen as the vessels become ectatic with age.
- The right border of the superior mediastinum should not be lobulated.
- The right tracheal stripe should be of uniform width, usually less that 2-3 mm, and ends in the right tracheo-bronchial angle in an elliptical opacity, not a round one (Figures 24.1 and 24.2).
- The elliptical opacity (the azygous arch) is normally less than 10 mm wide in an erect film.
- The trachea and bronchi have uniform parallel walls – it is important to examine them regularly – also the sub-carinal area where adenopathy can displace the bronchi and widen the carinal angle or indent the airways.
- The hila should be of equal size, shape and density. The left hilum is often partially hidden by the mediastinal structures, and its size must be 'judged'. It can be difficult to assess whether large hilar opacities are big vessels or if they are enlarged nodes or a mass. Masses or nodes usually increase the density of the hila. Compare the two sides (but remember that adenopathy can be bilateral). Increased density can also be caused by an overlying opacity – a lateral projection film is helpful here.
- If vessels cross the edge of the hila opacity by more than 1 cm it suggests that the opacity is not only vascular (the 'overlay sign'). (But remember that the right superior pulmonary vein crosses the pulmonary artery on its way to the left atrium). In a vascular structure the vessels usually join the edge of the 'mass' and 'come off it' (Figure 24.3). Vessels visibly crossing an opacity indicates that the opacity is mass lesion (Figure 24.4).
- Vessels have one convex and one concave border and masses usually have two convex borders (Figures 24.5 and 24.6).
- On the right the pulmonary artery runs along the lateral border of the bronchus intermedius (Figure 24.7). There should not be soft tissue between the bronchus and the right heart border (except for the right superior pulmonary vein on its way to the left atrium)

On the lateral film:

- Determine that the tracheal and bronchial walls are regular and parallel.
- Adenopathy can be seen behind the posterior tracheal wall (note the azygous vein can form an opacity here).
- The most important area is the sub-carinal region (Figure 24.8). The carina is higher than expected – the start of the subcarinal region can be localised by identifying the two upper lobe bronchi 'on face' (i.e. running towards/away from the viewer).
- The right pulmonary artery runs towards the viewer and is larger than its left counterpart. It is situated in front of the trachea, with the middle lobe bronchus running forward just below it.
- The left pulmonary artery courses inferiorly within the arch of the aorta (forming a 'miniature aorta'), behind the trachea and above the right pulmonary artery (Figure 24.9).
- The two arteries are separate structures and there should not be an opacity crossing the trachea from front to back (Figure 24.10).

Figure 24.1

Figure 24.2

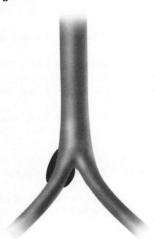

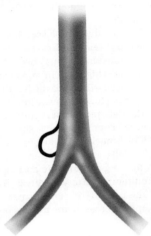

Normal azygous

Paratracheal lymph node (add widened
right paratracheal stripe)

Figure 24.3

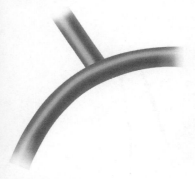

Vessel 'coming off' vessel

Figure 24.4

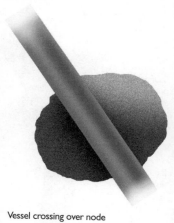

Vessel crossing over node

Figure 24.5

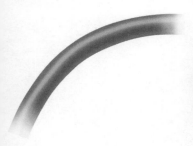

Vessel with convex and concave border

Figure 24.6

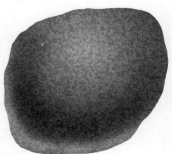

Mass with two convex borders

Figure 24.7 Relationships adjacent to the right heart border (PA view)

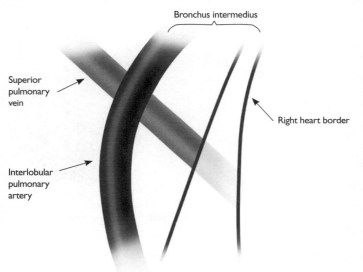

Bronchus intermedius

Superior pulmonary vein

Interlobular pulmonary artery

Right heart border

Figure 24.8 Sub-carinal region (lateral view)

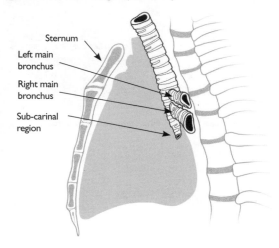

Sternum

Left main bronchus

Right main bronchus

Sub-carinal region

Figure 24.9 Right and left pulmonary arteries (lateral view)

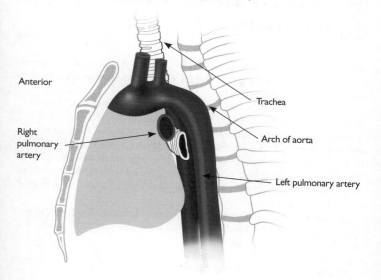

Anterior

Right pulmonary artery

Trachea

Arch of aorta

Left pulmonary artery

Figure 24.10 Mass crossing (lateral view)

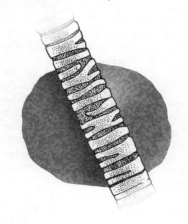

Sexually transmitted infections

Sexually transmitted infections (STIs) represent some of the most common illnesses in the world and have far-reaching health, social and economic consequences.

The majority of adult HIV infections in South Africa are acquired through heterosexual contact. A strong correlation exists between the spread of conventional STIs and HIV transmission exists. Both ulcerative and non-ulcerative STIs increase the risk of sexual transmission of HIV. Furthermore atypical presentations of STIs can occur in HIV-infected individuals. The treatment of persons co-infected with HIV has a worse prognosis. Effective treatment may require either longer or repeated courses of medication.

The effective management of STIs is multi-faceted. The focus is not only on appropriately identifying and treating affected individuals in a confidential manner but also on:

- primary sexual health education;
- partner notification and treatment;
- promotion and provision of condoms; and
- offering HIV counselling and testing.

The consultation for a possible STI presents an invaluable opportunity for sexual health promotion initiatives. Such initiatives aim to reduce the spread of STIs and enable targeted education about HIV prevention. Partner notification and treatment, by breaking the chain of transmission, is an essential component of the effective management of STIs.

Challenges facing clinicians treating STIs include the increasing antimicrobial resistance of several sexually transmitted pathogens. Some widely used and low cost antimicrobial regimens have now been rendered ineffective. The cost of newer, effective antimicrobial regimens must be weighed against the longer term costs of treatment failures, complications, referrals and possible erosion of trust among patients attending sexual health services. Another challenge facing clinicians in the developing world is the emergence of herpes simplex virus type 2 as the main cause of genital ulceration in their clients.

A syndromic approach to STIs in developing countries has been advocated by the WHO. This approach has been validated for the management of urethral discharge in men and genital ulcers in both men and women. The shortfall of the syndromic approach is its use in women presenting with vaginal discharge. The main cause of vaginal discharge, especially in adolescents and in areas with low prevalence of STIs, is endogenous vaginitis rather cervicitis. Risk factor assessments aimed at identifying subsets of women at risk for cervical infection have so far failed to increase the sensitivity and specificity of the vaginal discharge syndromic approach to diagnose cervical infection.

It is important also to note that the syndromic approach proposed by the WHO does not dispense with the need for the investigation and referral of problematic cases.

Due to the sensitive nature of symptoms associated with STIs for many people, clients should be treated non-judgementally, compassionately and respectfully. Every effort should be made to ensure confidentiality when triaging clients, taking a sexual history and during clinical examinations. Sexual history testing ideally should involve the use of easily understandable, open-ended questions.

Sexual history

Sexual history taking should encompass the following areas:
- reassurance regarding confidentiality;
- details of sexual contacts (last sexual contact, other sexual contacts in the last three months who will require contact tracing);
- past STIs;
- contraceptive history;
- current/recent drug history/drug allergies.

Counselling

The following key counselling issues should be covered during STI clinic consultations:

• HIV counselling

All clients with STIs should be counselled on the increased risk of HIV and encouraged to test for HIV.

• Specifics of the STI

The nature of the STI should be explained to the patient as well as the possible complications of an untreated infection and how to prevent future infections. Patients should be taught to recognise symptoms of a suspected STI, encouraging early treatment.

• Condom use

Condom use should be promoted and demonstrated to all STI patients.

• Treatment adherence

The importance of treatment adherence and the need to complete the full course of prescribed antibiotics should be emphasised. Common drug side effects and drug interactions (metronidazole and alcohol, oral contraceptive pill and antibiotics) should be highlighted.

• Partner notification

Patients should be encouraged to notify all sexual partners. The possibility of asymptomatic infections in partners should be explained to clients.

Treatment of STI syndromes

Urethral discharge syndrome

Presenting symptoms include urethral discharge, urethral pruritus, dysuria and urinary frequency although the patient may be asymptomatic. Urinary tract infection should be excluded.

The two commonest causative organisms are *Neiserria gonorrhoae* and *Chlamydia trachomatis*. *C. trachomatis* is a common cause of non-gonococcal urethritis (NGU). As gonococcal and chlamydial infections often occur simultaneously, patients should receive therapy for both these organisms. Trichomonal infection is another cause that can lead to asymptomatic or recurrent urethritis. Treatment should be syndromic and target all three infections. Ideally, in order to improve compliance, treatment should be administered in the STI clinic. Patients should be advised to return for assessment if symptoms do not clear after seven days of treatment.

Treatment of urethral discharge

The syndromic management of urethral discharge includes:
- cefixime 400 mg stat (gonorrhoea); and
- doxycycline 100 mg 12 hourly for 7 days (*Chlamydia*); and
- metronidazole 2 g stat (trichomoniasis).

Patients taking metronidazole should be advised to avoid alcohol.

Persistent or recurrent urethritis should prompt further investigation into the cause of the symptoms. It can be caused by poor treatment adherence, re-infection or drug resistance.

The following two investigations are of diagnostic use:
- the two-glass urine test;
- a urethral swab together with a wet slide and Gram stain.

Microscopy findings of five or more polymorphonuclear leukocytes/high power field are diagnostic of NGU. The presence of Gram-negative diplococci on Gram stain indicates gonorrhoeal infection.

The two-glass urine test

Method
- Patients should not void urine for two hours prior to the test.
- Two glasses are required: the first for the initial 10mL urine; the second for the following 20 mL.
- Threads of pus floating in the first glass but not present in the second glass are indicative of urethritis.

The following text box indicates treatment alternatives for gonorrhoeal, chlamydial and trichomonal infections.

Treatment alternatives for gonorrhoea:
- spectinomycin 2 g IM stat; or
- cefixime 400 mg stat.

Treatment alternatives for *Chlamydia*:
• azithromycin 1 g stat;
• erythromycin 500mg 6 hourly for 7 days (if doxycycline is
  contraindicated);
• ofloxacin 400 mg 12 hourly for 7 days;
• amoxycillin 500 mg 8 hourly for 7 days;
• tetracycline 500 mg 6 hourly 7 days.

Treatment alternatives for trichomoniasis:
• metronidazole 400 mg 12 hourly for 7 days;
• tinidazole 500 mg 12 hourly for 5 days.

Scrotal swelling

In men younger than 35 years of age, STI is the most likely cause of
infection. The differential diagnosis includes: testicular torsion, trauma,
tumour or hydrocoele. Once these alternative diagnoses have been
excluded, patients should be treated for epididymo-orchitis. Relevant
investigations include Gram stain of urethral smear, screening for *N.
gonorrhoeae*, *C. trachomatis* and other STIs where possible, and a MSU.
Further investigations include Doppler ultrasonography, which can be a
useful adjunctive diagnostic tool. Treat for gonorrhoea and *Chlamydia*,
and prescribe analgesia, scrotal support and/or bed rest. Severe cases
may require hospital admission and prolonged or parenteral antibiotic
therapy.

Vaginal discharge syndrome

STIs in women can present with the following: increased vaginal discharge,
dysuria without frequency, intermenstrual bleeding and/or menorrhagia,
postcoital bleeding and lower abdominal pain. It is important to note
that 50–70% of women with gonorrhoea and up to 80% of women with
chlamydia are asymptomatic. The symptom of vaginal discharge is highly
indicative of vaginal infection but poorly predictive of cervical infection.
T. vaginalis, *C. albicans* and bacterial vaginosis are the commonest causes
of vaginal infections. All women presenting with vaginal discharge should
also receive treatment for bacterial vaginosis and trichomonas vaginalis
infection according to WHO guidelines.

Risk assessments might be useful in identifying women presenting with vaginal discharge who should be treated for cervicitis. Knowledge of prevalence rates of *Chlamydia* and gonorrhoea in local communities can also prove a useful guide to deciding which patients receive treatment for cervicitis. Where resources permit, laboratory screening tests should be considered for women presenting with vaginal discharge.

The syndromic management of cervical infection includes:
- cefixime 400 mg stat (gonorrhoea);
- doxycycline 100 mg 12 hourly for 7 days (*Chlamydia*);
- metronidazole 2 g stat (trichomoniasis).

Note:
- cefixime is contraindicated in pregnancy and not recommended for children or adolescents (use ceftriaxone 125 mg IM);
- doxycycline and other tetracyclines are contraindicated in pregnancy and during lactation (use erythromycin).

The syndromic treatment of vaginal infections includes treatment for both *T. vaginalis*, bacterial vaginosis and, where indicated, *C. albicans*.

Please refer Chapter 26: Gynaecology for further details on the management of vaginal infections and the important diagnosis of pelvic inflammatory disease.

Genital ulceration

Herpes virus type 2 (HSV2) is fast becoming the commonest cause of genital ulcer disease in developing countries. The clinical differential diagnosis of genital ulcers is inaccurate, especially in the presence of more than one causative organism. Furthermore, genital ulcers may have atypical presentations in HIV-infected individuals and may require prolonged treatment. Treatment algorithims provide a reasonable approach to this problem. Treatment decisions in patients presenting with genital ulceration should also be guided by local epidemiological data.

Figure 25.1 Genital ulcer syndrome

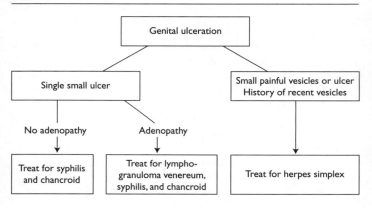

The WHO recommends the following syndromic treatment strategy for the treatment of genital ulceration:
- Syphilis therapy *plus either* treatment for:
  o chancroid, where it is prevalent; *or*
  o granuloma inguinale, where it is prevalent; *or*
  o lymphogranuloma venereum (LGV), where it is prevalent; *or*
  o HSV if indicated.

Herpes simplex virus (HSV)

The major public health implications of HSV relate to its potential role in the transmission of HIV. There is no known cure for HSV infection but prompt antiviral treatment can prevent the erruption of new vesicles and reduce healing times, viral shedding and symptoms such as pain. Prompt, appropriate treatment does not appear to affect recurrences of HSV infection.

Genital herpes simplex infection in the immunosuppressed patient may lead to persistent ulceration requiring both prophylactic and therapeutic antiviral treatment.

Antiviral treatment options for herpes simplex genital ulceration include:
• aciclovir 200 mg orally 5 times daily for 7 days; or
• aciclovir 400 mg orally 3 times daily for 7 days; or
• valaciclovir 1 g orally twice daily for 7 days; or
• famciclovir 250 mg orally 3 times daily for 7 days.

Intravenous therapy is recommended for severe disease (aciclovir 5–10 mg/kg IV every 8 hours for 5–7 days or until clinical resolution is obtained).
Topical treatment of genital herpes in any instance is not recommended.

General management of patients presenting with HSV2 infection also includes:
• adequate analgesia;
• hospital admission of patients who are unable to pass urine;
• basic care of the lesion – lesions to be kept clean and dry;
• health education and counselling regarding the recurrent nature of the infection, its natural history, sexual mode of transmission, asymptomatic shedding and the risk of perinatal transmission;
• advice to represent to a health provider should the lesions not heal or worsen during the seven days of treatment;
• referral for syphilis and HIV testing wherever possible;
• partner notification and treatment where appropriate;
• promotion of condom use.

Syphilis

Syphilis is a systemic disease caused by infection with the spirochaete *Treponema pallidum*. Acquired syphilis can be divided into early and late syphilis. The category of early syphilis comprises primary, secondary and early latent stages of syphilis infection. Late syphilis encompasses late latent syphilis, gummatous, neurological and cardiovascular syphilis.

The classical lesion described in primary syphilis is an initial painless papule at the inoculation site. This lesion then expands and ulcerates to form a round or oval painless chancre. This classical presentation has been confounded by HIV co-infected patients with primary syphilis who have presented with multiple painful and indurated ulcers that mimic genital herpes.

Of note is the fact that, in early primary syphilis, cardiolipin/non-treponemal tests such as the Venereal Disease Research Laboratory (VDRL) and rapid plasma reagin (RPR) tests may be negative and can not be interpreted as indicating the absence of syphilis.

Recommended treatment regimens for early syphilis (primary, secondary and early latent):
- benzathine benzylpenicillin, 2.4 million IU by IM injection at a single session, usually given at 2 separate injection sites because of the volume injected.

Alternative:
- procaine benzylpenicillin, 1.2 million IU intramuscular injection, daily for ten days.

Regimens suitable for non-pregnant penicillin allergic patients:
- doxycycline 100 mg twice daily for 14 days; or
- tetracycline 500 mg orally, four times daily for 14 days.

Suitable regimen for penicillin-allergic pregnant patients:
- erythromycin 500 mg orally, four times daily for 14 days.

Chancroid

Haemophilus ducreyi, a gram negative facultative anaerobic bacillus, is the causative agent. Antimicrobial resistance is widespread so penicillin and tetracycline therapy is not recommended. Chancroid presents as an initial painful papule, which progresses to a pustule forming between one and three ulcers after two to three days. Atypical chancroid lesions have been reported in the literature in patients co-infected with HIV.

Recommended treatment regimens:
- ciprofloxacin 500 mg orally twice daily for 3 days; or
- erythromycin 500 mg orally four times daily for 7 days; or
- azithromycin 1 g orally as a single dose.

Alternative therapy:
- ceftriaxone 250 mg IM stat.

Lymphogranuloma venereum (LGV)

Literature on suitable treatment options remains limited. The WHO recommends the following treatment regimens and advocates consultation of an expert. Fluctuant lymph nodes should be aspirated.

> Recommended treatment regimens:
> - doxycycline 100 mg orally twice daily for 14 days; or
> - erythromycin 500 mg orally 4 times daily for 14 days.
>
> Alternative therapy:
> - tetracycline 500 mg 4 times daily for 14 days.
>
> Please note that tetracyclines are contraindicated in pregnancy.

Inguinal bubo

Inguinal and femoral buboes are frequently associated with LGV and chancroid. They represent localised enlargements of the lymph nodes in the groin area. They are painful in nature and can be fluctuant. Where there are no ulcers on examination, patients should still receive treatment for LGV and chancroid. Fluctuant buboes may require aspiration. Patient follow-up is essential. Diagnostic biopsy may be required.

> Recommended treatment regimen:
> - ciprofloxacin 500 mg orally, twice daily for 3 days; and
> - doxycycline 100 mg orally twice daily for 14 days; or
> - erythromycin 500 mg orally, four times daily for 14 days.

Granuloma inguinale (Donovanosis)

This STI is rare in sub-Saharan Africa. The diagnosis is suspected when genital ulceration fails to respond to treatment for syphilis and chancroid. It is caused by the intracellular Gram-negative bacterium *Klebsiella granulomatis*. Granuloma inguinale presents with progressive, typically granulomatous, red, painless and haemorrhagic ulcers. There is no regional lymphadenopathy. Treatment should continue until all lesions have epithelialized.

Recommended treatment regimens:
- azithromycin 1 g orally, on 1st day, then 500 mg orally, once a day; or
- doxycycline 100 mg orally, twice daily.

Alternative regimen:
- erythromycin 500 mg orally, four times daily; or
- tetracycline 500 mg orally, four times daily.

Treatment should be continued until all lesions have healed.

References

Centers for Disease Control. 2006. 'Sexually Transmitted Diseases Treatment Guidelines.' *Morbidity and Mortality Weekly*; 55 (RR11): 1–94.

Centers for Disease Control. 2007. 'Update to CDC's Sexually Transmitted Diseases Treatment Guidelines , 2006: Fluoroquinolones no longer recommended for treatment of gonococcal infections.' *Morbidity and Mortality Weekly*; 56(14):332–336.

Lewis, D.A. et al. 2008. 'Escalation in the relative prevalence of ciprofloxacin resistant gonorrhoea among men with urethral discharge in two South African cities – association with seropositivity. *Sexually Transmitted Infection*; July (in press).

Pattman, R. et al. (Eds). 2005. *Oxford Handbook of Genitourinary Medicine, HIV, and AIDS*. Oxford University Press.

WHO. 2003. *Guidelines for the management of sexually transmitted infections*.

Gynaecology

Gynaecological problems are common among HIV-infected women, and are frequently present at the time HIV infection is diagnosed. Gynaecological and reproductive health care will, therefore, play an increasingly important role in the overall care of HIV-infected women.

Abnormal vaginal discharge

Abnormal vaginal discharge is one of the commonest complaints of HIV-infected women, is often recurrent, and may be resistant to the usual treatments.

Key elements of the history include the:
- duration and characteristics of the discharge;
- associated symptoms, e.g. odour, pruritus, burning, pelvic pain, dyspareunia, or dysuria;
- sexual history (including condom use);
- prior history of sexually transmitted infections;
- recent antibiotic use;
- concurrent illnesses; and
- Pap smear history.

The physical examination should include a full genital examination, with visualization of the cervix and bi-manual palpation of the pelvis. Document the characteristics of the discharge, as well as the presence of erythema, oedema, and tenderness.

Important side-room tests include:
- saline wet mount looking for motile *Trichomonas* and clue cells;
- adding 10% potassium hydroxide (KOH) for the whiff test; and
- swab for fungal culture in cases of recurrent candidiasis.

Bacterial vaginosis

This is the commonest cause of vaginal discharge, due to replacement of normal vaginal flora with anaerobic bacteria, *Gardnerella vaginalis*, and *Mycoplasma hominis*. Its prevalence is not known to be higher among HIV-infected women. However, some studies suggest that it may be associated with enhanced HIV transmission. Diagnosis is confirmed if there is a watery, greyish, foul-smelling discharge (usually without concomitant inflammation of the vaginal epithelium), clue cells on microscopic examination, a vaginal pH of more than 4.5, and a positive whiff test (a fishy odour after the addition of KOH to a slide). The treatment is oral metronidazole 2 g stat or metronidazole 400 mg twice daily for seven days (which has a higher cure rate).

Vulvovaginal candidiasis

This troublesome infection is caused by *Candida albicans*, but the prevalence of infection by non-albicans species is increasing. Classic symptoms are thick, white, cheesy discharge associated with pruritus, burning, dyspareunia, and dysuria. An increased rate of infection is found among HIV-positive women, owing either to increased use of antibiotics or to immune compromise. Treatment consists of a range of topical vaginal anti-fungal creams. Patients should be advised to complete the full course, and to abstain from sex during treatment. Some creams are oil-based and may weaken latex condoms. Fluconazole or itraconazole can be used for refractory candidiasis.

As neither bacterial vaginosis nor candidiasis is sexually transmitted, there is no need for routine treatment of partners.

Other common causes of vaginal discharge

Other pathogens include *Trichomonas vaginalis*, *Neisseria gonorrhoea*, and *Chlamydia trachomatis*. (See also Chapter 25: Sexually transmitted infections.)

Pelvic inflammatory disease

Primary pelvic inflammatory disease (PID) is an ascending sexually transmitted disease, usually caused by acute infection with *N. gonorrhoea* and *C. trachomatis*. Once infection is established, there may be infection with 'secondary invaders', usually bowel organisms such as *E. coli*, *Bacteroides fragilis*, and *Streptococcus faecalis*. HIV infection should be considered in all women presenting with PID.

The minimum criteria for diagnosis of PID include vaginal discharge, lower abdominal tenderness, and cervical excitation tenderness. In addition, pyrexia, a raised ESR, and raised white cell count support the diagnosis. Always exclude pregnancy and concomitant urinary tract infection.

The differential diagnosis of women presenting with symptoms of PID is long, but common conditions to be considered include:

- complications of pregnancy (especially ectopic pregnancy);
- rupture or torsion of ovarian cyst;
- severe endometriosis;
- acute appendicitis; and
- urinary tract infection.

HIV-positive women may present with more severe disease, particularly tubo-ovarian abscesses that often require surgical management. In addition, patients may take longer to respond to the usual antibiotic therapies. In these situations, the possibility of pelvic tuberculosis (TB) should be considered. Pelvic TB is a difficult diagnosis to make, and often is only made at laparotomy or laparoscopy. Menstrual washings with normal saline may be useful.

Treatment

Treatment assumes polymicrobial infection in most cases of PID.

Grade 1 pelvic inflammatory disease (evidence of pelvic infection without signs of peritonitis)

- cefixime 400 mg stat po or ceftriaxone 250 mg IMI stat; *and*
- doxycycline 100 mg 12 hourly for 14 days; *and*
- metronidazole 400 mg 12 hourly for 14 days.

Grade 2 pelvic inflammatory disease (pelvic infection with evidence of peritonitis)

- Admit the patient to hospital.
- Administer:
  - cefuroxime 750 mg eight hourly intravenously; *and*
  - metronidazole 400 mg eight hourly or rectal metronidazole 1 g 12 hourly; *and*
  - doxycycline 100 mg 12 hourly; *and*
  - a stat dose of cefixime or ceftriaxone.

- An alternative regime is benzylpenicillin 2 million units six hourly, a daily dose of gentamicin (6 mg/kg) and metronidazole, with oral doxcycline and a stat dose of cefixime or ceftriaxone.
- Intravenous antibiotics may be stopped once the patient has been apyrexial for 24 hours.
- Parenteral opioid analgesia may be required, with non-steroidal anti-inflammatories and paracetamol.
- If there has been no significant response in 24–48 hours, the diagnosis should be reconsidered.
- Laparoscopy may be of value. Laparotomy may be indicated if there is clinical evidence of deterioration and laparoscopy is not an option.

Grade 3 pelvic inflammatory disease (evidence of pelvic abscess)

Commence intravenous antibiotics and monitor the response. Surgical intervention should not be delayed for longer than 12–24 hours, unless there is a good response to antibiotic therapy.

On discharge, the patient should be made aware of:
- the short-term and long term consequences of pelvic infection, i.e. pain, dyspareunia, and possible infertility;
- the use of barrier contraception;
- notification of the partner; and
- the necessity of completing the course of antibiotics.

In women with recurrent disease, chronic intermittent antibiotic therapy may be useful (e.g. with menses).

Genital warts

Genital warts develop more frequently in immunocompromised women. Lesions in HIV-infected women tend to be more extensive and resistant to conventional therapies, and may be associated with vulval intraepithelial neoplasia or squamous carcinoma of the vulva. Women with genital warts are more likely to have concomitant cervical intraepithelial neoplasia and anal intraepithelial neoplasia.

Diagnosis

Diagnosis is made on clinical inspection. A biopsy should be performed if the lesions have an atypical appearance, if the warts are resistant to treatment, and if there are areas that are hyperpigmented, indurated, fixed, or ulcerated. All women should undergo a Pap smear and a careful inspection of the perianal area and the anus.

Treatment

Treatment is aimed at removing symptomatic lesions, as there is no evidence that any of the available therapies can eradicate human papillomavirus (HPV), or that the infectivity of HPV is decreased by the removal of visible warts.

The treatment modality depends on the size and location of the warts. Small, discrete lesions can be treated with weekly applications of topical agents such as 90% trichloroacetic acid or 10–25% podophyllum resin (the latter is contraindicated in pregnant women). Imiquimod 5% cream, applied to the lesions three times a week for up to 16 weeks, is effective in up to 70% of cases.

For larger lesions, covering more extensive areas of the vulva, surgical therapies such as laser therapy or cautery are indicated. Laser therapy is associated with less scarring and less damage to healthy skin. All modalities of treatment are associated with high recurrence rates (up to 80% in immune-compromised HIV-infected women), and repeat treatments are frequently required.

Genital warts are associated with significant psychosexual dysfunction, and careful counselling is essential.

Other vulval conditions

Bartholin's gland abscess

This is a common finding, and the usual cause is infection with *N. gonorrhoea*. Treatment is surgical: aspiration, incision and drainage, or marsupialization. Oral antibiotics are indicated if there is surrounding cellulitis.

Molluscum contagiosum

See Chapter 40: Dermatology.

Herpes simplex

See Chapter 25: Sexually transmitted infections.

Management of abnormal cytology and cervical cancer

Premalignant and malignant disease of the cervix is more common, progresses more rapidly, and occurs at a younger age in HIV-infected women. Screening with cytology should ideally begin at the time of the diagnosis of HIV. Previous recommendations have been to perform yearly screening but more recent data suggests that in women with a normal smear, this can be repeated at three yearly intervals. In women with abnormal smears, even low grade smears, referral for a baseline colposcopy should be done. If this confirms a low grade lesion (i.e LSIL) she requires yearly follow up until either progression or regression. If the lesion progresses to a high-grade lesion (HSIL) then treatment should be offered. Recommended treatment is with LLETZ (large loop excision of the transformation zone) that is performed under local anaesthetic in an outpatient setting. In spite of treatment, premalignant lesions of the cervix in immunocompromised HIV-infected women commonly recur (up to 50% in some series), and long-term follow up is essential. Recurrence and persistence of disease are related to viral load and CD4 count, which should be measured while following women up with abnormal Pap smears.

Women with cervical cancer are preferentially treated with surgery, however, women with more advanced disease, normally treated with radical chemoradiation, may require modification of anti-cancer therapy, as this is also immunosuppressive.

Table 26.1 The management of abnormal cytology

Cytology	Management
Atypical squamous cells of unknown significance	Repeat after 6 mo. If persistent, refer for colposcopy and biopsy
Atypical glandular cells of unknown significance	Treat empirically with doxycycline for 7 d. and repeat in 6 wk. If persistent, refer for colposcopy and biopsy
Low-grade squamous intraepithelial lesion HPV infection or CIN1*	Repeat every 6 mo. If persistent, refer for colposcopy and biopsy
High-grade squamous intraepithelial lesion CIN2 or CIN 3	Refer for colposcopy and biopsy/treatment
Invasive cancer	Refer immediately for colposcopy

* CIN1: cervical intraepithelial neoplasia 1.

References and further reading

Anderson, J. ed. 2000. *A guide to the clinical care of women with HIV.* Preliminary edition. Womencare: Maryland.

Van der Spuy, Z. and J. Anthony. 2002. Eds. *Handbook of obstetrics and gynaecology.* Oxford University Press: Cape Town.

27 Contraception

Contraception is a vital public health intervention for all women. Use of an effective contraceptive allows women to control their fertility, to optimally space children and to avoid unwanted pregnancies. In the case of HIV-1 infected women contraceptives prevent mother-to-child transmission by preventing unplanned pregnancies.

The ideal contraceptive method provides dual protection against pregnancy and sexually transmitted infections (STIs) including HIV. Currently the only methods that provide dual protection are the male and female condom. The diaphragm gives some protection against pregnancy and upper genital tract STIs but has not been shown to protect against HIV. In addition, the diaphragm is often used with the spermicide Nonoxynol-9 which increases a woman's risk of acquiring HIV if applied frequently.

Review of the evidence suggests that while hormonal contraceptive methods do not increase the risk of acquiring HIV in a general population, there may be an increased risk of acquiring HIV among women at higher risk of infection (sex workers) and among teenagers. In these groups use of hormonal methods is permitted but it is important to stress condom use in combination with the method. While fitting an intrauterine device (IUD) is not recommended in women at high risk of an STI, potential exposure to HIV or being HIV-infected is not a contraindication to fitting or ongoing use of the IUD. This advice applies to both the copper IUD and the levonorgestrel IUD.

There is conflicting evidence about whether any contraceptive method increases disease progression in HIV infected women. This remains a research question and at the present time all hormonal methods and intrauterine devices continue to be acceptable contraceptive choices for HIV-infected women. Caution should be applied to women on antiretroviral therapy or on TB treatment because of potential drug interactions as outlined below. Further, women on antiretroviral therapy may get pregnant as their health and fertility improves, so contraceptive counselling is imperative.

Contraceptive counselling

The general rules of contraceptive counselling apply to all consultations with a woman requesting a contraceptive method, irrespective of her HIV status. Prescribers should always take note of co-existing diseases or conditions that might influence contraceptive prescribing, and of all medications being taken that might interact with hormonal contraception. Counselling should include:

- the choice of available methods and what using them entails;
- the suitability of these methods to her social situation, including an assessment of how important it is for her to avoid pregnancy ;
- the effectiveness of each method and how it works;
- the risks and benefits of each method and how it works;
- advice on how to use a particular method;
- a risk assessment for STI and HIV exposure;
- HIV status including use of antiretrovirals and/or TB treatment.

For women known to be HIV-infected, the benefits of using contraception to avoid unwanted pregnancy and therefore mother-to-child transmission must be stressed.

Although contraceptive technologies are available mainly to women, it is important to engage men in discussions about their sexual health including their roles and responsibilities in contraceptive decision making with their partners.

Emergency contraception

Emergency contraception can be offered to both HIV-negative and HIV-positive women. Accepted regimens are:

- Before 72 hours:
  o Combined high dose oestrogen – progestogen (50 mcg ethinyl oestradiol pill) two tablets as soon after unprotected intercourse as possible, followed by two tablets 12 hours later.
  o Progestogen only: levonorgestrel 0.75 mg as soon after unprotected intercourse as possible repeated 12 hours later.
- Before 120 hours: a copper intrauterine device may be inserted provided the woman does not have an established STI. This may be inserted irrespective of the woman's HIV status and may be left in after this period as a permanent method of contraception.

- Consideration should be given to the co-administration of post exposure prophylaxis with antiretrovirals and of antibiotics to cover possible STIs.

Drug interactions with hormonal contraceptives

Rifampicin

Rifampicin induces cytochrome p450 enzymes and is likely to reduce the efficacy of combined oestrogen-progestogen pills or injectables, of progestogen only pills and of long acting progestogen implants. Concurrent use of these drugs is not recommended. Long acting progestogen injectables (DMPA or norethisterone acetate) may be used provided the woman comes back on time for her repeat injections. There is no need to reduce the time between injections or to increase the dose of injections. Use of other contraceptive methods, e.g. copper or levonorgestrel IUDs, or sterilization is also recommended.

Nucleoside reverse transcriptase inhibitors (NRTIs)

NRTIs can be used with all hormonal methods of contraception, and with copper and levonorgestrel IUDs.

Non-nucleoside reverse transcriptase inhibitors (NNRTIs)

Nevirapine induces cytochrome p450 enzymes and efavirenz both induces and inhibits p450 enzymes. Both may reduce the efficacy of combined oestrogen-progestogen pills or injectables, of progestogen only pills and of long acting progestogen implants. However, provided the woman takes a minimum of a 30 mcg ethinyl oestradiol pill and is able to take her contraceptive pills on time, it is acceptable for women taking NNRTIs to use all these hormonal methods. However, because of the higher dosage, DMPA may be the preferred hormonal method for women taking NNRTIs.

Current knowledge does not suggest that hormonal contraceptives have an impact on antiretroviral efficacy. Efavirenz is considered teratogenic and it is important that women taking this drug are advised to avoid pregnancy.

Table 27.1 Contraceptive choices in the era of HIV

Contraceptive method	User failure rates in first year of use (%)	Recommendations for use
Male and female condoms protect against STI/HIV. Other contraceptive methods do not protect against STI/HIV. If there is a risk of STI/HIV the correct and consistent use of condoms is recommended either alone or with another contraceptive method. The choice of method should take into account contraceptive efficacy and how important it is for the woman not to become pregnant		
Male condom	2–15. Provides dual protection against STI/HIV and pregnancy	Decreases HIV transmission if used consistently and correctly
Female condom	5–15. Provides dual protection against STI/HIV and pregnancy	Decreases HIV transmission if used consistently and correctly
Diaphragm	4–18. Provides dual protection against STI/HIV and pregnancy	Reduces upper genital tract infections but no evidence to support use for HIV prevention
Combined oestrogen-progestogen contraceptives (pills, injectables)	0.2–3	Drug interactions with some antiretrovirals and rifampicin
Progestogen only pills (POPs)	1–4	Must be taken at approximately the same time each day. Can be used when lactating
Long-acting progestogens (injectables, implants)	0–1	Some concerns about increased HIV acquisition in higher risk groups and in teenagers
Copper IUD	0.3–1	Safe to initiate and continue to use in HIV-positive women
Levonorgestrel IUS	0–0.2	Limited data suggest safe to initiate and continue to use in HIV-positive women
Female sterilization	0–0.2	Special care must be taken when performing sterilization on HIV-infected women because of risks of infection
Fertility awareness	2–20	Recommended only in couples able to negotiate consistent use of method

Protease inhibitors (PIs)

PIs are potent inhibitors of cytochrome p450. They may reduce the efficacy of combined oestrogen-progestogen pills or injectables and of progestogen only pills. Long-acting progestogen implants or injectables are the hormonal methods recommended for women using PIs. Use of other contraceptive methods, e.g. copper or levonorgestrel IUDs, or sterilization is also be recommended.

Current knowledge does not suggest that long-acting progestogen implants or injectables affect antiretroviral efficacy.

28 Sexual assault

Sexual assault is common in southern Africa in women, men and children, and poses complex management issues to the attending clinician. The risk of HIV transmission after sexual assault is presumed to be higher in children, when multiple partners are involved, after anal penetration, or where significant trauma is present. Given the high background prevalence of HIV, all sexual assailants should be assumed to be infected with HIV, and rape survivors should be counselled accordingly and offered post-exposure prophylaxis if they present within 72 hours of the assault.

Special issues surrounding sexual assault:

- As with all post-exposure prophylaxis (PEP), a careful assessment of the nature of the injury should be done, and PEP introduced appropriately. Exposure varies, from penetration with objects, to forced oral, vaginal and anal sex, as well as dermal exposure to ejaculate. Assailants may even use condoms. Commonly, other injuries, for example, bites, should be evaluated when considering PEP. Decisions concerning no, dual or triple therapy antiretroviral therapy should take this into account (See Chapter 52: Occupational post-exposure prophylaxis).
- Side effects of medication are a major contributor to failed adherence and these must be actively managed. HIV medication, especially AZT and protease inhibitors, are associated with significant gastrointestinal side-effects. Similar side-effects are encountered with sexually transmitted infections (STI) and pregnancy prevention drugs, and careful explanation, with the use of anti-emetics may be needed. Alcohol must be avoided, especially if taking metronidazole.
- Note that the high background prevalence of HIV means that the survivor may test HIV-positive (i.e. was HIV-positive prior to exposure). This can be devastating, after the considerable psychological trauma due to the assault itself. In some cases, testing may need to be deferred. Survivors commonly misunderstand the HIV result in this scenario, and it must be carefully explained.
- Sexual assailant survivors may not be in a state to have pre-test HIV counselling. In these cases, testing should be deferred and the survivor treated as HIV negative and offered PEP.
- Children may not be in a position to give a good history, either due to age, shock or inability to describe the sexual nature of the assault. PEP

must be guided by common sense and careful assessment of probable injuries. A common presentation is an anxious parent who believes their child may have been assaulted, but where objective evidence of assault is not present. Using drawings or pictures may assist the child in detailing injuries.

- Legal mechanisms are evolving in certain countries for compulsory HIV testing of alleged assailants. However, this legal process, if introduced, is likely to take significant time, and treatment should be initiated without waiting for the result. If the assailant is found to be HIV-negative, HIV PEP should be stopped.
- Condoms should be used during sex at all times in the three months after the assault in HIV-negative survivors, prior to confirming HIV-negative status.

Objectives

The key medical objectives in a post-rape situation are the following:
- Perform a rapid and thorough clinical assessment.
- Provide emergency care for injuries.
- Collect appropriate forensic evidence.

Take measures to prevent:
- unwanted pregnancy in women of child-bearing potential;
- acquisition of STIs; and
- the development of rape trauma syndrome and other psychological sequelae of rape.

Treat the survivor's:
- physical injuries; and
- emotional and psychological trauma.

History

This is essential in terms of determining treatment, and may be critical in any legal proceedings that follow. All clinical notes should be carefully written and signatures should be legible.

Critical factors

The clinician should do the following:

- Record the date, time, circumstances surrounding and place of the assault.
- Record the date, time, and place of the examination.
- Determine the number of assailants.
- Establish whether the survivor was conscious.
- Establish the surface on which the rape took place (e.g. ground, carpet, car seat).
- Find out about the use of violence, i.e. the type of weapon used and how it was used (e.g. threateningly, inserted into the vagina).
- Ask whether the assailant used a condom.
- Determine whether the survivor has douched, urinated, or bathed since the rape.
- Establish the type of sexual acts performed, including sodomy.
- In cases of oral penetration establish if the survivor has been taking anything by mouth after the assault.
- Take the relevant gynaecological history (to assess the pregnancy risk) from women.
- Establish whether the survivor had consensual sex within 72 hours of the rape (for DNA testing of semen).

Examination

The examination should include:
- careful documentation of all injuries, including bruises, lacerations, and fractures;
- an anatomical drawing of all injuries; and
- a detailed examination of the vulva, vagina, and anus.

In some countries, specific forms are available for documenting medico-legal cases, and these should be used.

Investigations

Critical post-sexual assault clinical investigations are:
- an HIV test (with appropriate pre-and post test counselling, noting the concerns above);
- syphilis serology;
- hepatitis B serology;
- pregnancy test in women of child bearing age; and
- toxicology, where appropriate.

Forensic specimens

- Prior to examination, the survivor should undress over a large piece of paper, to collect foreign debris, hair etc. Label, fold, and place this paper in an envelope.
- Keep the clothing, if possible – or only the underwear – and place it in a paper (not a plastic) bag.
- Take swabs of the mouth, anus, labia majora, labia minora, vaginal fornices, and endocervix.
- Swab any area of possible ejaculation or saliva.
- Swab under the survivors's fingernails.
- Take pubic hair combings.
- Seal all swabs and specimens.
- Give the forensic evidence directly to the police, or keep them in a specially designated and secured cupboard. If the chain of evidence is broken, investigation results cannot be used in court.

Treatment

Treatment consists of the following:
- Provide pregnancy prophylaxis with emergency contraception. (See Chapter 27: Contraception.)
- Prevent STIs using cefixime, doxycycline, and metronidazole, or ceftriaxone, erythromycin, and metronidazole for pregnant women. (See Chapter 25: Sexually transmitted infections.)
- Assist in the prevention of rape trauma syndrome by:
  o adopting a sensitive, patient-centred approach to care at the time of the initial examination; and
  o referring all survivors for counselling or intensive psychotherapy.

Ideally, ongoing psychological support should be provided by trained counsellors with experience in dealing with sexual assault survivors. Children should receive careful evaluation.

Prevention of HIV transmission

Data on the efficacy of antiretrovirals in the prevention of HIV transmission is equivocal, but there is biological plausibility, and large observational studies suggest efficacy of AZT-based regimens. A suggested regimens for adults is zidovudine (AZT) 300 mg 12 hourly and lamivudine (3TC) 150 mg 12 hourly for 28 days, and a protease inhibitor in high-risk cases, i.e. obvious disruption of the skin, mucosal integrity and cases involving anal penetration. Stavudine and tenofovir are often used instead of AZT, although there is little evidence to support their efficacy. Nevirapine should not be used due to toxicity; efavirenz should also be avoided as it may cause further psychological disturbance (see Chapter 44: Adult antiretroviral therapy).

Loss to follow up is high after sexual assault, and 'starter packs' of antiretrovirals for three days while awaiting HIV results, are inappropriate.

AZT and protease inhibitors have poor side effect profiles in the first few weeks of administration, and side effects must be actively managed.

Survivors should be counselled regarding the risk of seroconversion, the need for adequate follow up, and the need to use condoms in order to protect their partner.

Please always consult with the hospital protocol regarding treatment of survivors of sexual assault.

Further information

Rape Crisis 24-hour counselling line: 021 4479762
Rape Crisis KZN counselling line: 082 495 3261
LifeLine 24-hour counselling line: 086 132 2322

In South Africa

NB: only forensic evidence submitted in the Sexual Assault Evidence Collection Kit (SAECK) provided by SAPS can be admitted in court. The kit and its content is barcoded and contain a J88 form that must also be filled in and signed by the medical practitioner. Sexual assault of children must be reported to SAPS and Department of Social Welfare. For medical treatment please consult the hospital protocol. There is a Sexual Assault Evidence Collection Kit developed especially for child survivors.

PART 4

Systemic approach to HIV infection

29	Cardiology	293
30	Haematology	303
31	Nephrology	311
32	Pulmonology	322
33	Intensive care management	342
34	Endocrinology and metabolic abnormalities	346
35	Neurology	354
36	Psychiatry	381
37	Ophthalmology	389
38	Gastroenerology and hepatology	400
39	Oral medicine	413
40	Dermatology	426
41	Oncology	443
42	Rheumatology	448

Paediatric cardiology

Cardiac morbidity is an important consequence of HIV infection and may be due to HIV itself, opportunistic infections, drugs or nutritional impairment. Some manifestations are subclinical and have been identified by echocardiography. However, there is no role for echocardiography in the absence of signs or symptoms of cardiovascular disease. The most common cardiac lesions are cardiomyopathy, myocarditis, pericardial effusions and pulmonary hypertension. Drug induced hyperlipidaemia is also a concern.

Myocarditis and cardiomyopathy

Cardiomyopathy and subacute or chronic myocarditis are similar and present as subclinical left ventricular dysfunction (detected on echocardiography) or overt heart failure. Causes include opportunistic infections or myocardial injury induced by HIV. Micronutrient deficiencies may play a role.

The clinical manifestations, when present, are those of dilated cardiomyopathy with cardiomegaly and signs of left or right sided congestion. A gallop rhythm may be present. Left ventricular dilatation leads to functional mitral incompetence and a pansystolic apical murmur. The pulse may be of low volume with tachycardia or arrhythmias. The chest radiograph may show cardiomegaly and pulmonary venous congestion or oedema. ECG abnormalities include left ventricular hypertrophy, ST segment and T wave changes. An echocardiogram will confirm dilated ventricles with reduced myocardial contractility.

The important clinical differential diagnosis is a large pericardial effusion.

Heart failure should be treated with a combination of diuretics (furosemide and/or spironolactone), afterload reducing agents (angiotensin converting enzyme inhibitors) and inotropes (digoxin, dopamine, dobutamine) according to the clinical response. Digoxin should be used with caution if myocarditis is suspected.

Myocarditis or cardiomyopathy is associated with early mortality; but antiretroviral therapy may improve the condition.

Pericardial effusions

Effusions are common but mostly small and asymptomatic, not requiring specific therapy. Large and symptomatic effusions are often due to infective pericarditis, mainly TB. Clinically there may be features of congestive heart failure. The cardiac apex may be impalpable with marked precordial dullness on percussion. The heart sounds may be soft. A low volume pulse with palpable pulsus paradoxus is characteristic of tamponade. The chest X-ray can show marked cardiomegaly with a globular heart shadow. Pulmonary venous congestion and oedema occur with tamponade. The ECG may show low voltage QRS complexes. The diagnosis is confirmed on echocardiography.

Symptomatic pericardial effusion requires pericardiocentesis as both a diagnostic and therapeutic procedure. Pericardial fluid should be sent for microscopy and culture (viral, bacterial, tuberculous and fungal). The use of digoxin and afterload reducing agents are contraindicated. Depending on the cardiac output and the presence of congestive failure a fluid bolus to augment preload may be helpful while the pericardiocentesis is being arranged. There should be a high index of suspicion for tuberculous pericarditis and empiric therapy should be started if this diagnosis cannot be confidently excluded. Pericarditis due to other organisms should be treated according to culture and sensitivities and a formal pericardial drainage may be indicated.

Pulmonary hypertension

Pulmonary hypertension may be the result of changes in the pulmonary vascular bed (primary pulmonary hypertension), chronic upper airway obstruction, left ventricular dysfunction or chronic lung disease. Clinically there may be right sided congestion. A parasternal heave may be palpable. Auscultation reveals loud P2. A regurgitant murmur of pulmonary incompetence occurs at the mid-left sternal border. A pansystolic murmur may be heard at the lower left sternal border if tricuspid incompetence is present. There may be cyanosis, clubbing and signs of chronic lung disease. The chest X-ray may show right atrial and right ventricular enlargement with evidence of lung disease in cases of secondary pulmonary hypertension. The ECG shows right ventricular and right atrial enlargement. Echocardiography will show right ventricular hypertrophy and dilatation and right atrial enlargement. Doppler studies may confirm pulmonary hypertension.

Treatment should be directed at the primary cause (usually chronic lung disease). Oxygen supplementation should be provided. Diuretics and digoxin can be used to reduce right sided congestion. The role of vasodilators is controversial and these should only be initiated in consultation.

Cardiovascular therapy

Hyperlipidaemia is a side effect of protease inhibitor therapy, as well as other agents, and may require regular monitoring. Due to a lack of evidence regarding efficacy, there are no firm recommendations for lipid lowering agents in children.

The benefit of cardiac surgery in the HIV infected child needs to be weighed up against the possible harmful effects of surgery on the HIV infection and the prognosis of the HIV infection itself. Several studies in adults have not demonstrated any deleterious effect of heart surgery on HIV disease progression and the introduction of antiretroviral therapy has substantially improved the life expectancy of HIV infected children. Therefore all HIV-infected children with congenital heart disease should be referred to a paediatric cardiology centre where surgery may be undertaken if appropriate.

Adult cardiology

HIV-infected patients are living decades longer with the onset of more effective and safer antiretroviral therapy, meaning that the consequence of both HIV-related, as well as age-related cardiovascular disease will increase. As the background prevalence of southern African HIV increases, it has become difficult to differentiate HIV-related cardiac disease from the normal cardiac disease profile existing in the community. The commonest HIV-related cardiac diseases seen in southern Africa are pericardial effusions and cardiomyopathy. The presentation of these diseases is variable, but is often similar to that of HIV-negative patients. However, other concomitant disease may complicate the clinical picture. Therapy for all forms of cardiovascular disease is usually similar to that for non-HIV infected individuals, although clinicians should consider the potential for drug interactions with antiretrovirals and with drugs used to treat opportunistic infections (OIs).

Pericardial disease

Pericardial disease is the commonest cardiac manifestation of HIV in southern Africa, predominantly because of the signifcant incidence of tuberculous pericardial effusion.

Aetiology

Asymptomatic effusions of uncertain aetiology are very common and many do not progress to symptomatic disease. However, patients with effusions have a poorer prognosis than those without, irrespective of stage of disease and cause of effusion, and should be followed up closely. Tuberculosis (TB) is by far the commonest cause of overt pericardial effusions in southern Africa, although various tumours and OIs may involve the pericardial space. Lymphoma can mimic TB and is often associated with myocardial invasion. Kaposi's sarcoma (KS) can also invade the pericardium.

Clinical features

Patients only experience symptoms once a critical volume of fluid is present in the pericardial space. Pericardial tamponade presents with the classic triad of:

- low blood pressure;
- raised jugular-venous pressure; and
- soft heart sounds.

These features may mimic right-sided cardiac failure. A friction rub or pulsus paradoxus is only occasionally present. An electrocardiogram (ECG) may show small complexes, electrical alternans, tachycardia, and diffuse T-wave changes; the chest radiograph will show a large cardiac silhouette. Severe cardiomyopathy can present in an identical manner, but an echocardiogram or ultrasound scan can quickly differentiate between them, especially if a pericardial tap is being considered.

In tuberculous pericardial effusion, constitutional symptoms, including weight loss and drenching sweats, are often the most prominent presenting feature. The diagnosis may only be suspected when the chest radiograph shows an enlarged cardiac shadow. (See Photographs 1 and 2.)

Diagnosis

Diagnosis of the cause of a pericardial effusion can be a problem. Facilities may not exist for pericardial taps or biopsies (the best way of establishing a diagnosis), or the effusion may not be large enough to tap. In both cases, consider alternative diagnostic procedures, as aggressively investigating pericardial effusions only yields a diagnosis in a minority of cases. Look for other sites for histology or culture, particularly if empiric therapy is being considered for TB. (See Chapter 21: Evaluation of fever.)

Useful tests on pericardial fluid include:

- biochemistry;
- microscopy;
- culture (especially for TB);
- cytology; and

ADA testing is controversial. Elevated levels may suggest TB, but this is non-specific. None of the above investigations assist in the diagnosis of pericardial KS. Biopsy for KS is often diagnostic, but requires cardio-thoracic expertise, as the risk of bleeding from the biopsy site is high.

Treatment

Pericardiocentesis becomes necessary if the patient is haemodynamically compromised. This procedure is ideally done with the aid of echocardio-graphy. If these facilities do not exist, the tap can be done with clinical monitoring alone. Response may be dramatic, even after removing a small volume of fluid.

A drain can be left in situ to allow excess fluid to drain completely. A pericardial window, if cardiothoracic expertise is available, may assist if recurrent effusions cause haemodynamic compromise. Once the danger of tamponade has passed, treatment should be directed at the cause. In the absence of symptoms, remember that small, asymptomatic effusions are common, and are usually not the result of TB.

In areas of high TB prevalence in patients with significant effusions and constitutional symptoms, the clinician may decide to start empiric anti-tuberculous treatment, based on the assumption that TB is the most likely cause. However, the clinician should attempt to make the diagnosis from another site, before committing patients to prolonged anti-tuberculous therapy. The role of steroids in the treatment of tuberculous pericardial effusion is controversial, but may be useful to hasten the resolution of a large effusion that has not been tapped. Prednisone is given at a dosage of 60 mg daily for two weeks; TB treatment is given according to national protocols.

Dilated cardiomyopathy

Cardiomyopathies are diseases of the heart muscle. Here, the term refers to any disease of the heart muscle not caused by significant hypertension, valvular or other structural diseases.

Aetiology

The cause of dilated cardiomyopathy (CMO) is unclear, and may result from direct HIV infection of the myocardium. Nutritional deficiencies may also play a role, especially of selenium and thiamine.

Clinical features

Asymptomatic left-ventricular dysfunction is very common in HIV-positive patients, particularly in advanced disease, and overt cardiac failure is not uncommon. Underlying cardiac dysfunction and myocarditis both predispose patients to arrhythmias, which are commoner in HIV-positive patients. Symptoms usually develop gradually. Fatigue and weakness are common. Features of right-heart failure occur late and have a very poor prognosis.

Physical examination

A physical examination reveals cardiac enlargement and congestive cardiac failure. A low blood pressure with a narrow pulse pressure is common. Pulsus alternans is often present in the late stages of the disease. As right-sided heart failure develops, distended neck veins, peripheral oedema, liver engorgement, ascites, and tricuspid regurgitation occur. Heart sounds are often soft, and extra sounds (S3 and S4 gallops), are almost universal in advanced cases. Murmurs are common, owing to ventricular enlargement and loss of annular architecture.

The chest radiograph usually shows pulmonary congestion and a large cardiac shadow with multi-chamber enlargement. The patient may have pleural effusions, and prominent superior venae cavae and azygous veins. The ECG varies from being almost normal to showing gross abnormalities. Sinus tachycardias are common in cardiac failure and torsades de pointes has been reported. Echocardiography is useful to exclude potential remediable causes that commonly mimic cardiomyopathy, especially pericardial effusion and primary valve disease. Other causes of fluid overload include cor pulmonale, renal disease (renal failure, acute glomerulonephritis or nephrotic syndrome), and portal hypertension.

Treatment

The management of cardiac failure in HIV-positive patients is conventional, once all possible remediable causes have been addressed. Non-pharmacological measures include:

- smoking and alcohol cessation;
- salt restriction;
- fluid restriction, if necessary;
- contraception for women; and
- regular exercise (except in cases of acute heart failure).

First-line therapy comprises:

- an angiotensin-converting enzyme inhibitor (ACEI), or angiotensin receptor blocker (ARB), titrated to maximum doses;
- careful diuretic use; and
- digoxin.

ACE inhibitors, ARBs, spironolactone, hydralazine with nitrate therapy and β-blockade have all now been shown to improve survival in patients with heart failure. All these drugs, as well as digoxin, carry significant potential toxicity and must be used with care. Many require dose titration. Elevated blood pressure should be controlled. Thiamine, given for a limited period to patients with a possible nutritional or alcoholic history, is safe and cheap. Anticoagulation should be considered if there is evidence of embolism or mural thrombi, or a very low ejection fraction on echocardiogram. Anticoagulation is often complex, due to the large number of potential drug interactions with warfarin. All patients should receive annual influenza vaccinations.

Cardiac transplants (with antiretroviral therapy) would ideally be offered, but this option is not generally available in southern Africa.

Pulmonary hypertension

Cardiologists have described a form of unexplained pulmonary hypertension that is similar to primary pulmonary hypertension found in HIV-negative individuals. This is thought to arise from diseased T-cells. The disease has a similar clinical presentation to primary pulmonary hypertension and has a similarly poor prognosis. Exclude other potentially treatable conditions, such as pulmonary thromboembolic disease, cor pulmonale (often due to chronic TB-related lung disease), and cardiac shunts.

Infective endocarditis

Valvular heart disease secondary to rheumatic heart disease was a common problem in southern Africa before the advent of HIV. Both diseases have a high enough prevalence now for a significant number of patients to present with both incidentally. There is no evidence that HIV adversely interacts with rheumatic heart disease.

Clinical features

The clinical presentation of infective endocarditis in HIV-positive patients is similar to that of non-HIV-infected patients, although sequelae tend to be more severe as the CD4 count drops. Common features include:
- fever, drenching sweats, weight loss, myalgia;
- cardiac murmur;
- active urine sediment or haematuria;
- petechiae and splinter haemorrhage;
- embolic phenomena, including pulse deficits; and
- splenomegaly.

Intravenous drug abusers and patients with central venous catheters are prone to staphylococcal and fungal endocarditis, which are usually right sided. Nosocomial endocarditis carries a very high mortality. The most essential investigation is at least three sets of blood cultures from different sites, obtained before parenteral antibiotics are started. See Chapter 21: Evaluation of fever: Appendix 21.1.

Treatment and prophylaxis

Treatment and prophylaxis in HIV-positive infective endocarditis patients are the same as for HIV-negative individuals. There is no evidence that HIV-infected individuals with normal cardiac architecture require prophylaxis.

Myocarditis

Myocarditis is a very common finding at autopsy in HIV-infected patients, even in the absence of clinical and echocardiographic abnormalities.

Aetiology

Occasionally, OIs cause myocarditis, including *Pneumocystis*, all the common fungal pathogens, mycobacteria, toxoplasma, herpes simplex and cytomegaloviruses, and any other cause of endocarditis. Patients can also show a myocardial lymphocytic infiltrate, with no overt evidence of a specific cause.

Clinical features

The acute syndrome can range from an incidental ECG finding to catastrophic cardiac failure. Subsequent sequelae are variable, ranging from full recovery, to changes resembling dilated CMO. The clinical examination should direct the investigation of the causes of myocarditis, as most cases will not yield a diagnosis.

Treatment

The management of myocarditis is supportive, unless a treatable cause is found. Routine steroids do not seem to help. Cardiac failure is managed conventionally.

Cardiovascular and ischaemic heart disease

Most classes of antiretroviral therapy have now been associated with a broad number of morphological and biochemical abnormalities commonly associated with atherosclerosis. These include increased intra-abdominal fat deposition, hypertension, glucose intolerance, and lipid abnormalities (See Chapter 34: Endocrinology and metabolic abnormalities). It is still not yet clear, in southern Africa, whether these abnormalities will translate into increased rates of future myocardial infarction, stroke, and peripheral vascular disease, or that treatment will alter this progression, but it seems prudent to monitor and treat these complications along conventional lines. It is important to remember that lifestyle modification, especially smoking, has a far more profound impact on cardiovascular risk than drug selection for optimum improved metabolic profile.

Attention has been drawn to increased cardiovascular and other complications of patients with regular interruptions of their antiretroviral therapy. This is now not recommended. Abacavir has recently been implicated in increased cardiovascular events, and, despite the evidence being observational, is generally avoided if possible in patients with other risk factors for cardiovascular disease.

Drug interactions in HIV-cardiology

The following drug interactions are relevant to the treatment of cardiac patients:

- Co-trimoxazole can cause hyperkalaemia and hyponatraemia. Monitoring of electrolytes is occasionally necessary, especially if the patient is taking digoxin, ace-inhibitors, spironolactone, or loop diuretics.
- Pentamidine, now rarely used, can cause electrolyte disturbances and is pro-arrhythmic.
- Cisapride and terfenadine/astemizole are associated with life-threatening arrythmias, especially when used with certain PIs, azole-antifungals, and macrolides (as these all inhibit hepatic metabolism).
- Theophylline levels can increase in the presence of ritonavir and cause arrhythmias. Monitoring is important.

Certain statin drugs interact with the protease inhibitors. Simvastatin and lovastatin are contraindicated, with pravastatin being a preferred choice in most cases. Atorvastatin has also been used, and appears safe, although counselling patients regarding symptoms of myositis is important. Fibrates may be used as an alternative. Efavirenz may decrease statin levels.

Calcium channel blockers may have increased concentrations when combined with protease inhibitors, and should be titrated gently.

Warfarin has potent interactions with antiretroviral therapy and INR monitoring during changes in the drug is essential.

References and further reading

Braunwald, E. 2012. *Heart disease: A textbook of cardiovascular medicine.* 9th edition. Philadelphia: W. B. Saunders Company.

Dolin, R. et al. 2007. *AIDS therapy.* 3rd edition. Edinburgh: Churchill Livingstone.

Merigan, T. C. et al. 1999. *Textbook of AIDS medicine.* Baltimore: Williams and Wilkins.

Haematology

Haematological abnormalities in HIV infection may result from a host of diverse influences on the haematopoeitic tissue.

It is useful to consider haematological abnormalities as being due to:
- decreased cell production due to bone marrow abnormalities;
- increased cell destruction outside the marrow;
- increased cell sequestration due to hypersplenism;
- extramedullary haematopoiesis.

Effects of HIV infection on blood cell production

Dysregulation in haematopoiesis function due to HIV infection can result from:
- direct HIV infection of haematopoietic progenitor cells;
- HIV replication in marrow stromal cells;
- alteration of the cellular and cytokine milieu (e.g. release by HIV-infected monocytes of transforming growth factor β, tumour necrosis factor-α, interleukin-1);
- viral gene products, inhibitory glycoproteins, and antibody-mediated cytotoxicity;
- deregulation of T-cell subpopulations.

Suppression of haematopoietic function can also be due to invasion of the marrow by a variety of opportunistic infections such as *Mycobacterium tuberculosis*, *Mycobacterium avium* complex, *Cryptococcus neoformans*, and malignancies such as lymphoma.

Anaemia

Anaemia is the commonest haematological abnormality. The incidence increases significantly over the course of the disease, ultimately affecting 70%–95% of HIV-positive individuals. Anaemia is associated with a significantly increased risk of death, and is reversed by highly active antiretroviral therapy.

Useful tests in determining the aetiology of anaemia

These are usually cheap and easy to perform, and with a good clinical history can 'characterize' the anaemia, allowing for judicious use of more expensive or less available tests, such as red cell folate and B12 levels, iron studies, haptoglobin, haemosiderin antibody, and bone marrow aspirates and biopsy. This is particularly important, as HIV can induce anaemia in a variety of scenarios, but anaemia is very common and may be a separate clinical problem from the HIV status. Tests include:

- *Full blood count* – assessment of other cell lines may allow for determining whether there is a common process, or whether just the red cell lines are involved.
- *Corrected reticulocyte production index (RPI)* – the RPI is a very useful and underutilized test that can be done with the full blood count, and allows rapid assessment of whether the bone marrow is responding to the anaemia appropriately.
- *Mean cellular volume (MCV)* – this may allow for rapid correlation with a clinical history, e.g. a history of chronic blood loss or repeated pregnancies with a low MCV may strongly suggest iron deficiency.
- *Blood smear* – this is invaluable, and allows for, among other things, the assessment of haemolysis, presence of malignancies, and bone marrow infiltration.
- *Lactate dehydrogenase (LDH)* – this may indicate haemolysis. Raised bilirubin levels may also indicate haemolysis.

Anaemia of chronic disease

Anaemia of chronic disease (ACD) is a cytokine-mediated response to chronic infections that results in the sequestration of iron in macrophages. Interleukins-1 and -6, and tumour necrosis factor-α cause the release of hepcidin from hepatocytes, which causes the degradation of macrophage ferroportin (a transmembrane iron transporter protein). This response limits the access of invading microorganisms to iron and restricts microorganism growth. ACD usually resolves with effective treatment of the infection.

Note that routine prescription of iron supplementation to patients with tuberculosis is contraindicated, as the anaemia is probably due to ACD.

Nutritional deficiency anaemia

Iron deficiency anaemia (IDA) can be due to:
- poor dietary intake of iron;

- pregnancy-related blood loss and menorrhagia;
- gastrointestinal blood loss due to parasites (such as hookworm), dysentery, peptic ulcer disease, Kaposi's sarcoma cancers and cytomegalovirus colitis.

Evaluation of red cell parameters and iron studies can help to distinguish IDA from ACD (Table 30.1)

Table 30.1 comparison of the laboratory features of ACD and IDA

Parameter	ACD	IDA
Mean red cell volume*	Normal	Low
Mean haemoglobin concentration	Normal	Low
Ferritin**	Normal/raised	Low
Serum iron	Low	Low
Total iron binding capacity	Normal	Raised

* Mean cell volume can be low in genetic disorders such as thalassaemia.

** Ferritin is a hepatic acute phase protein that can be increased by inflammatory disorders. The ratio of soluble transferrin receptor to $\log_{10}$ ferritin may provide a more accurate assessment of iron stores, but this methodology needs to be validated in HIV-infected populations.

In resource-limited settings where iron studies are not readily available, the mean haemoglobin concentration (MHC) is probably the most useful parameter. If the MHC is very low and there are no cytokine-mediated constitutional symptoms (weight loss, fever or drenching sweats) or active infections, it may be reasonable to give a trial of iron supplementation and assess the haemoglobin response after two weeks.

Poor dietary intake or reduced absorption of folate, and vitamin B12, will also reduce red cell production. Subnormal vitamin B12 levels have been described in a large proportion of HIV-infected individuals.

Infections

Disseminated opportunistic infections such as *M. tuberculosis*, *M. avium* complex, *Cryptococcus neoformans*, *Histoplasma capsulatum*, *Pneumocystis jirovecii*, or viral infections with CMV or Epstein-Barr virus can all decrease red cell production. Parvovirus B19 can cause erythroid hypoplasia. Parvovirus B19 has also been associated with neutropenia, thrombocytopenia, and the haemophagocytic syndrome. The diagnosis of parvovirus is suspected morphologically on bone marrow histology and confirmed using polymerase chain reaction (PCR) testing.

Myelosuppression

Chronic renal failure is a common cause of anaemia, due to decreased renal production of erythropoietin. Many drugs used in the treatment of HIV infection can cause myelosuppression, including:

- zidovudine (anaemia, common, and neutropenia; macro cytosis without anaemia may occur);
- stavudine (anaemia and neutropenia, rare; macrocytosis without anaemia may occur);
- lamivudine (pure red cell aplasia, rare);
- amphotericin B;
- antineoplastic agents;
- co-trimoxazole;
- foscarnet;
- ganciclovir;
- interferon-a;
- pentamidine; and
- pyrimethamine.

Red cell destruction

Increased red cell destruction may contribute to anaemia:

- Microangiopathic haemolytic anaemias such as thrombotic thrombo-cytopenic purpura (TTP) or the haemolytic uraemic syndrome (HUS) are well described in HIV infection. Disseminated intravascular coagulation (DIC) may be precipitated by sepsis or malignancies. Fragmented red cells (schistocytes) and thrombocytopaenia are seen in all these conditions, but usually only DIC causes an abnormal prothrombin time or partial thromboplastin time. Pre-eclampsia causing the HELLP syndrome (haemolysis, elevated liver enzymes, low platelet count) is an important consideration in pregnant women.
- Coombs-positive haemolysis due to red cell autoantibodies (un-common).
- Haemolysis may result from G6PD deficiency in patients taking dapsone, sulphonamides, or other oxidant drugs. Screening for G6PD deficiency should be considered for patients born in regions where this condition is common (e.g. West Africa).
- Malaria is an important cause of haemolytic anaemia associated with fever.
- Haemophagocytosis (destruction of blood cells by bone marrow macrophages) may contribute to cytopenias.

Haemolysis should be considered in patients with:
  anaemia;
  raised serum lactate dehydrogenase (LDH) and unconjugated bilirubin;
  low serum haptoglobin;
  raised corrected reticulocyte count (less likely if there is a co-existing bone marrow abnormality).

Classically the diagnosis of TTP is suspected if the following pentad of features is present:
  microangiopathic haemolytic anaemia;
  thrombocytopenia (usually <20 000 × 10^9/l);
  neurological abnormalities;
  renal failure;
  fever.

However, TTP is common and can occur at any stage of HIV infection, with a very heterogeneous clinical presentation that may vary from low-grade, asymptomatic thrombocytopenia with mild renal insufficiency, to severe neurological deficits and renal failure. Multimeric Von Willebrand's factor and ADAMTS13 metalloproteinase deficiency have been implicated in idiopathic TTP, but the role of these proteins in HIV-associated TTP is uncertain. Early diagnosis and conventional management (with plasma-pheresis and infusion of fresh frozen plasma) are essential to ensure a favourable outcome.

Management of anaemia

Management involves identifying possible contributing conditions and taking one or more of the following steps:
  Treat nutritional deficiencies.
  Treat OIs and sepsis aggressively.
  Stop myelosuppressive drugs, where feasible.

Mild anaemia (Hb >8 g/dl) is well tolerated and should not be used as a reason to stop essential drugs. Consider transfusion for life-threatening blood loss or clinically symptomatic anaemia. Patients should clearly understand the inherent risks of transfusion such as transmission of other blood-borne infections, development of allo-antibodies, and iron overload. Recombinant erythropoietin (rEPO) reverses HIV-related anaemia when the erythropoietin (EPO) blood level is <500 IU/l. Most patients will show a response by at least week eight using doses of 100–

200 IU/kg subcutaneously three times per week. Iron reserves need to be monitored during the course of EPO therapy. Wide-scale EPO use is unlikely to be affordable or practical in resource-poor settings, and recent safety concerns regarding EPO use mean that the drug should probably be reserved until all other interventions have been tried.

Leucopenia

A low white-cell count is a common finding during the course of HIV infection, but is less clearly related to the stage of the disease than anaemia. Lymphopenia and granulocytopenia may both contribute to leucopenia. A monocytopenia is noted in up to 10% of individuals. Peripheral blood smear white-cell abnormalities may include very atypical lymphocytes, vacuolated monocytes, and dysplastic changes in the granulocytic series.

Neutropenia

Neutropenia occurs in approximately 10% of patients with early infection and between 50% and 75% of patients with more advanced disease. As with the anaemia, multiple aetiologies are thought to contribute. Drug-induced neutropenia is common. Zidovudine, stavudine, and high-dose co-trimoxazole are usually implicated. Vitamin B12 and folate deficiency should be excluded. Provided the absolute neutrophil count is greater than $1 \times 10^9/l$, the risk of infection is not increased. Use of colony-stimulating factors (e.g. filgrastim) reduces hospitalizations and the risk of infection, but is very costly, and has been associated with rare but serious side effects. In clinical practice, it is rarely necessary.

Lymphopenia

This is a hallmark of advancing HIV disease, and is partially or fully reversible with antiretroviral therapy. (See Chapter 3: The immune system and HIV infection.)

Thrombocytopenia

Thrombocytopenia occurs with increased frequency in HIV-seropositive individuals and occurs in 5%–40% of patients. Thrombocytopenia may be the first presenting feature in as many as 10% of individuals.

The mechanism of thrombocytopenia remains a controversial topic and may include:

- Platelet destruction, owing to anti-platelet antibodies (e.g. directed against GP IIb/IIIa and GP1b/IX);
- Platelet consumption, which is a feature of TTP, HUS (haemolytic uraemic syndrome), and DIC – all of which cause haemolysis and red cell fragments;
- Impaired thrombopoiesis, due to stem cell damage, altered regulation of platelet production, and reticuloendothelial dysfunction; and
- Secondary thrombocytopenias resulting from associated bacterial, viral, fungal, or parasitic infections, or marrow infiltration by a neo-plastic process, or drugs, or hypersplenism.

Management of thrombocytopaenia

Management consists of excluding secondary causes (i.e. a bone marrow biopsy should be performed if the peripheral blood megakaryocyte is not elevated) and prescribing:

- antiretroviral therapy (zidovudine should be included in the regimen if possible);
- high-dose IV gamma globulin;
- corticosteroids; and
- splenectomy (for refractory cases).

Bone marrow examination

A bone marrow examination may be helpful when investigating a fever of unknown origin (see Chapter 10: Evaluation of fever) or a progressive cytopenia. A bone marrow aspirate is less useful than a trephine biopsy since cytological findings are generally reactive and non-specific. The aspirate is better used for mycobacterial and fungal culture.

Hypercellularity and dysplasia are characteristic of HIV infection. The CD4 count is not a good predictor of these differences or progression in morphology. A mild to moderate plasmacytosis or eosinophilia is a relatively common feature. Lymphoid aggregates represent a reaction to viral insult and do not suggest underlying lymphoma. PCR testing for the immunoglobulin heavy chain locus may distinguish benign bone marrow lymphoid aggregates from malignant ones.

The greatest advantage of trephine biopsy is in the rapid diagnosis of tuberculosis, *M. avium* complex, cryptococcosis, and haematological malignancies. (See photo 3.)

Disorders of haemostasis

The risk of deep-vein thrombosis is at least 10 times higher in HIV-infected patients, with the greatest risk occurring when the CD4 count is less than 200 cells/µl, and in the period after initiating antiretroviral therapy. Concurrent infectious and neoplastic diseases, and the presence of the lupus anticoagulant and other anti-phospholipid antibodies, may also predispose patients to thrombosis. Indinavir, now rarely used, has been associated with portal-vein thrombosis.

Deep vein thrombosis typically presents as unilateral painful warm swollen lower leg. The diagnosis is confirmed by Doppler ultrasound scanning of the leg, demonstrating non-compressible veins. Pulmonary thromboembolism is a life-threatening complication (See Chapter 32: Pulmonology)

Interactions can occur between warfarin, rifampicin, the protease inhibitors (PIs), and non-nucleoside reverse transcriptase inhibitors. Frequent, careful monitoring of the prothrombin index/INR is recommended.

Haemophilia

Many people with haemophilia were infected by blood products prior to routine HIV testing of blood donors. Infection often occurred in childhood or adolescence and disease progression is slow. Co-infection with hepatitis B or C is common and causes significant morbidity (See Chapter 38: Gastroenterology and hepatology). KS is infrequently seen. PIs have been associated with an increased risk of bleeding. In other respects the course of HIV infection is similar.

References and further reading

Bain, B. J. 1999. 'Pathogenesis and pathophysiology of anaemia in HIV infection'. *Current Opinion in Haematology*; 6 (2):89–93.

Karstaedt, A. S. et al. 2001. 'The utility of bone-marrow examination in HIV-infected adults in South Africa'. *Quarterly Journal of Medicine*; 94:101–105.

Southern African HIV Clinicians Society. 2012. A review of the use of blood and blood products in HIV-infected patients. *South African Journal of HIV Medicine*; 13(2):87–103.

Volberding P, A. et al 2003. 'Human immunodeficiency virus haematology'. *Haematology*; 294–313.

Nephrology

HIV infection is associated with many forms of kidney disease, both acute (reversible) and chronic (irreversible). Patients of African descent are more susceptible to kidney disease, and the incidence of HIV-related kidney failure in sub-Saharan Africa is exceptionally high. Due to the enormous costs of renal replacement therapy many countries actively exclude HIV-infected patients from dialysis and transplantation. Whenever possible, it is essential to correctly diagnose and treat HIV-related kidney disease in order to prevent end stage renal failure.

Importantly, medical conditions such as diabetes, hypertension and auto-immune disorders causing kidney disease are equally common in HIV-positive and -negative patients.

Assessment of kidney disease

Screening

Kidney disease is usually asymptomatic until an advanced stage, and carefully designed screening programmes could prevent irreversible end stage disease. Initial assessment of *all* HIV-positive patients should include the following:

- a clinical history asking about previously known kidney disease, or diseases known to cause kidney failure (e.g. diabetes), or a family history of kidney disease;
- blood pressure measurement;
- urine dipstick for proteinuria;
- serum urea and creatinine.

Urine testing and creatinine testing should be performed on an annual basis on all patients.

History

A detailed history should to be taken once blood or urine analysis results reveal renal dysfunction. This includes attention to the specifics of HIV infection regarding WHO staging and associated opportunistic infections, as well as a history of swelling, rashes and arthralgia.

A detailed drug history should be taken with specific note of:
- sulphur containing compounds (e.g. co-trimoxazole);
- aminoglycosides;
- non-steroidal anti-inflammatory drugs;
- amphotericin;
- tuberculosis medications;
- non-prescription medications including traditional medications.

Examination

Carefully assess the hydration status of the patient. No one sign is sufficient and instead this is a composite 'guestimate' using:
- skin turgor;
- blood pressure with or without postural drop (>10 mmHg);
- heart rate;
- jugular venous pressure (both at 45° and with the patient flat when underhydrated);
- oedema.

As well as a general HIV examination looking for evidence of stage of infection, together with opportunistic infections, it is also important to look for rashes and evidence of other medical illnesses.

Investigations

These should include:
- Urine dipstick testing: a qualitative assessment of *proteinuria* is vital, as is the detection of blood and white cells. Usually, if there is more than 2 g/day (~2+ on a dipstick) of proteinuria, the kidney disease is glomerular. Anything less can come from tubulointerstitial or glomerular disease. Patients with isolated *haematuria* should have urine sent off for microscopy (including schistosoma ova) bacterial culture and sensitivity and, importantly, tuberculosis (TB) culture.
- Urine microscopy: to detect the presence of blood cells, casts and crystals.
- Urine spot protein creatinine ratios: these are a good substitute for the traditional, but more complicated, 24 hour urine collection.
- Serum urea and electrolytes, calcium, albumin, phosphate, glucose, full blood count. A normal haemoglobin (>11g/dl) points towards an *acute* kidney illness, while a low haemoglobin, in the setting of HIV

infection could be due to a number to causes including chronic renal failure (See Chapter 30: Haematology).

- Serum creatinine should be converted into calculated glomerular filtration rates (GFR) in patients whose levels are in a steady state using the Cockcroft Gault equation:

$$GFR = \frac{(140\text{-age}) \times \text{weight (kg)}}{\text{serum creatinine}(\mu mol/l)) \times 1.23 \text{ (men) or } 1.04 \text{ (women)}}$$

- Serum anti-nuclear antibody, anti-neutrophil cytoplasmic antibody, complement levels, hepatitis B and C virus antibodies, syphilis serology (if a biopsy is contemplated).
- Ultrasound scan: to detect kidney size (normal 10–12 cm) and presence of obstruction. Small kidneys (<9 cm) point towards *chronic* disease, while normal or big kidneys may be difficult to assess as many HIV-1-related nephropathies cause increased size initially.
- Renal biopsy: the two most important indications are: heavy proteinuria and acute kidney failure where the cause is not immediately apparent (e.g. ATN).

This approach will help identify whether the kidney disease is:

- *Reversible* (treatable) versus *irreversible* ('non-treatable', chronic – small kidneys)
- *Glomerular* versus *non glomerular* (tubulo-interstitial)
  (See Figure 31.1)

Figure 31.1 An approach to HIV-related kidney disease

ACUTE	Crescentic GN (e.g. HIVICK)	ATN AIN Obstruction	**1. haemoglobin** >11 g/dl = acute (low Hb = acute or chronic)
CHRONIC	HIVAN HIVICK OTHER GNs	ATN/AIN Obstruction Reflux	**2. ultrasound** <9 cm = chronic (Normal/big kidneys = acute or chronic **3. urine dipstix protein** >2+ = glomerular, usually chronic (minimal/no proteinuria = glomerular or tubulointerstitial

Key: HIVICK: HIV immune complex kidney disease; ATN acute tubular necrosis; AIN acute interstitial nephritis; HIVAN HIV-associated nephropathy; GN glomerulonephritis.

An approach to HIV-related kidney disease

In HIV-related kidney disease the virus can be either *directly* or *indirectly* involved in the disease process.

Indirect renal involvement

HIV can result in kidney disease via numerous indirect mechanisms, which probably account for the majority of cases of renal failure. Most of these diseases occur in the tubulointerstitial compartment and, for the most part, can be reversed if detected early enough.

Acute tubular necrosis

Urine reabsorption in the tubulointerstitial compartment is an energy requiring process. Any cause of decreased renal perfusion (e.g. hypotension, hypovolaemia, renal vasoconstriction secondary to sepsis or drugs) will mean that this large energy demand is not met. This causes tubular cell death, a process known as acute tubular necrosis (ATN). In the context of advanced HIV infection ATN is a common cause of renal failure secondary to opportunistic infections, diarrhoeal illnesses and dehydration. Fortunately this can be reversed with correct management.

Treatment consists of re-establishing renal perfusion:
- Correcting fluid losses using clinical monitoring of blood pressure, heart rate, jugular venous pressure and skin turgor. More precise measurements of venous pressure may be required using an indwelling central venous catheter.
- Restoring blood pressure using inotropes once the patient is euvolaemic (See Chapter 33: Intensive care management).
- Treatment of sepsis using appropriate parenteral antibiotics, and surgery for abscess collections. Note that aminoglycosides should be avoided in renal failure.
- Stopping drugs that interfere with renal perfusion (e.g. angiotensin converting enzyme inhibitors and non-steroidal anti-inflammatory drugs).

These simple measures, if instituted promptly, can reverse ATN and restore renal function.

Indications for dialysis are:

- fluid overload and pulmonary oedema that does not respond to diuretics;
- potassium overload (hyperkalaemia) that does not respond to insulin, intravenous dextrose and/or bicarbonate and gastrointestinal transfer gels such as sodium polystyrene sulphonate (Kexelate);
- uraemia syndrome defined by encephalopathy, bleeding, serositis (usually pericardial effusion) and acidosis. This is not dependent on a set biochemical 'cut off' point.

Acute interstitial nephritis

HIV-positive patients are at increased risk of acute interstitial nephritis (AIN), due to an increased incidence of allergic drug reactions. There may be associated fever, rash, eosinophilia and transaminitis. The urine findings are non-specific and may include protein, blood, granular casts, and white cells. Biopsy findings are characterized by the infiltration of inflammatory cells such as lymphocytes and plasma cells in the tubulointerstitial component. Any drug can cause AIN but the sulphur containing drugs and anti-TB medication are common offenders. HIV may itself cause inflammation.

Treatment is to stop any drugs that might be responsible where possible. If this does not reverse the renal disease, steroids can be considered in consultation with a nephrologist.

Urological tract tuberculosis

The kidneys, ureters and bladder are common sites for TB infection, particularly in the setting of immune compromise. This can result in obstruction secondary to the associated scarring and fibrosis associated with granulomata. Diagnosis can be made by culturing the urine, especially in the presence of haematuria, while ultrasound evaluation is helpful. Cystoscopy and biopsy of affected areas may even be necessary.

Crystalluria

This may be associated with use of certain antiretrovirals, especially the protease inhibitors (e.g. indinavir).

Direct renal involvement

In these HIV-related kidney diseases, it is felt that the virus is directly involved in the pathogenesis. Most of these diseases occur in the glomerular compartment of the kidney and cause chronic renal failure.

HIV-associated nephropathy

HIV-associated nephropathy (HIVAN) is perhaps the best known of all the HIV-related kidney diseases, although it accounts for only a proportion (~30% to 80%) of those who are infected and have renal involvement. It is thought to be caused by direct viral infection of podocytes in patients who have a genetic predisposition.

HIVAN can occur at any stage of HIV infection, although it seems to be more common in those with advanced infection and low CD4 counts. It would appear to occur almost exclusively in Africans. Clinically it is characterized by heavy proteinuria (often above 10 g per day) associated with hypoalbuminaemia and swelling. However, unlike typical nephrotic syndrome, the cholesterol levels are often low, probably reflecting patient malnutrition. Renal ultrasound typically shows normal to large sized kidneys, even when the kidney disease has been present for a long period of time. Although most patients tend to have advanced renal failure, the disease can occur at any stage of renal (dys)function.

HIVAN can mimic any glomerulopathy clinically. Therefore biopsy is essential to make an accurate diagnosis. Histology is characterized by the following features:

- podocyte swelling;
- segmental collapse of glomerular tuft;
- focal segmental scarring;
- interstitial inflammation;
- interstitial microcyst formation;
- negative immunofluorescence.

Alternative names for HIVAN are focal segmental glomerulosclerosis or collapsing HIV-associated glomerulopathy.

Once the diagnosis has been made, the progression to end stage kidney failure is usually rapid, occurring within months.

Management

This remains very controversial. Unfortunately many of the therapeutic trials contain small numbers and are often retrospective. The following treatment strategies are in use:

- Angiotensin converting enzyme inhibitors (ACEI): these diminish the degree of proteinuria in a non specific fashion and have proven benefits in many other forms of kidney disease. Maximum doses should be used, blood pressure and potassium permitting. If the patient develops side effects such as angioneurotic oedema or a persistent cough, substitute angiotensin receptor blockers.
- Antiretrovirals: there is accumulating evidence which suggests that HIVAN is the result of direct viral infection of the renal cells. HIV-1-associated nephropathy is a WHO Stage 4 diagnosis and antiretroviral therapy should be started regardless of the CD4 count. Importantly some antiretroviral drugs need dose adjustments when renal function is abnormal (see Table 31.1).
- Blood pressure control: many patients tend to be hypotensive, but, when blood pressure is elevated add standard anti-hypertensive drugs to achieve a systolic pressure of ≤130mmHg.
- Statins: many patients tend to have normal to low cholesterol, but if this is not the case, add standard statin therapy to achieve a cholesterol of <5.5 mmol/L.

As HIVAN is thought to be a result of HIV infection of renal cells, corticosteroids may not have a therapeutic role although some small trials suggest benefit.

HIV immune complex kidney disease

This disease entity accounts for almost the same number of those with HIV-related kidney disease as those with HIVAN, in some series. It is thought to be more common in those of non-African origin but can occur in all demographic groups. HIV infection is often associated with poly-clonal immunoglobulin production resulting in the formation of immune complexes. It is envisaged that these complexes are either deposited in the kidney glomerulus (which deals with 25% of the cardiac output in normal circumstances) or else are created in situ. The resultant complement and cytokine activation results in inflammation and eventual kidney damage in a manner analogous to lupus nephritis.

Clinically HIV immune complex kidney disease (HIVICK) can present in a manner indistinguishable from HIVAN, namely, heavy proteinuria, hypoalbuminaemia, varying cholesterol levels and degrees of renal dysfunction.

Renal biopsy reveals the following changes:
- immune complex deposition in the glomeruli in varying patterns:
  o diffuse mesangial (lupus like),
  o subendothelial,
  o subepithelial 'ball in cup' pattern,
- interstitial infiltration.

These changes are often accompanied by those seen typically in HIVAN (e.g. glomerular collapse and interstitial microcyst formation).

Management of this condition is almost completely without guidance from clinical trials and is based at this stage mainly on anecdotal evidence. Consider treatment with ACEIs, blood pressure control and statins. As HIV is directly involved in the generation of immune complexes antiretroviral therapy should probably be used regardless of CD4 count, especially when there is concomitant evidence of podocyte inflammation on biopsy (e.g. swelling or collapse such as in HIVAN).

Consideration can be given to the use of steroids and/or cyclophosphamide in HIVICK-associated severe crescentic nephritis, together with antiretroviral therapy.

Other glomerulonephritidies

Many other forms of glomerulonephritis can occur in patients who are HIV-positive, (e.g. post infectious, membranous, minimal change, IgA nephropathy). As it is unknown what the aetiological agent is in these diseases, it is not clear whether HIV can cause these histological variants. These diseases should receive standard treatment (as for HIV-negative patients) and antiretroviral therapy should only be added when the usual indications are present.

Hepatitis B infection can cause membranous nephropathy and co-infected patients should be treated with lamivudine as a component of antiretroviral therapy (See Chapter 38: Gastroenterology and hepatology). Lamivudine monotherapy should not be used.

Holistic management of renal disease

HIV-positive are as likely as HIV-negative patients to contract a number of other kidney diseases that are clearly unrelated to their HIV infection including diabetes, polycystic kidney disease and reflux nephropathy. Even though HIV may not have an aetiological role in these kidney diseases, it is important that these patients are carefully monitored in terms of both HIV and chronic kidney disease staging.

Table 31.1 Holistic management of renal disease

Stage	Description	GFR (ml/min)	Management
1	Kidney damage with normal GFR	>90	Screening, CKD risk reduction, diagnosis and treatment, slow progression of CKD, treat co-morbidities, cardiovascular disease risk reduction
2	Mild kidney dysfunction	60–89	Estimate progression
3	Moderate kidney dysfunction	30–59	Evaluate and treat complications
4	Severe kidney dysfunction	15–29	Prepare for dialysis and/or transplantation
5	End stage kidney failure	<15	Start renal replacement therapy if uraemic

Renal failure is in itself a form of immunosuppression.

Patients with declining renal function should be referred through to a specialist centre where antiretroviral therapy can be started promptly and the various aspects of chronic kidney disease (e.g. anaemia, bone disease) can be managed by a multi-disciplinary team of nephrologists and infectious disease physicians.

When progression to end stage disease appears inevitable, it is important that patients are properly prepared for eventual renal replacement under a nephrology service. In the USA, HIV-related kidney disease is the third most important cause of permanent renal failure requiring dialysis amongst Black Americans. Currently there are many centres in Africa where maintenance dialysis and transplantation are not offered to HIV-positive patients, but this is changing. Some centres in the USA and Europe perform renal transplantation in HIV-positive patients. Although there are many potential pitfalls when balancing the effects of antiretroviral therapy and antirejection medication initial reports are encouraging.

References and further reading

Gerntholtz, T.E. et al. 2006. 'HIV-related nephropathy: a South African perspective.' *Kidney International*; 69(10):1885–1891.

Appendix 1 Nucleoside reverse transcriptase inhibitor dose adjustments for renal failure

Table 31.2 Nucleoside/nucleotide reverse transcriptase inhibitors

Generic name	Usual dose	Dose for reduced GFR (CrCl)
Emtricitabine	200 mg/d	30 to 49 ml/min: 200 mg q48h 15 to 29 ml/min: 200 mg q72h <15 ml/min and HD: 200 mg q96h
Lamivudine	150 mg bid or 300 mg/d	30 to 49 ml/min: 150 mg/d 15 to 29 ml/min: 150 mg LD, 100 mg/d 5 to 14 ml/min: 150 mg LD, 50 mg/d <5 ml/min: 50 mg LD, 25 mg/d
Zidovudine	300 mg bid or 200 mg tid	HD or PD: 100 mg q6–8h
Didanosine	≥60 kg: 200 mg bid <60 kg: 125 mg bid EC: ≥60 kg: 400 mg/d <60 kg: 250 mg/d	30 to 59 ml/min: >60 kg: 100 q12h or EC 200/d <60 kg: 75 q12h or EC 125/d 10 to 29 ml/min: >60 kg: 150/d or EC 125 mg/d <60 kg 100/d or EC 125/d <10 ml/min, HD: >60 kg: 100/d or EC 125 mg/d <60 kg: 75/d or EC: Avoid
Tenofovir	300 mg/d	30 to 49 ml/min: 300 mg q48h 10 to 29 ml/min: 300 mg twice weekly <10 ml/min without HD: No data HD: 300 mg every 7 d
Abacavir	300 mg bid or 600 mg/d	No dosage adjustment

| Stavudine | ≥60 kg: 40 mg q12h
 <60 kg: 30 mg q12h | 26 to 50 ml/min:
 ≥60 kg: 20 mg q12h
 <60 kg: 15 mg q12h
 10 to 25 ml/min, HD (administer after HD):
 ≥60 kg: 20 mg/d
 <60 kg: 15 mg/d |

Modified from: Highly Active Antiretroviral Therapy and the Kidney: An Update on Antiretroviral Medications for Nephrologists. *Clinical Journal of the American Society of Nephrologists*; 1: 117–129, 2006 with permission.

NOTE: HD haemodialysis; LD loading dose; PD peritoneal dialysis; EC enteric coated

32 Pulmonology

HIV-associated pulmonary diseases in children

Respiratory illness is a major cause of morbidity and mortality in HIV-infected African children. A respiratory problem is often the first sign of HIV, with pneumonia predominating. *Pneumocystis* pneumonia (PCP) prophylaxis and antiretroviral therapy have led to a substantial decline in HIV-associated respiratory infections. Improved survival will allow HIV-infected children with HIV-associated chronic lung disease to live longer. The spectrum of disease includes infectious and non-infectious conditions (Table 32.1).

Acute respiratory disease

Upper and lower respiratory tract infections are the most common cause of HIV-related pulmonary disease.

Upper respiratory tract infections

Otologic diseases

These include otitis media, otitis externa, serous otitis media and mastoiditis. The aetiology of infections is similar to that in HIV-uninfected children. Otitis externa is frequently caused by *P. aeruginosa*. Treatment involves cleansing and dry mopping of the auditory canal and topical acidifying agents (e.g. 1% acetic acid or 2% boric acid) or antibiotic drops. Systemic antibiotics are indicated for extensive local inflammation, tender adenopathy or systemic symptoms. Chronic fungal infection may cause persistent otitis externa – treatment involves topical acidifying agents and systemic antifungal medication.

Recurrent acute otitis media and chronic otitis media are very common in HIV-infected children. *S. pneumoniae*, *H. influenzae* and *M. catarrhalis* predominate in acute otitis media while gram negative bacteria and *S. aureus* occur more frequently in chronic infection. Amoxicillin at 90 mg/kg/day is recommended for otitis media. Failure to respond may indicate a β-lactamase producing organism – use either cefuroxime or amoxicillin-clavulanate.

Sinusitis and rhinitis

Chronic sinusitis and rhinitis are common. Causative organisms are similar to those causing otitis media. First line treatment is amoxicillin at 90 mg/kg/day. A decongestant nasal spray, e.g. phenylepinephrine for 5–7 days may reduce mucosal oedema and improve sinus drainage.

Epiglottitis

Bacterial epiglottitis presents with a high fever and dysphagia and may rapidly progress to airway obstruction. *H. influenzae, S. pyogenes, S. viridans* and *S. aureus* predominate. Empiric therapy is intravenous cefuroxime. *C. albicans* may occasionally cause hoarseness, sub-acute airway obstruction and clinical disease resembling epiglottitis; treat with fluconazole.

Laryngotracheobronchitis and upper airway obstruction

Recurrent upper airway obstruction due to persistent laryngeal candidiasis or lymphadenopathy secondary to tuberculosis (which can be exacerbated by immune reconstitution inflammatory syndrome) requires antifungal or antituberculosis therapy. Nebulized adrenaline and corticosteroids are recommended. The outcome is good, even for children requiring intubation.

Lower respiratory tract infections

Pneumocystis jirovecii pneumonia

Pneumocystis jirovecii pneumonia (PCP) is common in HIV-infected infants not on chemoprophylaxis and is frequently the presenting illness in a child with undiagnosed HIV. Infants aged 3–6 months are at highest risk.

Clinical presentation

PCP usually presents as an acute illness. There are no specific distinguishing features of PCP. The major symptoms are tachypnoea, fever, cough and dyspnoea. Cough is characteristically dry. Auscultation of lungs is usually normal although crepitations or wheezing may occur. The clinical course is frequently characterized by progressive hypoxia.

Investigations

Arterial saturation by pulse oximetry or blood gas may show low oxygen saturation or PaO_2. The alveolar-arterial oxygen gradient is high, usually above 12 mmHg. Serum lactate dehydrogenase (LDH) may be markedly elevated (greater than 1 000 IU/L) but is non-specific. Chest X-ray (photo 4) usually shows a diffuse interstitial pattern but hyperinflation, focal infiltrates, cavities, a miliary pattern, pneumothorax or a normal appearance may occur.

A presumptive diagnosis can be based on a history of acute respiratory decompensation, lack of auscultatory signs, hypoxia and diffuse interstitial infiltrates. Definitive diagnosis is dependent on identification of cysts or trophozoites from lower respiratory tract secretions (either induced sputum or bronchoalveolar lavage fluid) or from lung tissue. Nasopharyngeal aspirates may yield the organism in severe infection. Staining methods include silver methenamine, modified Giemsa, toluidine blue or immunofluorescence.

Treatment

The treatment of choice is intravenous trimethoprim-sulfamethoxazole (TMP-SMX) with a loading dose of 10 mg/kg TMP followed by a maintenance dose of 20 mg/kg/day TMP component in four divided doses for two to three weeks. Intravenous therapy is preferable for severely ill children, but oral treatment can be substituted in mild illness or after clinical improvement. If initiating oral therapy, give a loading dose of 20 mg/kg TMP component.

Corticosteroids (prednisone 2 mg/kg for seven to 10 days, then tapered over 10 to 14 days) improves survival and should be co-administered in moderate to severe illness. Oxygen should be given to all hypoxic children (room air arterial oxygen saturation <92%). The response to therapy may be slow, requiring three to five days.

Morphine may alleviate symptoms of severe respiratory distress (see Chapter 56: Palliative care).

Prophylaxis

Prevention is initiated in HIV-exposed infants within the first weeks of life. Oral TMP-SMX is the most effective. In the only randomized controlled study of TMP-SMX prophylaxis in HIV-infected Zambian children, mortality was reduced by 43% and morbidity, including hospitalization, by 23%. The impact on mortality occurred at all ages, suggesting that prophylaxis may also protect against bacterial infections.

Current recommendations for PCP prophylaxis include:

- all HIV-exposed children from four weeks (until six months); thereafter discontinue if HIV infection has been excluded and breastfeeding has been discontinued for at least six weeks.

all HIV-infected children from four weeks of age irrespective of age or CD4 count when antiretroviral therapy is unavailable; prophylaxis may be discontinued when older than a year if the CD4 is greater than 25% and if without symptomatic HIV disease; prophylaxis may however protect against bacterial illnesses.

discontinuation of prophylaxis may be considered when on antiretroviral therapy for at least six months once immune reconstitution has occurred. However, WHO recommendations are for prophylaxis to be continued even where immune reconstitution has occurred due to a potential protective effect against bacterial infections. Discontinuation of prophylaxis with confirmed immune restoration for six months or more as indicated by two measurements of CD4% >25% at least three to six months apart in children two to six years has been validated in USA.

lifelong prophylaxis should be given after an episode of PCP.

The recommended regimen is daily oral co-trimoxazole 5 mg/kg/day of the trimethoprim component (1 ml of the suspension contains 8 mg trimethoprim). An alternative is 5 mg/kg on three days of the week. The two regimens are probably equivalent and interchangeable. For children unable to tolerate TMP or SMX, use dapsone (2 mg/kg once daily or 4 mg/kg per week).

Bacterial infections

HIV-infected children are at risk for recurrent, severe bacterial pneumonia.

S. pneumoniae is the most common. Additional organisms include *H. influenzae, S. aureus, K. pneumoniae* and other gram-negative bacteria. Tuberculosis can present as acute pneumonia. There is an increased incidence of bacteraemia in HIV-infected patients with pneumonia. Co-infection with viral, fungal or mycobacterial pathogens is common.

Investigations

Acute phase reactants, erythrocyte sedimentation rate (ESR), C-reactive protein (CRP)), white cell count (WBC) and procalcitonin cannot distinguish bacterial, viral and mixed infections in children. A blood culture may be useful in hospitalized children. Sputum culture cannot distinguish colonizing from pathogenic bacteria. Pleural fluid should be cultured.

Treatment

Empiric antibiotic therapy should cover the common community-acquired bacteria. Oral or intravenous therapy depends on the severity of illness. High dose oral amoxicillin (30 mg/kg/dose eight hourly) is recommended for outpatient treatment. For hospitalized children, intravenous ampicillin and an aminoglycoside, or a cephalosporin, or amoxicillin-clavulanate is recommended. Add cloxacillin if staphylococcal pneumonia is suspected (if there has not been response to therapy in 48 hours, or if suggestive chest X-ray changes such as a pneumatocoele, empyema or abscess). Consider vancomycin if recent history of hospitalization. Pyogenic pleural effusions should be drained via an intercostal drain. For treatment of mycobacterial infections see Chapter 16: Paediatric tuberculosis.

Viral infections

Respiratory syncytial virus (RSV), parainfluenza virus, metapneumovirus, influenza virus and adenovirus cause pneumonia, which may be more severe than in immunocompetent children. Bronchiolitis is less common. Prolonged shedding of virus poses a risk for nosocomial transmission. Measles may produce a severe respiratory illness without the typical skin rash. High dose vitamin A will reduce severity of the measles.

The herpes viruses, including herpes simplex virus (HSV), varicella-zoster virus (VZV) and Epstein-Barr virus (EBV), occasionally cause pulmonary infection. Aciclovir should be given for VZV and HSV. Varicella-zoster immunoglobulin (VZIg) may prevent chickenpox if given within 72 hours of exposure.

Cytomegalovirus (CMV) can cause primary pneumonitis or severe, disseminated disease in HIV-infected children. CMV may occur in association with other pathogens especially PCP. Ganciclovir is most widely used, with an induction and maintenance dosage. Prophylaxis with oral ganciclovir or valganciclovir should be provided to severely immuno-suppressed children or those with a history of disseminated CMV disease until immune restoration on antiretroviral therapy.

Annual vaccination against influenza virus may be protective. Appropriate infection control and isolation policies for respiratory viruses are essential to prevent nosocomial transmission. Most spread is via contact with secretions: hand washing and equipment disinfection between patients is the most important preventative measure. Where possible, patients with viral respiratory infections should be segregated. Visitors and staff with any respiratory infection should avoid contact with hospitalized patients.

Fungal infections

Fungi are relatively uncommon causes of pneumonia in HIV-infected children except for *P. jirovecii*. Pulmonary candidiasis is unusual, occurring late as part of disseminated disease. *Cryptococcus neoformans, Histoplasma capsulatum, Coccidioides immitis* and *Aspergillus* species occasionally cause pneumonia as part of systemic infection.

Chronic lung disease

Chronic lung disease is common in HIV-infected children with increasing age, particularly in the absence of antiretroviral therapy. The spectrum includes chronic infections, lymphocytic interstitial pneumonia (LIP), immune reconstitution inflammatory syndrome (IRIS) bronchiectasis, malignancies, bronchiolitis obliterans and interstitial pneumonitis. Gastro-oesophageal reflux occurs commonly and may exacerbate respiratory disease. Children with chronic lung disease are candidates for antiretroviral therapy.

Chronic infections

These include:

- persistent pneumonia with or without collapse;
- recurrent pneumonia;
- destructive pneumonia with or without pleural space disease;
- tuberculosis;
- bronchiectasis.

Persistent pneumonia

HIV-infected children often have lung infections persisting for more than one month. Mucous plugging or lymphadenopathy contribute to atelectasis. Broncho-alveolar lavage (BAL) with physiotherapy may help to re-expand the lobe while antibiotics help to clear infection. Common causative pathogens include *S. pneumoniae, H. influenzae,* and occasionally *M. tuberculosis*.

Recurrent pneumonia

Children with LIP have increased susceptibility to recurrent bacterial infections, caused by the same organisms responsible for acute disease. Amoxillicin is given for least seven days. Non-responders should receive amoxicillin-clavulanate (combined with additional amoxicillin for penicillin-resistant *S. pneumoniae*) or cefuroxime. Failure to provide adequate treatment may promote drug resistance. Radiology may help to differentiate persistent from recurrent pneumonia.

Destructive pneumonia with or without pleural space disease

This occurs with partially treated infections or severe immunosuppression. There is breakdown in the lung parenchyma with or without cavity formation. Cavities may be thin or thick walled. Pneumatocoeles and bulging of the inter-hemispheric fissures may occur, with associated pleural effusions or empyema. Besides the common pathogens, *S milleri*, *S. viridans*, anaerobes and fungi are found. A straw-coloured effusion with parenchymal lung involvement suggests tuberculosis. Repeated antibiotic use predisposes to methicillin resistant *S. aureus* (MRSA). Patients at high risk for MRSA include those with recent hospitalization, treatment with cloxacillin, prolonged hospitalization and malnutrition. Treatment may be initiated with cloxacillin but non-responders should be changed to vancomycin. A search for the specific pathogen is mandatory. Pleural fluid should be drained with an intercostal drain for pyogenic effusions. Surgery should be considered early for unilateral localized disease or for thick pus.

Tuberculosis

See Chapter 16: Paediatric tuberculosis.

Bronchiectasis

Follicular and cystic changes within the lung and bronchial tree are seen in advanced HIV disease. Lymphocytic interstitial pneumonitis (LIP), TB, fungi and repeated bacterial infections are implicated. The common bacteria are *S. aureus, H. influenzae* and *K. pneumoniae*. Signs associated with bronchiectasis include clubbing, halitosis, cyanosis, chest deformity and persistent chest signs. Diagnostic evaluation includes chest radiographs, high resolution CT scan and lung function tests. Induced sputum samples or BAL fluid may identify secondary infections. Treatment includes physiotherapy, bronchodilators and antibiotics. There is no benefit from prophylactic antibiotics. Nebulized saline to encourage sputum production may relieve symptoms. Oxygen is sometimes required in advanced disease. Localized areas may be treated with surgery.

Chronic non-infectious diseases

Non-specific interstitial pneumonitis

This self-limiting disease presents as an interstitial lung disease secondary to viral infections, commonly respiratory syncitial virus (RSV) or adenovirus. The presentation is similar to other viral infections and the diagnosis is suggested by high resolution CT scan and confirmed by lung biopsy. No therapy is required as the clinical and radiological changes improve with time.

Lymphocytic interstitial pneumonitis (LIP)

LIP resulting from chronic lymphocytic infiltration of the lungs is common. The aetiology may be associated with Epstein-Barr virus. Clinical presentation includes clubbing, parotid enlargement, hepato-splenomegaly and generalised lymphadenopathy. Lung manifestations include slowly progressive dyspnoea with persistent cough and occasional wheeze. Radiological features include reticular, reticular-nodular or nodular infiltrates and lymphadenopathy (photo 5). Non-specific eleva-tion of serum globulin and LDH has been described. Lung biopsy is seldom performed. Prednisone 1 mg/kg/d for two wks, followed by a tapering dose for further four to six weeks may help if the child is very symptomatic. LIP is a WHO stage 3 condition requiring antiretroviral therapy.

Immune reconstitution inflammatory syndrome (IRIS)

See Chapter 50: Immune reconstitution inflammatory syndrome.

Malignancy

Kaposi's sarcoma is the commonest pulmonary malignancy in HIV-infected African children, and may produce upper airway obstruction. Pulmonary dissemination causes chronic progressive dyspnoea, cough, and fever; haemoptysis occurs with endobronchial lesions. Chest radio-graphs are non-specific, revealing bilateral interstitial patterns, nodular infiltrates, focal opacification with mediastinal lymphadenopathy or pleural effusions. Diagnosis can be made at bronchoscopy where multiple purple flat lesions are seen, or on histology.

HIV-infected children have a higher incidence of lymphoma than immunocompetent children. Lymphoma may involve the respiratory tract. Chest radiographs may show focal parenchymal opacities, mediastinal lymphadenopathy or pleural effusions. Diagnosis is by biopsy.

Table 32.1 Pulmonary diseases occurring in HIV-infected children

INFECTIOUS DISEASES

Bacterial

S. pneumoniae
H. influenzae
S. aureus
M. tuberculosis
M. avium complex
K. pneumonia
P. aeruginosa

Viral

RSV
Adenovirus
Parainfluenza
Influenza
Metapneumovirus
Measles virus
CMV
HSV
VZV
EBV

Fungal

P. jirovecii
Candida species
Aspergillus species
C. immitis
C. neoformans
H. capsulatum

NON-INFECTIOUS COMPLICATIONS

Interstitial pneumonia

Lymphocytic interstitial pneumonia
Non-specific interstitial pneumonia

Malignancies

Kaposi's sarcoma
Lymphoma
Leiomyoma

Other

Reactive airways
Bronchiolitis obliterans
Congestive cardiac failure with cardiomyopathy

HIV pulmonary disease in adults

As in children, pulmonary disease is a major cause of illness and death in adults with HIV infection. Approximately 70% of HIV-positive patients will have at least one respiratory episode during the course of their disease. At postmortem, the lungs are affected in about 90% of cases. Pulmonary complications in HIV/AIDS are best considered as either infectious or non-infectious. Abnormalities in pulmonary function tests can occur in the absence of clinical disease. The CD4 count may be useful as a correlate with the development of specific diseases (see Table 32.2). Appendix 32.1 gives details of chest radiograph findings in HIV-associated lung disease.

Table 32.2 Selected disease conditions listed by usual CD4 count at the time of diagnosis

CD4 count	Disease condition
<500 cells/μl	Sinusitis/mastoiditis/otitis
	Bronchitis
	Bacterial pneumonia
	Pulmonary TB
<200 cells/μl	PCP
	KS
	Disseminated TB
<100 cells/μl	Disseminated MAC
	CMV disease
	Disseminated fungal infections

Note: Conditions listed in higher CD4 categories continue to present with increased frequency at lower CD4 counts.

Infectious complications

Upper respiratory tract infections

Otitis media and sinusitis occur with increased frequency in HIV patients. The clinical features are the same as those in non-HIV-infected patients. Symptomatic chronic sinusitis affects up to 16% of HIV-positive patients and is especially common in advanced disease. A chronic cough with purulent post-nasal discharge suggests this diagnosis. In this setting, opportunistic pathogens may be responsible. Initial treatment is with amoxicillin 1.0 g three times daily and metronidazole 400 mg three times daily.

Community-acquired pneumonia

Bacteria, *Pnuemocystis jirovecii*, atypical organisms and TB can all present as community-acquired pneumonia in HIV-infected adults.

Bacterial pneumonia occurs very commonly, and is more frequent in the HIV population than in the general population. *Streptococcus pneumoniae* and *Haemophilus influenzae* are the most common pathogens. *Staphylococcus aureus* and Gram-negative organisms including *Klebsiella pneumoniae* are seen in advanced disease. The clinical presentation is usually that of a typical, community-acquired pneumonia. Bacterial pneumonia in HIV patients has a higher rate of complications, including intrapulmonary cavitation, abscess formation, and empyaema. The overall mortality, however, is similar to that of the non-HIV-infected population.

Pneumocystis jirovecii pneumonia (PCP) occurs after re-infection with airborne organisms. The clinical presentation of PCP depends on the severity of the infection. (See Table 32.2.)

Table 32.3 Clinical assessment of the severity of *Pneumocystis* pneumonia

	Mild	Moderate	Severe
Symptoms	Dyspnoea on exertion	Dyspnoea on mild exertion	Dyspnoea at rest
Arterial PaO2*	>11 kPa	8.1–11 kPa	<8 kPa
Arterial oxygen* saturation at rest	>94%	90–94%	<90%
Chest radiograph	Normal or perihilar shadowing	Interstital shadowing	Extensive alveolar shadowing

*In room air

Appendix 32.2 shows a diagnostic strategy for patients with community acquired pneumonia.

Treatment of community-acquired pneumonia

Patients with uncomplicated pneumonia, without respiratory distress and normal oxygen saturations in room air can be managed as outpatients. Bacterial pneumonia should be treated with:

amoxicillin-clavulanate with additional amoxicillin or 2nd generation cephalosporin; and

macrolide, azalide or tetracycline.

Table 32.4 summarizes drug treatment for PCP.

Patients with any of the following factors should be hospitalized:

physical frailty or advanced age (>65 years);

multilobar opacification;

respiratory rate >30 breaths/minute;

arterial oxygen saturation <92% in room air;

poor socio-economic circumstances;

altered mental status (confusion);

urea >7.0 mmol/L ;

systolic blood pressure <90 mmHg, diastolic blood pressure <60 mmHg.

The decision on whether to treat in an intensive care unit can be difficult: see Chapter 33: Intensive care management.

Hospitalized patients should be treated with:

intravenous amoxicillin-clavulanate or 2nd generation cephalosporin or 3rd generation cephalosporin;

macrolide, azalide or tetracycline.

All patients with PCP and hypoxia should receive adjunctive cortico-steroids as this decreases the likelihood of respiratory failure, deteriora-tion, and death. The largest controlled trial showing corticosteroids to be beneficial used the following dosages of prednisone (or an equivalent):

days 1–5: 80 mg/day;

days 6–10: 40 mg /day; and

days 11–21: 20 mg/day.

See Chapter 22: Adult tuberculosis, for details on diagnosing and treating HIV-associated tuberculosis.

Pneumocystis jirovecii pneumonia prophylaxis

See Chapter 22: Primary prophylaxis and immunization.

Table 32.4 Drug treatment of *Pneumocystis jirovecii* pneumonia

Treatment	Drug	Dose/route	Comments	Side-effects
First-line	Co-trimoxazole	15/75 mg/kg d. IV or oral (in divided doses)*	Any grade of pneumonia	Rash GIT disturbance Bone marrow toxicity
Second-line	Pentamidine	4 mg/kg/d. slow IV infusion	Severe PCP	Hypotension Hypoglycaemia Pancreatitis Cardiac arrythmias
Second-line	Dapsone-trimethoprim	Dapsone 100 mg (oral) daily and trimethoprim 300 mg (oral)	Mild to moderate PCP	Bone marrow toxicity Rash GIT disturbances Avoid in G6PD† deficiency
Third-line	Clindamycin-primaquine‡	Clindamycin 450–600 mg 3x/d.(oral) and primaquine‡ 15 mg/d. (oral)	Mild to moderate PCP	Maculopapular rash *C. difficile* diarrhoea Avoid in G6PD† deficiency
Fourth-line	Atovaquone	750 mg 2x/d.	Mild to moderate PCP	Rash GIT intolerance

*Typical adult dose: co-trimoxazole 80/400 mg—4 tablets 8 hourly.

† G6PD: glucose-6-phosphate dehydrogenase.

‡ Available in South Africa on named patient basis only.

Table 32.5 Prophylaxis of *Pneumocystis jirovecii* pneumonia

Prophylaxis	Drug	Dosage	Side-effects
First-line	Co-trimoxazole 80/400 mg	2 tablets/d.	Rash Bone marrow suppression GIT disturbances
Alternatives	Co-trimoxazole 80/400 mg Co-trimoxazole 80/400 mg	2 tablets 3 x/wk. I tablet/d.	
Second-line	Dapsone	100 mg/d.	Rash GIT disturbance Haemolytic anaemia in G6PD deficiency*
Third-line	Atovaquone	750 mg 2x/d.	Rash Deranged liver function tests
Fourth-line	Nebulized pentamidine	300 mg/mo. via jet nebulizer	Bronchospasm Metallic taste Renal impairment Hypoglycaemia Pancreatitis

*G6PD: glucose-6-phosphate dehydrogenase.

Tuberculosis prophylaxis

See Chapter 22: Primary prophylaxis and immunization.

Fungal infections

These include cryptococcosis, histoplasmosis, blastomycosis, aspergillosis sporotrichosis, and coccidioidomycosis.

- Cryptococcal pneumonia usually presents as part of a disseminated infection with meningitis and fungaemia. Chest radiograph patterns include large nodules, non-confluent opacification, and cavitation (see photo 6). Enlarged nodes or pleural effusions are uncommon.
- Aspergillus pulmonary infections are rare and occur in patients with advanced disease, who are often neutropenic. Aspergillomas may become locally invasive.

Disseminated histoplasmosis is rare in South Africa. It typically presents with nodular skin rash, oral ulcers, and a diffuse micro-nodular pattern on chest radiograph (see photo 7).

Treatment

The initial treatment for severe fungal infections is amphotericin B. For less severe disease, an alternative and less toxic therapy is fluconazole for cryptococcus and itraconazole for histoplasma and aspergillus. These agents are also used in maintenance therapy, as relapse rates are high following cessation of treatment.

Cytomegalovirus

Cytomegalovirus (CMV) This virus may cause retinitis, oesophagitis, gastritis, colitis, hepatitis, encephalitis, pneumonia, and death in patients with very low CD4 counts. Clinically significant pneumonia is unusual even though CMV is often isolated from the lung. CMV tends to co-exist with other pathogens such as *P. jirovecii*, and treatment directed at these pathogens often leads to resolution. Diagnosis rests on the demonstration of intranuclear or cytoplasmic inclusion bodies within lung cells (including alveolar macrophages) in the absence of other pathogens.

Treatment

The treatment of established CMV pneumonitis in AIDS is intravenous ganciclovir (5 mg/kg twice daily for 14 days). This drug can cause bone marrow suppression and the blood count should be monitored regularly. Intravenous foscarnet is an alternative, although this drug has associated nephrotoxicity.

Neoplastic diseases of the lung

Neoplastic diseases of the lung include:
- Kaposi's sarcoma (KS);
- non-Hodgkin's lymphoma (NHL);
- bronchial carcinoma.

Kaposi's sarcoma

This is the most common HIV-associated malignancy.
- Pulmonary KS is almost always accompanied by mucocutaneous or lymphadenopathic KS, but this is not always present.

- The presence of KS involving the soft palate or pharynx is strongly predictive of the presence of pulmonary KS.
- The usual presentation is one of progressive shortness of breath and cough.
- Haemoptysis is rare.
- The chest radiograph is non-specific, usually involving middle and lower zones bilaterally and symmetrically, with irregular nodules. Pleural effusions are common. (See photo 8).

Treatment

See Chapter 41: Oncology.

Non-Hodgkin's lymphoma

- NHL is usually high-grade, of B-cell origin, and occurs in late-stage disease.
- It may involve intrathoracic lymph nodes, pleura, and pulmonary parenchyma (multiple nodules or localized opacities are present on chest radiograph).
- The prognosis is generally poor despite chemotherapy, and median survival is <1 year.

Smoking and HIV infection

HIV-infection is associated with a 2.5 times increased risk of bronchial carcinoma in smokers. Smoking is also associated with worse HIV-associated symptoms and worse quality of life, which improve within three months of quitting.

Smokers should be encouraged at each visit to quit smoking. Strategies include:

- nicotine replacement therapy with patches or gum;
- motivational counselling and support;
- drug therapy (e.g. bupropion – note potential for interactions with non-nucleoside reverse transcriptase inhibitors and protease inhibitors).

Other pulmonary disorders

Chronic bronchitis and bronchiectasis

There is increased incidence of these conditions in patients with HIV. They are seen in advanced HIV infection, even in non-smokers. The reason for the increased incidence is unknown.

Treatment

Treatment is in the standard manner, but recurrences are common, especially when *P. aeruginosa* is isolated from the sputum.

Spontaneous pneumothorax

This is almost always caused by PCP, but has been described in patients with LIP and KS.

Treatment

Treatment is with intercostal drainage, with or without pleurodesis.

Non-specific interstitial pneumonitis

- may occur at any stage of disease;
- may be asymptomatic; and
- may be diagnosed by biopsy.

Patients usually present with increasing dyspnoea. Examination reveals late inspiratory crackles at both lung bases.

Treatment

Therapy is with corticosteroids in those who are symptomatic.

Bronchiolitis obliterans organizing pneumonia

The clinical presentation is similar to that seen in HIV-negative patients. This includes:
- cough;
- dyspnoea;
- constitutional symptoms;
- crackles on chest auscultation; and
- patchy infiltrates on the chest radiograph.

A lung biopsy is necessary for diagnosis.

Treatment

Treatment is with corticosteroids.

Primary pulmonary hypertension

This occurs more commonly among HIV-infected patients than in the general population. Treatment should be discussed with a pulmonologist.

References and further reading

American Academy of Pediatrics. 2003. *Human Immunodeficiency Virus Infection*. In Pickering, L.K. ed. Red Book: Report of the Committee of Infectious Diseases. 26th ed.

Cadranel, J. et al. 2006 'Lung cancer in HIV infected patients: facts, questions and challenges.' *Thorax*; 61:1000–1008.

Chintu, P.C., Bhat G., Walker, A., Mulenga, V., Sinyinza, F., Lishimpi, K. et al. 2004. 'Co-trimoxazole as prophylaxis against opportunistic infections in HIV-infected Zambian children (CHAP): a double-blind randomised placebo-controlled trial.' *Lancet*; 364(9448):1865–1871.

Guidelines for cotrimoxazole prophylaxis for HIV-related infections among children, adolescents and adults in resource-limited settings. Recommendations for a public health approach. WHO 2006. Available: http/www.who.int/hiv/pub/guidelines/ctx.

Jeena, P.M., Coovadia, H.M., Thula, S.A. et al. 1998. 'Persistent and chronic lung disease in HIV-1 infected and uninfected African children.' *AIDS*; 12(11) 81-87.

Mofenson, L.M., Oleske, J., Serchuck, L., Van Dyke, R., Wilfert, C. 2005. 'Treating opportunistic infections among HIV-exposed and infected children: Recommendations from CDC, the National Institutes of Health, and the Infectious Diseases Society of America.' *Clinical Infectious Diseases*; 40:S1–84.

Zar, H.J. 2003. 'Prevention of HIV-associated respiratory disease in developing countries: potential benefits.' *International Journal of Tuberculosis and Lung Disease*. 7(9):820–827.

Zar, H.J. 2004. 'Pneumonia in HIV-infected and uninfected children in developing countries – epidemiology, clinical features and management.' *Current Opinion in Pulmonary Medicine*; 10(3):176–182.

Appendix 32.1 Chest radiographic patterns and common diagnoses in HIV (in order of likelihood)

Radiographic pattern	Diagnoses
Focal infiltrates	Bacteria *Mycobacterium tuberculosis* Fungi *Pneumocystis jirovecii*
Diffuse infiltrates	*Pneumocystis jirovecii* *Mycobacterium tuberculosis* Kaposi's sarcoma Lymphocytic interstital pneumonitis Cytomegalovirus Bacteria
Diffuse nodular infiltrates	Kaposi's sarcoma (large nodules) *M. tuberculosis* (nodular or miliary) Fungi (small nodules)
Pneumothorax	*Pneumocystis jirovecii* Lymphocytic interstital pneumonitis
Mediastinal lymphadenopathy	*Mycobacterium tuberculosis* Kaposi's sarcoma Lymphoma Fungi
Pleural effusion	*Mycobacterium tuberculosis* Kaposi's sarcoma Bacteria Lymphoma Fungi Pulmonary oedema Hypoproteinaemia
Cavitation	*Mycobacterium tuberculosis* *Pneumocystis jirovecii* *P. aeruginosa* (low CD4 count) *Rhodococcus equii* (low CD4 count) Fungi (low CD4 count) Nocardia (low CD4 count)

Appendix 32.2 Diagnostic strategy for community acquired pneumonia

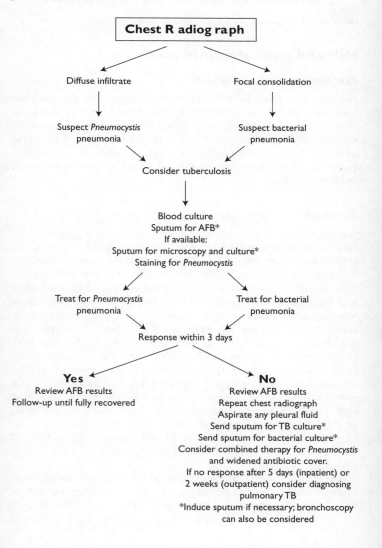

Intensive care management

HIV and paediatric intensive care

Ventilation in the newborn

The short-term outcome of mechanically ventilated HIV-exposed newborns is similar to that of HIV-uninfected children, so they should be offered ventilatory support. The aetiology of acute respiratory failure in newborns with HIV infection is similar to HIV-uninfected children but the spectrum of opportunistic infections is different: HIV-infected children acquire congenital tuberculosis and CMV more frequently *in utero* than uninfected children.

Ventilation in the older child

The availability of ICU services is extremely limited, especially in countries with the largest burden of HIV disease. In the USA children with HIV-1-related acute respiratory failure requiring mechanical ventilation have reported survival rates of between 50-81%. In HIV-infected children *Pneumocystis* pneumonia (PCP) is associated with a poorer outcome than with bacterial pneumonia. HIV-infected children with respiratory failure requiring mechanical ventilation have a higher mortality than those admitted to ICU for non-respiratory conditions. Since the introduction of corticosteroids for PCP, acute and long-term survival has improved. However, the benefits of corticosteroids for PCP in children on mechanical ventilation may not be as marked if children referred for mechanical ventilation have received prior corticosteroids. Factors predictive of a worse outcome in developed countries, such as CD4 counts <50 cells µl, LDH >1 000 IU, serum albumin <20 g/dl, serum creatinine >24 µg/dl, persistent hypoxaemia, pneumothoraces and a diagnosis of AIDS for <1 year duration have limited value in developing countries. Many of these tests are not routinely available; moreover, they are influenced by underlying malnutrition.

The outcome of HIV-infected ventilated children in Africa varies. Initial studies from Durban and Johannesburg confirmed a high mortality of between 87% to 100% among children with AIDS. HIV-negative children had outcomes similar to asymptomatic and symptomatic HIV-infected patients without AIDS. The commonest causes of death were PCP with associated cytomegalovirus (CMV) infection in Durban. Recent data from Cape Town have shown improved outcome of HIV-infected children admitted to a paediatric ICU with an in-hospital mortality rate of 29%, but the treatment regimes, ventilation strategies and selection criteria at entry were different to those in the previous studies. No specific factors could be identified to predict a better outcome in HIV-infected children.

In deciding whether to admit HIV-infected children to a paediatric ICU, many factors must be considered. These include the child's underlying illness, prognosis, social circumstances and the resources available. Such decisions are made increasingly difficult as the demand for ICU beds increases as a result of progression of the HIV epidemic. Where resources are scarce conservative management outside the ICU is warranted for children with a poor prognosis as a third may improve. Outcome of HIV-infected infants with PCP requiring mechanical ventilation is still unfavourable. Recent trends include empiric co-treatment for PCP and CMV together with initiating antiretroviral therapy in the ICU.

HIV and adult intensive care

Decision making can be difficult as the patient's right to health care needs to be weighed against medium-term prognosis and restricted ICU resources. Indications for mechanical ventilation include:

- community-acquired pneumonia;
- acute demyelinating polyneuropathy;
- severe sepsis and septic shock;
- trauma;
- obstetric conditions; and
- postoperative support.

HIV-infected patients who are not severely wasted, who have not had a prior AIDS-defining diagnosis or who have good antiretroviral options are usually suitable candidates for ICU management. Note that previous pulmonary or extrapulmonary TB should probably not be considered AIDS-defining in high TB prevalence areas. The prognosis of conditions not associated with HIV is usually much better than that of HIV-associated conditions.

Respiratory failure

Patients with advanced HIV disease who present with respiratory failure and diffuse pulmonary infiltrates on chest radiograph (suggesting PCP or disseminated TB) are usually not offered ventilation, as mortality rates exceed 50% even in the developed world. An exception may be patients who develop respiratory failure as a result of immune reconstitution inflammatory syndrome due to PCP after starting antiretroviral therapy, as prognosis seems to be good. Other conditions should be excluded and corticosteroids should be used with high dose co-trimoxazole.

Patients with respiratory failure who are not offered ICU admission should receive supplemental oxygen given with continuous positive airway pressure (CPAP), intravenous antibiotics, treatment for PCP, corticosteroids, and considered for antituberculous treatment. Difficult decisions should be discussed with an experienced colleague.

Management of severe sepsis

Severe sepsis and septic shock is common in HIV-infected patients and aggressive goal-oriented resuscitation before admission to the ICU can be life saving. (See Chapter 20: Common emergencies.)

Use of antiretroviral therapy in the ICU

In general antiretroviral therapy should be continued in patients admitted to ICU. This should be administered regularly in the pre-operative and post-operative period, using liquid formulations and the nasogastric route if necessary. If ileus develops antiretroviral therapy should probably be discontinued, using intravenous zidovudine for seven to 14 days to cover the long half-life 'tail' of nevirapine and efavirenz. Importantly, the non-nucleoside reverse transcriptase inhibitors and protease inhibitors interfere with the cytochrome P450-mediated excretion of drugs commonly used in the ICU, for example interfering with the pharmacokinetics of midazolam, amiodarone and the calcium channel blockers. Potential interactions can be checked on Internet sites such as www.hiv-druginteractions.org.

Antiretroviral therapy can be initiated in the ICU under specialist supervision after the risk-benefit ratio has been considered. Problems associated with antiretroviral therapy in the ICU include drug interactions, immune reconstitution, and poor absorption leading to viral resistance. The benefits of antiretroviral initiation are largely theoretical and include improved immune function, reduced HIV viral load, and more rapid recovery. Enteral feeding should be well established and diarrhoea controlled before therapy is initiated. Patients who recover will need intensive antiretroviral counselling and good social support.

References and further reading

Bedos, J.P. et al. 1999. '*Pneumocystis carinii* pneumonia requiring intensive care management: Survival and prognostic study in 110 patients with human immunodeficiency virus'. *Critical Care Medicine*; 27 (6):1109–1115.

Dellinger, R.P. et al. 2008. 'Surviving Sepsis Campaign: International guidelines for management of severe sepsis and septic shock: 2008.' *Critical Care Medicine*; 36 (1):296–327.

Dickson, S.J. et al. 2007. 'Survival of HIV-infected patients in the intensive care unit in the era of highly active antiretroviral therapy.' *Thorax*; 62:964–968.

Morris, A. et al. 2006. 'Current issues in critical care of the human immunodeficiency virus-infected patient.' *Critical Care Medicine*; 34 (1):42–49.

Walzer, P.D. et al. 2008. 'Early Predictors of Mortality from *Pneumocystis jirovecii* Pneumonia in HIV-Infected Patients:1985–2006.' *Clinical Infectious Diseases.*; 46:625–633.

Endocrinology and metabolic abnormalities

Endocrine abnormalities and metabolic disturbances can present in many different contexts in HIV-infected patients, most notably during advanced disease, while taking antiretroviral therapy, and during immune reconstitution. Fascinating links between HIV infection, the immune system and metabolic abnormalities are beginning to emerge.

Paediatric endocrine problems

Endocrinological problems in HIV-infected children are relatively uncommon. However good scientific data for the paediatric age group is limited. Endocrine dysfunction may not be readily apparent. The presentation may be non-specific and often similar to florid HIV disease. Conversely children with abnormal laboratory values may appear entirely asymptomatic

Poor growth and pubertal delay

Poor growth (in height) occurs in about 50% of HIV-infected children. The majority is due to non-endocrine causes, i.e. inadequate intake, enteropathy, the catabolic state or the non-specific effect of any chronic disease, commonly identified as 'failure to thrive'. Wasting is the hallmark of advanced infection. Anthropometric assessment including length/height, weight and (ideally) body mass index (BMI) is essential for proper diagnosis. The BMI (weight/(height)^2) is plotted on an age and gender specific BMI chart. Children with a low BMI have a high mortality. Management always includes correction of nutritional deficiencies and treatment of underlying infections. Consider endocrine causes, especially deficiency of growth, sex or thyroid hormones, when a low height velocity or short stature is associated with a high BMI. Remember that in children on antiretroviral therapy, weight increases out of proportion to height.

Girls should enter puberty not later than 13.5 years and boys not later than 14 years. The onset of puberty is delayed by up to two years in girls and by up to one year in boys with perinatal HIV infection possibly related to the chronic disease or to unfavourable environmental conditions. If the clinical picture for short stature or delayed puberty suggests an endocrine problem and the child is otherwise appropriately managed (i.e. on adequate nutrition, infections treated and on antiretroviral therapy), hypothyroidism should be excluded (see below) and the help of a paediatric endocrinologist should be sought. Lipoatrophy occurs commonly in children, most likely linked to stavudine. A single drug switch from stavudine to abacavir is indicated if viral suppression is confirmed.

Adult endocrine problems

Lipodystropy, the metabolic syndrome and atherogenesis

Patients with HIV appear to be at increased risk of premature atherosclerotic disease, especially myocardial infarction and stroke. The role of individual antiretrovirals in contributing to this risk is complex, and unfolding largely from observational cohorts. Atherosclerotic plaques are inflammatory lesions in the intima of large and medium sized arteries. The key inflammatory cell is the cholesterol-laden macrophage ('foam cell'). Plaques can limit arterial blood flow and, more seriously, can rupture, causing arterial occlusion from local thrombus formation or distal thromboembolisation. Clinical consequences of atherosclerosis include myocardial infarction, cerebral infarction and peripheral vascular disease.

This risk is partially mediated by changes linked to antiretroviral therapy such as:

- lipodystropy;
- an unfavourable lipid profile (elevated triglycerides (TG), elevated total cholesterol (TC), elevated low density lipoprotein cholesterol (LDL-C) and low high density lipoprotein cholesterol (HDL-C));
- insulin resistance and type 2 diabetes mellitus;
- endothelial dysfunction.

HIV is also associated with atherosclerosis by causing:

- endovascular inflammation and endothelial activation;
- high levels of LDL-C and triglycerides, and low levels of HDL;
- abnormal cholesterol metabolism in infected macrophages;
- low CD4 count (immune suppression associated with increased atherosclerotic risk).

Atherosclerotic risk is also determined by traditional factors such as: family history of (or genetic predisposition to) coronary artery disease; increased LDL-C, apolipoprotein B levels and triglyceride levels; low HDL-C; diabetes; male gender; older age; hypertension; and smoking history.

Three categories of antiretroviral-associated lipodystrophy are recognised:

- Lipoatrophy is the loss of subcutaneous fat tissue due to adipocyte apoptosis and involves the face, limbs, buttocks and abdominal wall. Lipoatrophy is usually associated with nucleoside reverse transcriptase inhibitors, especially stavudine, didanosine and zidovudine, and may be due to damage to adipose cell mitochondria.
- Lipohypertrophy is conventionally associated with the protease inhibitors and is the expansion of intra-abdominal visceral adipose tissue, and may be associated with a dorsocervical fat pad ('buffalo hump'). There is some evidence that visceral fat accumulation is actually simply a normal age and lifestyle side effect, and may be accentuated by lipoatrophy. The 'buffalo hump' is made up of brown fat, and the precise aetiology and causation is speculative.
- The presence of both subcutaneous lipoatrophy and visceral lipohypertrophy is known as fat redistribution.

Lipoatrophy causes reduced levels of the adipokine adiponectin, which is associated with insulin resistance, type 2 diabetes and atherosclerosis. Lipohypertrophy and increased intra-abdominal fat is also associated with insulin resistance and type 2 diabetes. Interestingly visceral adiposity is associated with reduced nocturnal secretion of growth hormone and insulin-like growth factor 1. Administration of a growth hormone-releasing hormone analogue corrects this abnormality, decreases abdominal visceral fat, reduces triglyceride levels and increases HDL-C levels. Long term effects on insulin resistance and atherogenic risk are unknown.

Clinically, metabolic abnormalities are translated into atherosclerotic risk by determining whether diagnostic criteria for the metabolic syndrome are present. The metabolic syndrome can be diagnosed using the 2006 International Diabetes Federation definition – these criteria were developed for the general population but can also be used for HIV-infected patients. For a person to be defined as having the metabolic syndrome the following must be present:

- central obesity (defined as waist circumference ≥94 cm for Europid men and ≥80 cm for Europid women – these values are also used for men and women of sub-Saharan decent until additional data become available);

Plus any two of the following four factors:
- raised TG level: ≥1.7 mmol/L, or specific treatment for this lipid abnormality;
- reduced HDL cholesterol: <1.03 mmol/L in males and <1.29 mmol/L in women, or specific treatment for this lipid abnormality;
- raised blood pressure: systolic BP ≥130 or diastolic BP ≥85 mmHg, or treatment of previously diagnosed hypertension;
- raised fasting plasma glucose ≥5.6 mmol/L, or previously diagnosed type 2 diabetes.

Waist circumference is measured by locating the top of the right iliac crest and placing a measuring tape in a horizontal plane around the abdomen at level of the iliac crest. Before reading the tape measure, ensure that the tape is snug but does not compress the skin and is parallel to the floor. Measurement is made at the end of a normal expiration.

Diabetes mellitus is diagnosed on two separate glucose blood samples of >7.0 mmol/L (fasting) or >11.1 (non-fasting or two hours after a 75 g glucose load).

Management of the metabolic syndrome is focused on:
- lifestyle modification including quitting smoking, moderate exercise, weight control, moderate alcohol intake, reduction in dietary salt, increased intake of fresh fruit and vegetables and low fat dairy products;
- reducing LDL-C to <3.4 mmol/L (<1.8 mmol/L for patients with diabetes, or coronary artery disease, or stroke or carotid artery stenosis >50%); low dose atorvastatin or pravastatin can be used for patients taking a protease inhibitor; simvastatin can be used for patients taking efavirenz or nevirapine but not a protease inhibitor;
- normalizing triglyceride and HDL-C levels using a fibrate (e.g. gemfibrozil) with or without niacin (photo 9);
- blood pressure reduction to <140/90 (non-diabetics) or <130/80 (diabetics or chronic kidney disease) initially using low dose thiazide diuretics and angiotensin converting enzyme inhibitors or angiotensin receptor blockers;
- treatment of diabetes mellitus with additional dietary measures, metformin and/or a thiazolidinedione (e.g. rosiglitazone), and insulin to achieve a haemoglobin A_{1C} of <7%. Detailed guidelines on the management of diabetes can be accessed at http://professional.diabetes.org/.

Note that:

- Cholesterol cannot be accurately measured if the triglyceride is >4.5 mmol/L.
- Undiagnosed alcohol abuse, diabetes, hypothyroidism, nephrotic syndrome or chronic renal failure can exacerbate lipid abnormalities, as can medications such as high dose thiazide diuretics, beta blockers, oral oestrogen, progesterone and testosterone.
- It is desirable to switch stavudine or zidovudine to tenofovir or abacavir for patients with lipodystrophy, hyperlipidaemia or the metabolic syndrome (this may not be possible in the state sector).
- Unlike nevirapine, efavirenz is associated with elevated LDL-C and triglycerides.
- Atazanavir is the only protease inhibitor not associated with lipid abnormalities (this advantage is lost when boosted with ritonavir).
- Antiretroviral treatment interruptions are associated with an athero-genic lipid profile, and increased risk of cardiovascular death.
- There is a theoretical risk of myopathy with combined statin and fibrate therapy.
- Cholestyramine should not be used due to unknown effects on antiretroviral absorption and risk of elevated triglyceride levels.
- Metformin and the thiazolidinediones reduce insulin resistance but do not improve lipodystrophy.

Other endocrine disorders

HIV infection can mimic endocrine disorders including:

- hyperthyroidism – weight loss, sweats, tachycardia, diarrhoea, tremor, lid retraction (see photo 9);
- hypothyroidism – fatigue, depression, slowed mentation, cold intoler-ance, dry skin;
- adrenal insufficiency – diarrhoea, hypotension, hyponatraemia, hyper-pigmentation.

However, true endocrine disorders are encountered in HIV-infected patients and the clinician should request appropriate testing if an alter-nate diagnosis is not readily apparent.

Immune reconstitution Graves' disease

Hyperthyroidism due to autoimmune production of thyroid stimulating hormone (TSH) receptor stimulating antibodies occurs 12 to 36 months after initiation of antiretroviral therapy, (i.e. later than immune reconstitution against opportunistic infections). The diagnosis is made by demonstrating elevated T4 and T3, suppressed TSH and uniformly increased uptake of radioactive iodine by the thyroid gland. Symptoms can be controlled by propranolol, and T4 and T3 levels by titrated doses of carbimazole. Further management should be in consultation with an endocrinologist or physician and may include prolonged treatment with carbimazole or ablation of the thyroid gland with radioactive iodine.

Hypothyroidism

Low T4 and T3 levels and elevated TSH have been linked to the use of stavudine, but the association has not been consistently demonstrated. However hypothyroidism is common in the general population (0.3%) and can occur in HIV-infected patients. Delayed relaxation of the tendon jerk is a useful clinical sign suggesting the diagnosis. Routine screening is not recommended. Treatment is with levothyroxine titrated to keep the TSH within the normal range.

Sick euthyroid syndrome

Thyroid hormone levels should not be checked during acute illness as the T4 and T3 levels can be transiently suppressed with elevation of TSH just outside the normal range. Elevated rT3 is typical but is not measured in routine practice.

Adrenal insufficiency

The adrenal glands have considerable functional reserve, and although affected by infections (tuberculosis, cytomegalovirus, fungi) and malignancies (lymphoma, Kaposi's sarcoma), adrenal insufficiency is seldom seen in HIV-infected patients. Clinical clues to the diagnosis include advanced HIV disease, treatment with rifampicin (which increases cortisol excretion), eosinophilia and hyperkalaemia. The diagnosis is made by demonstrating low serum cortisol or suboptimal response to synthetic corticotropin stimulation test.

Septic shock refractory to inotropic support suggests sub-clinical adrenal insufficiency, and some patients in the intensive care setting may benefit from hydrocortisone 50 mg intravenously eight hourly.

Recently, adrenal suppression has been described in patients taking ritonavir-boosted protease inhibitors with inhaled corticosteroids for the treatment of asthma. Excretion of exogenous corticosteroids is delayed by ritonavir-mediated inhibition of cytochrome P450, resulting in suppression of pituitary corticotropin and adrenal hypoplasia. Life-threatening cortisol insufficiency can occur during intercurrent infections.

Metabolic bone disease

HIV infection is associated with an increased incidence of osteopenia in children and young adults. Initiation of antiretrovirals is associated with short-term loss of bone density, presumably due to alterations in inflammatory cytokines. Long-term follow up data are required as the HIV-infected population ages. Antiretroviral therapy does not affect bone mineral density, although there is some data of bone demineralisation associated with tenofovir. Screening for osteoporosis should be focused on patients with multiple risk factors such as:

- history of low trauma fracture;
- low body mass index;
- smoking;
- being post-menopausal;
- HIV infection for more than seven years.

DEXA scanning and measurements of bone density in the lumber spine and hip are used to determine the need for treatment. Treatment with bisphosphonates, calcium carbonate 1.0 g daily and vitamin D 400 U daily increases bone mineral density.

Recommended reading and references

Alberti, G. et al. 2006. *The IDF consensus worldwide definition of the metabolic syndrome.* Available: http://www.idf.org/webdata/docs/IDF_Meta_def_final.pdf

Amorosa, V. et al. 2006. 'Bone disease and HIV infection.' *Clinical Infectious Diseases*; 42:108–114.

Blackman, M.R. 2007. 'Manipulation of the growth hormone axis in patients with HIV infection.' *New England Journal of Medicine.* 357:2397–2399.

Carr, A. et al. 2006 'Does HIV cause cardiovascular disease?' *PLoS Medicine*; 3 (11) e495–496.

DAD Study Group. 2007 'Class of antiretroviral drugs and the risk of myocardial infarction.' *New England Journal of Medicine*; 356(17): 1723–1735.

Fisher, S.D. et al. 2006. 'Impact of HIV and highly active antiretroviral therapy on leukocyte adhesion molecules, arterial inflammation, dyslipidemia, and atherosclerosis.' *Atherosclerosis*; 185:1–11.

Grundy, S.M. 2005. 'Diagnosis and Management of the Metabolic Syndrome: An American Heart Association/National Heart, Lung, and Blood Institute Scientific Statement.' *Circulation*; 112: 2735–2752.

Hoffmann, G.J. et al. 2007. 'Thyroid function abnormalities in HIV infected patients.' *Clinical Infectious Diseases*; 45:488–494.

Mayo, J. et al. 2002. 'Adrenal function in the human immunodeficiency virus-infected patient.' *Archives of Internal Medicine*; 162:1095–1098.

Meya, B.D. et al. 2007. 'Functional adrenal insufficiency among critically ill patients with human immunodeficiency virus in a resource-limited setting.' *African Health Sciences*; 7:101–107.

'Third report of the National Cholesterol Education Programme expert panel on detection, evaluation and treatment of high blood cholesterol in adults (Adult Treatment Panel III) executive summary.' *NIH publication* No. 01–3607 May 2001.

Sweeny, L.L. et al. 2007. 'The role of adipokines in relation to HIV lipodystrophy.' *AIDS*; 21:895–904.

Wohl, D.A. et al. 2006. 'Current Concepts in the Diagnosis and Management of Metabolic Complications of HIV Infection and Its Therapy.' *Clinical Infectious Diseases*; 43:645–653.

Neurological symptoms occur during all stages of HIV infection. Before the advent of highly active antiretroviral therapy, it was estimated that 40%-70% of people infected with HIV developed symptomatic neurological disturbances. All levels of the nervous system are variously affected by HIV-associated processes, including inflammation and neuronal damage, and by opportunistic infections and lymphoma. Neurological conditions are frequently debilitating, and often life-threatening. In addition, anti-retroviral therapy and other medications used in HIV treatment can have prominent neurological side-effects.

HIV is a neuro-invasive virus that enters the central nervous system (CNS) in infected monocytes that cross the blood-brain barrier to establish HIV infection in perivascular microglial cells and macrophages. Systemic inflammation makes the blood brain barrier more permeable and is associated with increased perivascular infiltration by infected monocytes. HIV replication in the brain can be minimal. Neurodysfunction is thought to be mediated by activated microglial cells and astrocytes producing toxic cytokines and viral proteins. Microglial cells have a long lifespan and the brain is a sanctuary site for HIV. Other long-term consequences include neuronal apoptosis, deposition of beta-amyloid, and increased risk of irreversible cognitive impairment.

Paediatric disease

HIV encephalopathy

HIV encephalopathy is the most common neurological manifestation of HIV in children and can be a presenting feature.

Clinical presentation

The disease can be static or progress as a subacute process with a rapid, relentless course, or can plateau with a more indolent course.

Clinical symptoms – cognitive, behavioural and motor dysfunction

Early signs of progressive motor dysfunction include bilateral tone normalities and the onset of pathological reflexes (hyperreflexia and clonus), chiefly affecting the legs (spastic diparesis). If untreated, progression to a spastic quadriparesis with pseudobulbar palsy will issue. Extrapyramidal symptoms such as rigidity, dystonia, tremors and ataxia are uncommon and seen in advanced disease. Focal neurological signs are rare.

Diagnosis

HIV encephalopathy is a clinical diagnosis. The American Academy of Neurology AIDS Task force recommends at least one of the following progressive findings for at least two months in the absence of other concurrent illness that could explain the findings:

Acquired microcephaly – head circumference measurement or brain atrophy on serial CT/MRI imaging in children younger than two years of age.

Acquired symmetrical motor deficits – ≥2 of the following: paresis, pathological reflexes, ataxia, gait disturbance.

Failure to attain, or loss of developmental milestones, or loss of intellectual ability verified by standard developmental or neuropsychological tests.

Cerebrospinal fluid analysis is not indicated in suspected HIV encephalopathy unless opportunistic infections require exclusion. Cerebrospinal fluid is usually either normal or non-specific (predominant lymphocytic pleocytosis and mildly elevated protein levels).

Changes observed on neuroimaging include global cerebral atrophy, calcifications and white matter abnormalities. Computed tomography is adequate for identification of cerebral atrophy and calcifications. Magnetic resonance imaging (MRI) is better for white matter changes. Radiographic findings may lag behind clinical symptoms.

Management

Early antiretroviral therapy with drugs that have good CSF penetration (lamivudine, stavudine, zidovudine, efavirenz, nevirapine and lopinavir) may avoid encephalopathy.

Immune reconstitution inflammatory syndrome (IRIS)

CNS infections may be exaggerated, e.g. CMV, TB meningitis, varicella zoster and cryptococcal meningitis.

Tuberculous meningitis

Clinical presentation

The neurological findings in HIV-infected children with TB meningitis are similar to those in uninfected children.

Diagnosis

The CSF findings in HIV-infected children with TB meningitis are also similar to those in uninfected children. The likelihood of radiographic evidence of pulmonary TB is higher in HIV-infected children, while classical signs of TB meningitis on computed tomography, such as obstructive hydrocephalus and basal meningeal enhancement are less prominent (compared to uninfected children). Hydrocephalus warrants air encephalography to determine whether obstructive (shunting required) or communicating nature (medical therapy).

Management

Isoniazid, rifampicin, ethionamide (20 mg/kg/day) and pyrazinamide 40 mg/kg, once daily in hospital for six months. Prednisone 4 mg/kg day (maximum dose 60 mg) is added during the first month of treatment. To minimize the risk of IRIS, the initiation of antiretroviral therapy, should be delayed. The extent of the delay depends on the degree of immunosuppression and varies from a few days to two months. Medical treatment of hydrocephalus consists of acetazolamide 50–100 mg/kg/day in three divided doses and furosemide 1 mg/kg/day in three divided doses for four weeks.

Cryptococcal meningitis

Cryptococcal meningitis is seen in older children with advanced HIV.

Clinical presentation

Symptoms at onset may be non-specific and are secondary to raised intracranial pressure (fever, nausea, vomiting, headache, visual disturbances, change in mental status). Clinical signs include meningism, cranial neuropathies and papilloedema. Focal neurological deficits are uncommon. The two most accurate predictors of poor prognosis are persistently raised intracranial pressure and alteration in mental status.

Diagnosis

CSF shows mononuclear pleocytosis with elevated protein and low glucose. Macroscopically it is clear or turbid. India ink often staining shows encapsulated yeasts, but the cryptococcal antigen test is more sensitive for the diagnosis. CSF culture is important to exclude fluconazole resistance. Monitoring the changes in cryptococcal antigen titre in serum or CSF is useful for evaluating the response to therapy. Computed tomography or MRI may reveal communicating hydrocephalus, pseudocysts or mass lesions (cryptococcomas). Most children will have an abnormal chest radiograph (bilateral alveolar or interstitial pneumonitis)

Management

Amphotericin B, IV, 0.5–1 mg/kg/dose once daily over four hours for 14 days, or longer depending on disease response. Total dose: 30–35 mg/kg over four to eight weeks, with an initial test dose – see package insert. Pre-loading with normal saline infusion before each dose (20 mL/kg) may minimize renal toxicity.

then

Fluconazole orally, 12–15 mg/kg once daily for a further six to eight weeks (maximum dose: 400 mg) *then* secondary prophylaxis.

Fluconazole, oral, 6–10 mg/kg/once daily.

For adolescents receiving antiretroviral therapy, maintenance fluconazole may be stopped if immune reconstitution occurs, i.e. CD4 count increases to between 100–200 cells/μl. There are insufficient data for stopping maintenance therapy in children.

elevated intracranial pressure, should be treated aggressively. Lumbar puncture allows determination of opening pressure and therapeutic CSF drainage. CSF diversion (shunting) should be considered (despite the increased risk of shunt infection) if there is no response to other forms of treatment. Medical management includes:

Acetazolamide, oral, 50 mg/kg/24 hours in three divided doses:
o maximum dose: 1 g/day.
o monitor for metabolic acidosis and potassium loss.

plus

furosemide, oral, 1 mg/kg/24 hours in three divided doses for the first month of treatment. Taper slowly over two weeks if the intracranial pressure has normalised, as indicated by clinical response.

Stroke

Stroke is uncommon in children with HIV.

Clinical presentation

Suspect stroke in any child with focal neurological signs/deficits (hemiparesis), seizures or altered sensorium. HIV-related strokes may be clinically silent in advanced HIV encephalopathy.

Diagnosis

If suspected, refer to a tertiary centre. Investigations must confirm stroke and determine underlying aetiology. Computed tomography (CT) differentiates between haemorrhagic and ischaemic stroke and excludes other diagnoses. CT imaging may miss an infarction less than 48 hours old. Rather use MRI (with diffusion weighted imaging) if presenting within 48 hours. Cerebrospinal fluid analysis is mandatory in children with unexplained fever or signs of intracranial infection, especially to rule out tuberculous meningitis. Cardiac echo excludes cardiomyopathy or endocarditis. Immune-mediated thrombocytopenia or other bleeding disorders should be excluded if there is an intracerebral hemorrhage.

Treatment

Supportive: There are no evidence-based guidelines for anticoagulants in children with ischaemic stroke. Children with haemorrhagic stroke should be referred for urgent neurosurgical opinion.

HIV myelopathy

Clinical presentation

Suspect in any child with a spastic paraparesis (lower limb spasticity) or spastic gait without cognitive decline. Other signs on clinical examination include ataxic gait, and bladder and bowel dysfunction.

Diagnosis

MRI of the spine (with T2 weighted imaging). The CSF profile in children with HIV-related vacuolar myeopathy is usually normal, but is needed to exclude other potential causes of myelopathy, i.e. cytomegalovirus, varicella zoster, herpes and *Mycobacterium tuberculosis*. Syphilis and vitamin B12 deficiency should be excluded.

Treatment

Treat the underlying cause where identified. Vacuolar myelopathy is treated with antiretroviral therapy. Baclofen 15 mg/day in three to four divided doses may attenuate leg spasticity and reduce leg cramps.

Seizures

HIV-associated CNS disease is largely a white matter disorder, therefore seizures occur infrequently.

Diagnosis

Simple febrile seizures occur in HIV-infected children. CSF analysis is indicated in any HIV-infected child under the age of two years presenting with febrile seizures, as the signs of meningism may be subtle or even absent. Neuroimaging is indicated in children with new onset focal seizures to exclude cerebral mass lesions (tuberculomas, toxoplasmosis).

Treatment

Anticonvulsants such as phenobarbitone and sodium valproate work well; carbamazepine should be avoided in children with severe lymphopenia.

Neurodevelopmental disorders in HIV-infected children

See Appendix 35.1.

Adult neurology

The spectrum of neurological disease in southern Africa is similar to that in the developed world. Brain imaging with CT or MRI is recommended in HIV-infected patients with meningitis or encephalitis, as focal lesions are more likely. All patients with focal signs or features of raised intracranial pressure should be imaged.

Meningitis

Meningitis is common in HIV infection. As meningism is relatively uncommon, a lumbar puncture (LP) should be performed on all patients with any combination of the following clinical features:

- headache;
- fever;

- photophobia;
- vomiting;
- altered mental status;
- neck stiffness.

Patients with cryptococcal meningitis may present with headache only, and this diagnosis should be considered in all patients with advanced HIV disease. A CT scan should be done before lumber puncture in patients with coma, focal signs or papilloedema to rule out midline shift. If bacterial meningitis is a significant possibility, and a LP cannot be performed immediately, it is acceptable to take a blood culture and give an immediate dose of a third-generation cephalosporin, before arranging a CT scan. CSF pressure should be measured in all patients undergoing LP (the normal pressure is <20 cm H_2O). The following investigations should be considered (at least 10 mL of CSF will be required):

- cell count and differential;
- protein and glucose concentrations;
- India ink smear, a stain for acid-fast bacilli (AFB), and a Gram stain;
- mycobacterial, bacterial, and fungal cultures;
- cryptococcal antigen test;
- syphilis serology (if indicated by positive RPR or TPHA in blood); and
- Herpes simplex, varicella zoster, cytomegalovirus, and HTLV-1 poly-merase chain reaction (PCR) (in patients presenting with meningo-encephalitis or myelitis).

Blood samples should always be taken for glucose and RPR or VDRL assays.

Cryptococcal meningitis (and occasionally also tuberculous meningitis) may be present without CSF pleocytosis and with normal protein and glucose levels. Severely immunocompromised patients may have dual infection, which makes it important to follow up the results of the myco-bacterial and fungal cultures.

Cryptococcal meningitis

Presentation

Cryptococcal meningitis is the commonest cause of community-acquired HIV-associated meningitis in sub-Saharan Africa. It is associated with high rates of morbidity and mortality and is uniformly fatal if left untreated. However, if treated aggressively, patients may have good outcomes when started on antiretroviral therapy after several weeks of maintenance of fluconazole. Typical symptoms and signs of meningitis such as headache or meningism may be absent. The clinical presentation is typically that of a subacute meningitis with varying combinations of fever, headache, nausea, vomiting, or cognitive dysfunction (irritability, behavioural changes, somnolence, or even psychosis). Focal signs and seizures may be present. Altered mental status and persistently raised intracranial pressure are the most significant marker for poor prognosis.

Diagnosis

An opening pressure above 20 cm water is often a clue to the diagnosis. Cell counts are often mildly raised or even in the normal range. CSF glucose may be low and protein raised. Approximately 10% of patients with HIV-associated cryptococcal meningitis will have normal biochemical CSF findings. A positive culture for *Cryptococcus neoformans* gives a definitive diagnosis, but this may take up to two weeks. A positive India ink smear is often helpful, but is too insensitive to exclude the diagnosis (see photo 10). By contrast, the CSF cryptococcal antigen test has a sensitivity of 95%. The presence of cryptococcal antigen in the serum is a good marker for HIV-associated cryptococcal meningitis. It is therefore essential to check the cryptococcal antigen titre of a patient with a negative India ink CSF smear to definitely exclude a diagnosis of cryptococcal meningitis. Cryptococcal culture is the investigation of choice in order to diagnose relapse, as the antigen and Indian ink remains elevated for long periods.

Management

The standard treatment for patients with cryptococcal meningitis is amphotericin B, 0.7–1.0 mg/kg/day IV for two weeks, followed by fluconazole 400 mg daily for eight weeks, and then 200 mg daily until the CD4 is >200 and VL undetectable for at least three months. Two weeks of amphotericin B and flucytosine is considered to be the gold standard therapy for cryptococcal meningitis; however, flucytosine is currently unavailable in South Africa.

- Amphotericin B should initially be given as a test dose of 1 mg over an hour, and if this is tolerated, the full dose can be given daily, infused over a four-hour period. The slow administration of the drug is essential to prevent arrhythmias. 1 L IV normal saline, unless contraindicated, should be given first to prevent nephrotoxicity. Electrolytes and creatinine should be measured on alternate days. Should the creatinine rises to above 220 µL miss one dose and check hydration and repeat every 24 hours. If the creatinine is stable or improving resume amphotericin B at 0.7 mg/kg on alternate days. If creatinine continues to rise change to fluconazole, adjusting the dose for the degree of renal impairment. Hypokalaemia and hypomagnesaemia are common and require aggressive replacement. Full blood count should be checked twice weekly as anaemia is a common. Amphotericin B at a dose of 0.7 mg/kg may be considered for patients with haemoglobin levels of nine or less. Paracetamol can be given for febrile reactions. Patients should be checked daily for signs of thrombophlebitis.

- Raised intracranial pressure is a common problem associated with cryptococcal meningitis. Effective management with repeated therapeutic LPs is as important as the patient receiving the correct, carefully monitored chemotherapy. Any pressure greater than 20 cm of water should lead to a therapeutic tap. The CSF pressure should ideally be measured at every lumbar puncture. Remove about 1 mL of CSF for every 1 cm of water pressure above 25 cm, up to 30–40 mL. Remeasure dosing pressure every 10 mL CSF. This should be either <50% of opening pressure or <20 cm water. Serial therapeutic LPs should be performed until CSF pressures are controlled.
- Wherever possible patients should receive intravenous amphotericin B for a total of two weeks. Where amphotericin B is not available fluconazole 800 mg daily for eight to 10 weeks may be an acceptable alternative.
- Secondary prophylaxis with fluconazole 200 mg daily should be continued until the CD4 count is >200 cells/µl and viral load undetectable for at least three months.

Tuberculous meningitis

Presentation

Meningeal tuberculosis is common in HIV-infected patients and is associated with high morbidity and mortality. As in HIV-seronegative individuals presentation is variable, and diagnosis is not clear-cut. Patients presenting with altered mental status have higher mortality rates and a greater risk of neurological sequelae. The diagnosis should be suspected in patients presenting with a gradual onset of headache. Meningism is a feature on examination. 'Breakthrough' tuberculosis meningitis (TBM) can develop while patients are on treatment for TB at other sites and there is an increased incidence of co-existing tuberculomas in HIV-positive patients, which may develop while the patient is on anti-tuberculous therapy.

Diagnosis

In practice, the diagnosis is based on clinical findings and lumbar puncture results. There may be elevated cerebrospinal fluid (CSF) pressures. The diagnosis is based on: duration of symptoms >5 days; pleiocytosis (usually with lymphocytic predominance); elevated protein and low glucose (gradient <0.5 calculated using blood glucose or capillary blood glucose *or* glucose <1.9).

CSF neutrophil predominance occurs in 40% of patients. Acellular fluid is not uncommon in elderly patients. The CSF is smear-positive for AFB in only 5% of cases.

The gold standard for diagnosing TBM is mycobacterial culture of the CSF, which may take four to six weeks. The result from PCR testing for mycobacterial DNA is available within days. However, the diagnosis is not excluded by a negative culture or PCR result. In-hospital mortality of TBM may be as high as 70%, so is reasonable, when there is a high clinical suspicion of TBM, to start empiric anti-tuberculous therapy. CSF adenosine deaminase levels are not very sensitive or specific for the diagnosis of TBM.

Treatment

The treatment is standard antituberculous therapy for a minimum of six months. See Chapter 24: Adult tuberculosis. Patients should be referred to the National Tuberculosis Programme.

Dexamethasone should be given, preferably intravenously, at a dose of 0.4 mg per kilogram per day for week one, 0.3 mg per kilogram per day for week two, 0.2 mg per kilogram per day for week three, and 0.1 mg per kilogram per day for week four. This is followed by oral treatment for four weeks, starting at a total of 4 mg per day and decreasing by 1 mg each week. Usual therapy would be 8 mg tds for seven days, then 6 mg tds for seven days, then 4 mg tds for seven days, then 2 mg tds for seven days, then 2 mg bd, decreasing by 1 mg per week for a total of 28 days. Lower doses of dexamethasone can be given for a total of six weeks for mild cases of TBM with normal mentation and no focal signs.

Meningovascular syphilis

Meningovascular syphilis is more common among HIV-positive individuals. Even if the CSF VDRL is negative, a positive serum VDRL or RPR in the presence of an otherwise unexplained pleiocytosis should lead to treatment for neurosyphilis. Treatment options are:

- benzylpenicillin 12–24 million units IV administered in doses of 2–4 million units every four hours for 14–21 days; or
- procaine penicillin 2.4 million units IM once daily, plus probenecid 500 mg six hourly, both for 10–14 days.

Either of the above regimens should be followed by benzathine benzyl-penicillin 2.4 million units weekly for three weeks.

Alternatives include:
- ceftriaxone 2.0 g IM/IV daily for 14 days;
- doxycycline 200 mg twice daily for 28 days;
- amoxicillin 2 g, 8 hourly, plus probenicid 500 mg, six hourly for 28 days.

After treatment the LP should be repeated every six months. The CSF cell count should be <10 cells/mL within 12–24 months. CSF VDRL and protein fall more slowly.

Pneumococcal meningitis

Pneumococcal meningitis occurs with increased frequency in patients with HIV. As HIV-positive patients have an increased incidence of bacterial sinusitis, all patients presenting with bacterial meningitis should have a clinical and radiological evaluation of the sinuses and middle ear. CT scanning is recommended.

Viral meningitis and encephalitis

Viral meningitis and encephalitis resulting from HIV itself can occur during the acute seroconversion illness or in later disease. Typical CSF findings are a lymphocytic predominance with a modest elevation of protein. Herpes simplex is rarely the cause. Zoster (shingles) is occasionally accompanied by symptomatic meningitis (but CSF is usually abnormal in all patients with shingles). Encephalitis due to varicella-zoster infection results from the involvement of small vessels, often presenting weeks after the shingles.

Parenchymal brain disease

HIV-associated dementia

Several different terms are used to describe the cognitive changes related to HIV infection. These include HIV-associated minor cognitive or motor deficit, and or HIV-associated dementia (HAD) for advanced disease. There is evidence that postponing the initiation of antiretroviral therapy until blood CD4 counts fall to <300 cells/µl may increase the risk of HIV-associated neurocognitive impairment. HAD improves with antiretroviral therapy, even with CD4 counts of <100 cells/µl.

HAD occurs in 20-30% of patients with advanced HIV and typically develops over a few months. Clinical features include subcortical dementia, with abnormalities in motor and cognitive functions, as well as behavioural changes. (See Chapter 36: Psychiatry.) Antiretroviral therapy can reverse cognitive deficits, and alter the progression of HAD – patients may experience 'static' forms of dementia. Risk factors for the development of HAD include: low CD4 counts, increasing age, female sex, anaemia and low body-mass index.

Important clinical features include:
- cognitive changes, including poor attention span, impaired recall, and slowed mental processes;
- altered behaviour, including social withdrawal, low mood and apathy;
- motor dysfunction including saccadic and pursuit eye-movement abnormalities, poor fine finger movements and difficulty with tandem gait.

Early in the disorder, the mini-mental state examination (MMSE) is usually normal. The International HIV Dementia Scale is a modification of the MMSE, developed to screen for HAD and includes a test of psychomotor speed (see Appendix 35.2).

Depression must always be considered as an alternative diagnosis, and may be present with HAD. Disease processes involving the frontal cortex need to be excluded, including progressive multifocal leuko-encephalopathy, primary CNS lymphoma and cryptococcal meningitis.

Over time, the cognitive abnormality interferes with work and social function, and the patient's gait deteriorates. End-stage disease is characterized by:
- global dementia;
- frontal lobe release signs;
- basal ganglia signs including rigidity and tremor;
- spasticity and paraparesis (10% of patients have a vacuolar myelopathy); and
- incontinence.

CT scan usually demonstrates cerebral atrophy and MRI findings reveal diffuse atrophy and diffuse or patchy periventricular white matter hyperintensities on T2-weighted images. CSF and EEG findings are usually non-specific. Drugs that penetrate the brain, though only backed by empirical evidence, include: zidovudine, abacavir, lamivudine, nevirapine and lopinavir. Protease inhibitor-containing regimens, both in developed and resource-poor settings, have been found to reverse neurocognitive deficits. Response to antiretroviral therapy, which should, if possible include zidovudine, may be impressive. Research currently focuses on treatments for CNS inflammation or oxidative stress as new adjunctive targets. Novel therapies may include antioxidants, tumour necrosis factor alpha antagonists and N-methyl-D-aspartate receptor antagonists.

Seizures

Seizures are a common and non-specific manifestation of neurological illnesses in adults with HIV. Most HIV-infected patients who develop new onset seizures have:

- a space-occupying lesion (most often because of cerebral toxoplasmosis or a tuberculoma);
- meningitis (most often cryptococcal);
- metabolic disturbances; or
- no identified cause other than HIV infection.

Intracranial pathology (mass lesion or meningitis) is present in 75% of patients.

Metabolic abnormalities, specifically hyponatraemia, hypomagnesaemia, hypocalcaemia, and renal failure are important reversible causes of seizures in HIV patients, with or without CNS disease. The seizure type is often related to the underlying cause, and may be generalized or focal. Treatment is aimed at the underlying disorder and seizure control is achieved through standard antiepileptic medication. However, drug interactions are a problem with antiretroviral therapy and, in patients on such therapy, valproate is the antiepileptic agent of choice.

Stroke

Cerebral infarction has been found in between 4% and 34% of AIDS cases in autopsy series and cerebral haemorrhage in 4%–10%. These pathologic findings are however frequently asymptomatic. Stroke-like presentations are not common, but may become more frequent due to premature onset of atherosclerosis in the cerebral circulation (see Chapter 34: Endocrinology and metabolic abnormalities). There are many possible causes of stroke in an HIV-infected patient and it is important to identify the potentially treatable causes. A careful cardiovascular examination, followed by brain imaging and LP, are often necessary.

Approach to intracranial mass lesions on scan

Brain scans of HIV-infected patients commonly show intracranial mass lesions (IMLs). In developed countries the IMLs are most often caused by toxoplasmosis, primary CNS lymphoma, and progressive multifocal leukoencephalopathy (usually a focal rather than a mass lesion). In KwaZulu-Natal, toxoplasmosis is the commonest cause of IML, followed by pyogenic abscess, and tuberculoma. Multiple mass lesions are usually due to toxoplasmosis. Histology is the gold standard for diagnosis of IML (as the aetiology cannot be accurately determined from the clinical features or scan characteristics), but is not always practical or available. A sensible approach is to treat patients empirically in a step-by-step manner, starting with the most likely cause suggested by the CT scan characteristics, CSF findings, and associated non-neurological illnesses. (See Figure 35.1 for a summary of the approach to a mass lesion on CT scan and Figure 35.2 for an alternative approach for facilities with access to an MRI scanner.)

Figure 35.1 Approach to a mass lesion on CT or MRI scan

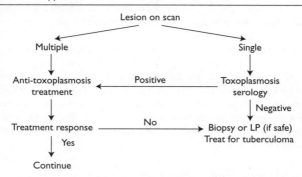

Toxoplasma encephalitis

Disease usually occurs as a result of reactivation of latent infection following immunosuppression. CNS reactivation of *Toxoplasma gondii* typically presents with focal signs and an impaired level of consciousness. Patients presenting in this way should undergo an urgent CT scan of the head, with and without contrast. If a CT scan is not immediately available empiric treatment should be started, with further treatment dependent on the CT result. Toxoplasmosis is unusual in patients with CD4 cell counts >200 cells or patients who have been reliably taking co-trimoxazole prophylaxis for PCP.

Diagnosis

A serological test for toxoplasmosis is usually IgG positive. An IgM response is seldom seen. CT brain typically shows multiple, hypodense contrast-enhancing mass lesions with oedema. MRI is the gold standard investigation and usually reveals multiple ring-enhancing lesions, often with oedema and mass effect (see photo 11).

Treatment

Treatment must be continued for 12 weeks, followed by secondary prophylaxis that should be continued lifelong or until the CD4 count is >200 cells/µl for six months with an undetectable viral load. Therapy in resource poor settings is with co-trimoxazole (80/400 mg) one tablet for each 8 kg of body weight per day, in two divided doses. The usual dosage is, therefore, four tablets 12 hourly, given for four weeks, followed by half the dose (i.e. two tablets) 12 hourly for eight weeks. A response to therapy is usually seen clinically in seven to ten days and CT scan appearances improve within three to four weeks.

Patients who cannot tolerate co-trimoxazole can be treated with clindamycin 600 mg eight hourly and pyrimethamine 100 mg 12 hourly for one day, followed by 50 mg daily for three to six weeks. Pyrimethamine should be combined with folinic acid at an initial dose of 15 mg daily to prevent marrow toxicity. Relapses are extremely common and all patients will require lifelong prophylaxis with co-trimoxazole, 80/400 mg two tablets daily or until immune reconstitution is successfully achieved on antiretroviral therapy.

Approach to a single lesion on CT scan

The differential diagnosis of single contrast-enhancing CNS lesions in HIV includes:

- toxoplasmosis;
- tuberculoma;
- primary CNS B-cell lymphoma; and
- cryptococcoma.

Progressive multifocal leukoencephalopathy (PMLE) and CNS infarct typically do not enhance with contrast, but may do so in the early stages.

Note that:
- Patients who have a CD4 count below 200 cells/μl and test positive for toxoplasma IgG should be treated for toxoplasma encephalitis.
- Patients who are toxoplasma IgG negative or who do not respond to therapy should be treated for tuberculoma.

If extra-neurological TB is suspected then anti-tuberculous treatment should be initiated first, with a repeat brain scan at around four weeks. Avoid steroids whenever possible, as the diagnosis is made by assessing the response to therapy. Patients not responding to therapy within seven to 14 days should undergo further investigations, preferably starting with a LP, if this is thought to be safe.

Primary CNS lymphoma

Primary CNS lymphoma is an uncommon form of extranodal non-Hodgkin's lymphoma. Patients may respond to antiretroviral therapy, whole brain radiation therapy or therapies directed against the Epstein-Barr virus. Patients seldom benefit from the aggressive pursuit of a diagnosis of CNS lymphoma, as the prognosis is very poor. CSF cytology may make the diagnosis (if LP is safe), as may CSF PCR testing for the Epstein-Barr virus. Dexamethasone, 8 mg eight hourly combined with radiotherapy provides effective palliation. (See Chapter 41: Oncology.)

Progressive multifocal leukoencephalopathy (PMLE)

PMLE has emerged as an important opportunistic infection occurring in up to 5% of patients. PMLE is caused by JC virus (JCV), a polyomavirus, and presents in advanced disease with progressive focal neurological deficits, often associated with visual and cognitive impairment. The presentation of PMLE in AIDS patients is variable, as lesions may occur anywhere in the CNS white matter.

Neuroimaging shows irregular non-enhancing white matter lesions without oedema or mass-effect. Brain biopsy has a sensitivity and specificity of between 64% and 96% and 100%, respectively. A diagnosis of PMLE may be established through polymerase chain reaction (PCR) detection of JCV DNA in the CSF. However, the advent of antiretroviral therapy has significantly reduced the sensitivity of this test and it is not uncommon for AIDS patients with PML to have negative CSF JCV PCR results.

At present there is no effective therapy. Optimizing antiretroviral therapy remains the best therapeutic option in HIV positive patients. 80% of PMLE survivors are left with severe neurological sequelae as remyelination does not occur in affected areas, despite increased survival rates with antiretroviral therapy.

Acute disseminated encephalomyelitis (ADEM)

ADEM is a rare condition presenting as a febrile illness with altered mental status, limb weakness, and blindness (due to retrobulbar neuritis). MRI scanning shows enhancing lesions in the subcortical white matter that may also involve the grey matter, brain stem and spinal cord, which correlates pathologically with demyelination. Herpes simplex encephalitis needs to be excluded with CSF PCR. Treatment includes high dose steroids and intravenous immunoglobulins and antiretroviral therapy.

Spinal cord involvement

The spinal cord is often involved in HIV infection. Common HIV-associated causes of cord disease include:

- spinal tuberculosis;
- herpes zoster, herpes simplex and cytomegalovirus myelitis;
- vacuololar myelopathy;
- toxoplasmosis;
- lymphoma.

Other important causes of cord pathology that need to be considered include:

- HTLV-1 infection (common in KwaZulu-Natal);
- syphilis;
- vitamin B12 deficiency.

Spinal column imaging with pre- and post-contrast MRI scan is essential in the evaluation of spinal cord lesions. Urgent imaging may be necessary to exclude extrinsic cord compression by a tuberculous cold abscess, bacterial abscess, or lymphoma. If these are excluded, CSF should be sent for neurotropic virus PCR, and cytology.

Vacuolar myelopathies

Vacuolar myelopathy is a slowly progressive painless spastic paraparesis, due to intralamellar vacuolation in the spinal white matter, especially in the lateral and posterior columns of the thoracic spinal cord. Vacuolar myelopathy typically presents late in the course of HIV infection, with slowly progressive weakness over a period of months associated with sensory ataxia, gait abnormalities and neurogenic bladder. Spasticity is not usually marked. Reflexes are typically brisk at the knee, but may be brisk or reduced at the ankle depending on whether there is coexisting neuropathy. Pain and temperature sensation remain relatively spared, and a clear sensory level suggests an alternative diagnosis. There is currently no specific treatment, but there may be substantial improvement with antiretroviral therapy. Supportive treatment focuses on relieving spasticity, physiotherapy and managing the neurogenic bladder.

Radiculopathy and neuropathy

Inflammatory demyelinating polyneuropathy

Acute inflammatory demyelinating polyneuropathy (AIDP), or Guillain-Barré syndrome, occurs during the stage of immune dysregulation and presents with distal motor neuropathy and neuropathic pain. If the neuropathy extends proximally, respiratory muscle function and the autonomic nervous system may be affected, and admission into the intensive care unit is indicated. The CSF usually shows elevated protein with minimal pleocytosis and nerve conduction studies show demyelination. As the condition occurs in patients in the early stages of the disease, aggressive treatment with intravenous immunoglobulin (0.4 g/kg/d for five days) or plasmapheresis is appropriate. Chronic inflammatory demyelinating polyneuropathy also occurs and, unlike AIDP, is steroid responsive. It presents with a gradual onset of sensory and motor limb weakness. In both conditions seek expert advice.

HIV-related neuropathy

HIV-related neuropathy is a troublesome condition that occurs in a third of patients with CD4 counts below 200 cells/µl. It presents with painful dysaesthesias and numbness in a 'glove-and-stocking' distribution.

Nerve conduction studies show an axonopathy. HIV-associated sensory neuropathies (HIV-SN) include distal sensory polyneuropathy and antiretroviral toxic neuropathy, which cannot be distinguished on clinical grounds. Several reversible factors including alcohol, vitamin deficiencies, and drugs exacerbate the neuropathy. Strongly encourage patients to abstain from alcohol completely. Patients should be given thiamine 100 mg daily. Patients taking isoniazid should be given pyridoxine (vitamin B6), 50 mg daily. Stavudine (d4T) and didanosine (ddI) can cause severe neuropathy, which may necessitate a change in the drug regimen. Zalcitabine (ddC) also causes severe neuropathy, but is no longer available. Pain can be severe and may respond to analgesics (paracetamol, NSAIDS, codeine) combined with amitriptyline, carbamazepine, gabapentin or lamotrigine. Morphine should be used in end-stage disease.

Polyradiculopathy

Polyradiculopathy is a rare condition, most often caused by cytomegalovirus (CMV) in advanced HIV. The condition presents with a flaccid paraplegia, numbness in the saddle area and bladder dysfunction, which may mimic myelopathy. The diagnosis of CMV is suggested by CSF neutrophil predominance and confirmed on PCR or viral culture. Ganciclovir is the standard treatment. HIV polyradiculopathy, unrelated to CMV occurs as a subacute flaccid paraparesis with sphincter involvement. The diagnosis is confirmed by negative CSF virology for neurotropic viruses, pleocytosis and normal CSF glucose. MRI demonstrates enhancement of the cauda equina. Treatment is with prednisolone 1 mg/kg with good response being anticipated within six weeks. Therafter, a tapering dose of steroids is recommended.

Bell's palsy

Acute-onset lower motor-neuron facial weakness occurs with increased frequency in HIV-infected individuals. It is often treated with prednisone 60 mg daily for five days.

VZV infection of the geniculate ganglion will cause the Ramsay-Hunt syndrome, which presents with vesicles on the external auditory meatus and an ipsilateral lower motor-neuron facial nerve palsy. (For the treatment of VZV, see Chapter 40: Dermatology.)

Myopathy

HIV-associated myopathy may be the result of direct effects of HIV on muscle or due to opportunistic infections or drugs (See Chapter 42:

Rheumatology.) Zidovudine has been associated with myopathy, but the extent to which histology and clinical findings are related to HIV infection rather than zidovudine is not clear.

Patients presenting with slowly progressive proximal weakness, with or without myalgia, should have the creatine kinase (CK) checked. If the CK is raised then the patient should undergo an EMG. If the EMG is abnormal (myopathic picture) a muscle biopsy is indicated. If the patient is on AZT, an off-treatment trial of four to eight weeks' duration may be indicated. Treatment of HIV-associated myopathy includes corticosteroids and intravenous immunoglobulin. Note that CK is often raised in patients on antiretroviral therapy and, in the absence of weakness, does not imply myositis.

References and further reading

Bhigjee, A.I. 2005. 'Neurological manifestations of HIV infection in Kwazulu-Natal South Africa.' *Journal of Neurovirology*; 11 Suppl 1:17–21.

Hoffmann, M. et al. 2000. 'Cerebrovascular disease in young, HIV-infected, black South Africans in the KwaZulu Natal province of South Africa.' *Journal of Neurovirology*; 6:229-236

Koralnik, I. 2006. 'Progressive Multifocal Leukoencephalopathy revisited: Has the disease outgrown its name?' *Annals of Neurology*; 60:162–173.

McArthur, J.C. et al. 2005. 'Neurological complications of HIV infection.' *Lancet Neurology*; 4:543–555.

Modi, G. et al. 2007. 'The frequency and profile of neurology in black South African HIV infected (clade C) patients – A hospital-based prospective audit.' *Journal of Neurological Sciences*; 254:60–64.

Power, C. et al. 1995. 'HIV Dementia Scale: A rapid screening test'. *Journal of Acquired Immune Deficiency Syndrome*; 3:273-278.

Rabinstein, A. 2003. 'Stroke in HIV-infected patients: a clinical perspective.' *Cerebrovascular Diseases*; 15:37–44.

Sacktor, N. 2002 'The epidemiology of human immunodeficiency virus-associated neurological disease in the era of highly active antiretroviral therapy'. *Journal of Neurovirology*; 8:115–121.

Sacktor, N. et al. 2005. 'The international HIV dementia scale: a new rapid screening test for HIV dementia.' *AIDS*; 19:1367–1374.

Sacktor, N. et al. 2006. 'Antiretroviral therapy improves cognitive impairment in HIV positive individuals in sub-Saharan Africa.' *Neurology*; 67:311–314.

Appenidix 35.1 Neurodevelopmental disorders in children and infants

Neurological disorders in children and infants may manifest as:
- failure to lose primitive reflexes;
- failure to attain age appropriate developmental milestones;
- failure to develop secondary protective reflexes;
- loss of previously attained milestones.

Any of the above should be clues for a more thorough neurological assessment. Only when the neurological examination is normal, can a systemic illness be assumed to be the cause of developmental delay.

The system developing most rapidly is the one most affected in a specific age group. In the young infant the gross motor system is the most affected and in the older child, language and fine motor are developing rapidly so these most affected.

Any clinical assessment of the young child and infant should include the assessment of milestones. Tables 35.3 and 35.4 give a quick and easy examination that should lead the clinician to important problems.

Appendix 35.2 International HIV Dementia Scale

Memory-Registration – Give four words to recall (dog, hat, bean, red) – one second to say each. Then ask the patient all four words after you have said them. Repeat words if the patient does not recall them all immediately. Tell the patient you will ask for recall of the words again a bit later.

1. Motor Speed: Have the patient tap the first two fingers of the non-dominant hand as widely and as quickly as possible.
4 = 15 in 5 seconds
3 = 11–14 in 5 seconds
2 = 7–10 in 5 seconds
1 = 3–6 in 5 seconds
0 = 0–2 in 5 seconds

2. Psychomotor Speed: Have the patient perform the following movements with the non-dominant hand as quickly as possible: 1) Clench hand in fist on flat surface. 2) Put hand flat on surface with palm down. 3) Put hand perpendicular to flat surface on the side of the 5th digit. Demonstrate and have patient perform twice for practice.

4 = 4 sequences in 10 seconds
3 = 3 sequences in 10 seconds
2 = 2 sequences in 10 seconds
1 = 1 sequence in 10 seconds
0 = unable to perform

3. Memory-Recall: Ask the patient to recall the four words. For words not recalled, prompt with a semantic clue as follows: animal (dog); piece of clothing (hat); vegetable (bean); color (red).
Give 1 point for each word spontaneously recalled.
Give 0.5 points for each correct answer after prompting
Maximum – 4 points.

Total International HIV Dementia Scale Score: This is the sum of the scores on items 1–3. The maximum possible score is 12 points. A patient with a score of ≤10 should be evaluated further for possible dementia.

Table 35.3 Neurodevelopmental screen for first six months

Lying on back: Keep head in midline: Undress completely (including nappy off)

Age	6 weeks	3 months	6 months	Worrying signs
Head control	Head falling to side Left/right	Head in midline		Asymmetry at 3–6 months
Communication	Smiling	Cooing and chuckling	"mmm" sound	
Fixing and following	Fixing and following: to midline	Fixing and following 180°		Squint Not fixing or following
Fine motor		Hands to mid-line/mouth/clothes	Reaching and grasping (From 4½ months)	Not reaching Only uses one hand
ATNR	ATNR present	ATNR present	No ATNR	Persistent ATNR at 6 months

Age	1–3 months	3–6 months	Worrying signs
Abduction of legs	40° to 80°	70° to 110°	Decreased angles Asymmetry
Straight leg raising	80° to 100°	90° to 130°	Decreased angles Asymmetry
Dorsiflex ankles	60° to 70°	60° to 70°	Decreased angles Asymmetry
Reflexes at knees	(R) (L)	(R) (L)	Brisk reflexes Crossed adductors – can be present till 7 months
Moro Reflex	Present	Present until 4.5 months	Asymmetry Fisting Persistent at 6 months

Pull to sit and sitting:

Age	3 months	6 months	Worrying signs
Pull to sit		No head lag on pull to sitting	Head lag after $4\frac{1}{2}$ months
Sitting	Head upright in propped sitting (wobble) (4 months)	Sits with support	No head control
Protective extension		Lateral protective reflex	Fisting Asymmetry

Prone:

Age	3 months	6 months	Worrying signs
	Elbow flexion support	Elbow extension support	Fisting Asymmetry

Table 35.4 Developmental milestones from six months to six years of life

Age	Gross Motor	Fine Motor/Vision	Hearing And Speech	Personal/Social	Warning Signs
6 months	Pull to sit: braces shoulders and pulls to sit; sits with support; prone: lifts head and chest well up; support on extended arms	Reaches for and grasps toy; transfers toy from one hand to other	Initiates "conversation"	Takes everything to mouth; responds to mirror image	Floppiness, failure to use both hands, squint; failure to turn to sound; poor response to people
9 months	Sits without support; attempts to crawl; pulls to stand	Immediately reaches out; holds a cube in each hand	Vocalizes deliberately; babbles	Stranger anxiety; holds bottle/cup	Unable to sit; hand preference; fisting; squint; persistence of primitive reflexes
10 months	Pulls to stand	Picks up small object between thumb and index finger	Shakes head for no; waves bye-bye	Plays peek-a-boo with mother	
12 months	Bear walks; walks around furniture lifting one foot and stepping sideways; may walk alone	Pincer grasp; releases object on request	Knows own name; 2–3 words with meaning	Finger feeds; pushes arm into sleeve	Unable to sit or bear weight; abnormal grasp; failure to respond to sound
15 months	Walks alone — uneven steps, arms out for balance	2 cube tower	Jabbers with expression	Holds and drinks from cup; attempts feeding with spoon, spills most.	
18 months	Walks well, arms down, pulls a toy; throws a ball, climbs onto chair	3 cube tower; scribbles	2-word utterances	Handles spoon and cup; indicates wet nappy	Failure to walk; no pincer grip; inability to understand simple commands; no spontaneous vocalization; mouthing; drooling

Age	Gross motor	Fine motor / vision	Speech / language	Social	Abnormal signs
24 months	Runs; up and down steps two feet per step	6 cube tower; train with cubes; imitates vertical line; hand preference usually obvious	Short phrases, uses pronouns	Spoon feeds without spilling, clean and dry by day	Unable to understand simple commands; tremor; incoordination
36 months	Rides a tricycle, up steps one foot per step and down two feet per step	9 cube tower; bridge with cubes; copies circle	Knows name and sex; talks incessantly	Toilet trained; dresses without supervision	Ataxia; using single words only
48 months	Up and down stairs one per step; stands on one (preferred) foot for 3–5 seconds and hops on preferred foot	Copies cross; gate with cubes	Full name, home address and (usually) age; recognizes colours	Eats with spoon and fork; washes and dries hands; dresses and undresses; make-believe play	Speech difficult to understand because of poor articulation or omission or substitution of consonants
60 months	Walks easily on narrow line; can hop on each foot separately	6–10 cube steps; copies square and triangle; draws a man with all features	Fluent speech; full name, age, (usually) birthday, address	Uses knife and fork competently; undresses and dresses alone; chooses own friends	Emotional immaturity
72 months	Sits without help of hands; walks backwards along straight line (10 paces)	10 cube steps; copies diamond but oddly shaped	Word definition (5); compositions – door, shoe, spoon	Cooperative play – leadership and division of labour	Clumsy; poor posture; poor pencil grip

Acknowledgements: Dr C Molteno, S Lingham and D Harvey Manual of Child Development.
Prepared by Dr Sharon Kling, Developmental Clinic, Child Health Unit

Figure 35.2 An alternative approach to a mass lesion on CT or MRI scan

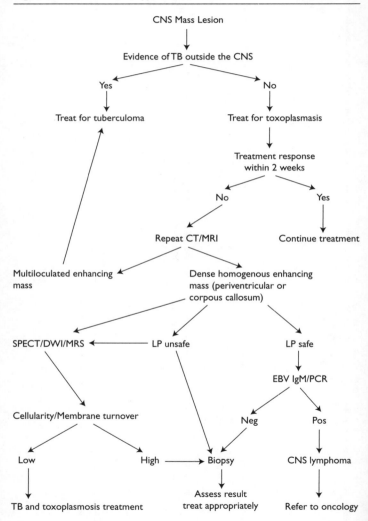

In the context of the HIV epidemic, health workers are increasingly encountering individuals with psychological and neuropsychiatric complications of HIV infection. Clinical presentations are varied and frequently complex. HIV has replaced syphilis as the 'great imitator' in the central nervous system. Both diagnosis with the disease and the morbidity and mortality associated with it have major consequences for the psychological and social functioning of individuals and their communities. The burdens resulting from chronic illness, social stigma, increasing numbers of orphans and loss of income are massive. Perhaps more than any other disease, HIV/AIDS calls for a truly holistic and biopsychosocial approach from health workers.

Context of psychiatric problems

HIV infection can interact with psychiatric illness in a number of ways:

- the 'worried well', i.e. individuals who are HIV-negative but who are concerned about being infected due to contact with HIV-positive sources/individuals;
- pre-test anxiety;
- the stress of diagnosis may precipitate a psychiatric illness, e.g. adjustment disorder, major depression or suicidality;
- living with the burden of being HIV-positive;
- those with pre-existing psychiatric problems may be more vulnerable to HIV infection due to impulsivity, disinhibition and increased risk-taking behaviours, e.g. unsafe sex;
- immunocompromised individuals are susceptible to secondary opportunistic infections and/or tumours of the CNS, which may manifest as neuropsychiatric disorders;
- antiretroviral medications can precipitate psychiatric disorders (see below);
- increasing social burdens of burnout in caregivers; loss of income; large numbers of AIDS orphans.

Figure 36.1 HIV/AIDS and mental illness – a problem relationship

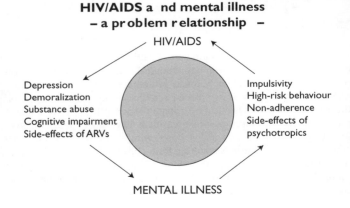

Depression and HIV/AIDS

Depression is extremely common (in up to 50% of individuals) and can occur at any stage of HIV infection. In this context, depression has many complex causes that should be identified and managed. Diagnosis itself can be difficult. For example, somatic symptoms of depression (weight loss, loss of energy, apathy) must be differentiated from physical effects of HIV infection. Another important differential diagnosis is HIV-associated dementia. Depression may reduce adherence to antiretroviral therapy and diminish attention to nutritional and other health needs.

Core symptoms include: changes in appetite, sleep pattern and energy levels; decreased libido; poor concentration and memory; suicidal ideation; tearfulness; poor self-esteem and deteriorating interpersonal relationships.

Antidepressant therapy

Serotonin reuptake inhibitors (SSRIs) such as fluoxetine, are safe in over-dose and free of sedating effects. However, side-effects such as headache, loss of appetite, diarrhoea and insomnia may exacerbate HIV-associated symptoms. Start at low doses (e.g. fluoxetine 10 mg daily) with slow increments, especially in patients with neuropsychiatric impairment.

Tricyclic antidepressents (TCAs) are dangerous in overdose, thus suicide risk must be carefully evaluated. Anticholinergic side-effects can be troublesome, especially in patients with cognitive deficits who are more sensitive to side-effects. However, other side-effects may in fact be useful in the context of HIV disease, e.g. increased appetite and weight gain; reducing diarrhoea; sedation at night. Low doses of amitriptyline (e.g. 25 mg nocte) may help with chronic pain, especially neuropathic pain due to HIV infection. Dosage: start at 25 mg nocte and slowly titrate up to 75–150 mg nocte.

Newer agents such as venlafaxine are useful for appetite stimulation and treatment of chronic pain. Dosage of venlafaxine starts at 75 mg nocte.

Electroconvulsive therapy (ECT) is not contraindicated in HIV-positive patients provided intracranial pressure is normal. Indications for ECT are the same as those in HIV-negative patients.

Suicide

There is a 30 times increased risk of suicide in individuals who are HIV-positive. High-risk periods are:
- at diagnosis;
- at the death of an HIV-positive friend or relative;
- during periods of relapse or deterioration;
- following losses (e.g. occupational or relational);
- when there is comorbid psychiatric illness;
- during end-stage AIDS.

Mania

Manic symptoms may develop in the context of HIV psychosis or as a side-effect of antiretroviral agents such as efavirenz.

Treatment

Mood stabilisers such as carbemazepine may be problematic. Hepatic enzyme inducing properties of carbemazepine may decrease efficacy of antiretrovirals. Lithium is preferable, but lithium levels and renal function must be monitored carefully, especially in patients with diarrhoea or any wasting syndrome.

HIV-related psychoses

The clinical presentation of HIV-related psychosis (due to direct viral effects on the brain) is often difficult to distinguish from schizophreniform and manic psychoses. The illness may be characterised by fluctuating symptoms, including bizarre and persecutory delusions, mixed mood symptoms and withdrawn apathetic states. Patients presenting with HIV psychosis are usually WHO Stage 3 or 4 (although the illness may occur as early as seroconversion) and most have some features of cognitive impairment, even if these are mild. Thus psychosis is a common early manifestation of subsequent HIV-associated dementia. Clinical evaluation together with appropriate special investigations such as CT scan, VDRL testing and a lumbar puncture are often indicated to exclude secondary CNS infection. While there are no specific investigations that can assist in differentiating manic or schizophreniform psychosis in an HIV-positive patient from psychosis due to HIV infection, it is important to make this distinction. Treatment, prognosis, psycho-education, rehabilitation and prevention all differ between these two groups of patients.

Treatment

Low-dose haloperidol (e.g. start with 0.5–1 mg bd and increase slowly) and atypical agents such as risperidone or olanzapine are preferred due to increased sensitivity in these patients to EPSEs. Chlorpromazine may be useful in the agitated patient for its sedating properties. Antiretrovirals may reduce psychotic symptoms.

Delirium

Delirium occurs in up to 30% of infected patients and has a high mortality rate. Core symptoms include:
- fluctuating level of consciousness;
- exacerbation at night;
- disorientation;
- prominent visual hallucinations.

Causes include:
- sepsis or fever;
- electrolyte abnormalities;
- hypoglycaemia;
- hypoxia;
- alcohol withdrawal;
- drug interactions/ side effects/ toxicity.

Note: delirium is often a first manifestation of HIV-associated dementia.

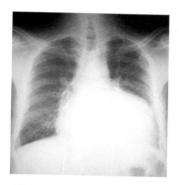

1 Tuberculous pericardial effusion: pre-aspiration.

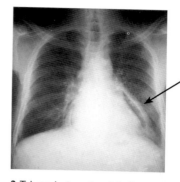

2 Tuberculosis pericardial effusion: post-aspiration, with the injection of air into the pericardial space to show thickened pericardium (arrowed).

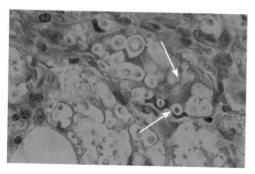

3 *Cryptococcus neoformans* on bone marrow trephine biopsy. Macrophages are seen with large numbers of intracellular encapsulated yeasts (arrowed). (Source: Dr Jill Finlayson.)

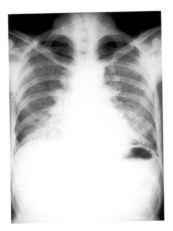

4 Extensive PCP – bilateral ground-glass opacification with areas of consolidation including the right middle lobe.

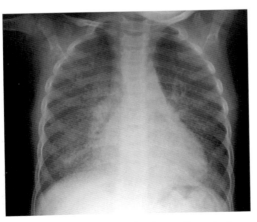

5 Diffuse nodular pattern on the chest radiograph of a child with lymphocytic interstitial pneumonitis. The differential diagnosis includes miliary tuberculosis.

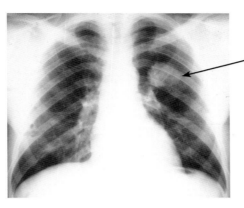

6 Cryptococcoma in the left upper zone (arrowed).

7 Bilateral miliary lung infiltrates. The most common cause is tuberculosis. This patient had disseminated histoplasmosis that was diagnosed on a biopsy of her skin rash.

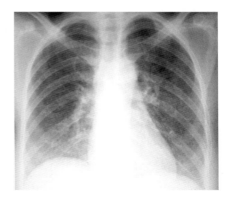

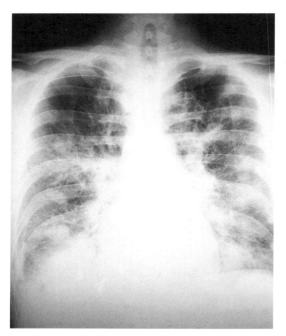

8 Pulmonary Kaposi's sarcoma with nodules and bilateral reticular pattern.

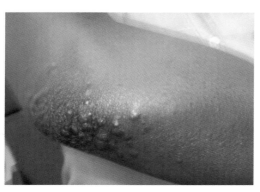

9 Eruptive xanthomata due to severe hyperlipidaemia in a patient taking lopinavir/ritonavir. The lesions resolved on treatment with gemfibrozil.

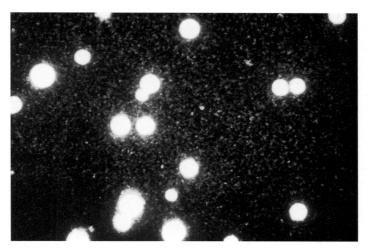

10 India ink stain of *Cryptococcus neoformans* in the cerebrospinal fluid. Note budding yeasts (arrowed).

11 Toxoplasmosis on MRI scan. Note multiple ring enhancing lesions with surrounding oedema and midline shift.

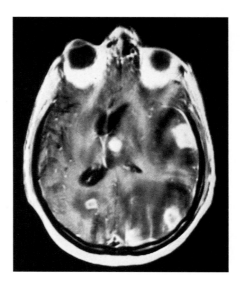

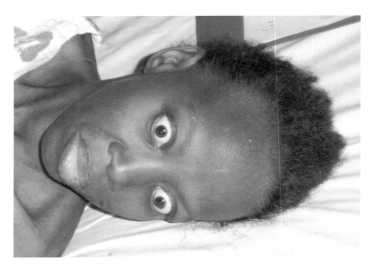

12 Lid retraction and mask-like face is due to HIV-associated dementia.

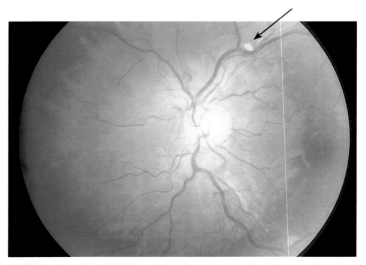

13 HIV retinopathy of the left eye. Note the cotton-wool spot (arrowed). This is a benign condition seen in late HIV disease.

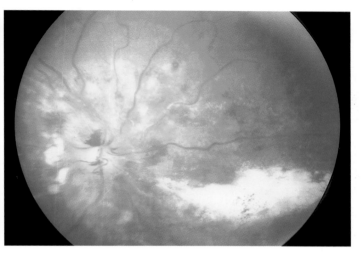

14 Cytomegalovirus retinitis of the right eye. Note the vascular sheathing.

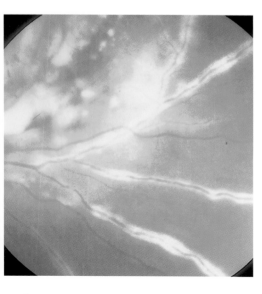

15
'Frosted branch' angiitis due to Cytomegalovirus retinitis.

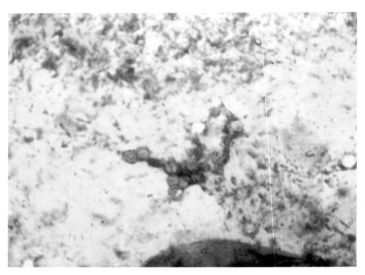

16 Modified Ziehl-Neelsen stain of *Cryptosporidium* oocytes in a stool specimen.

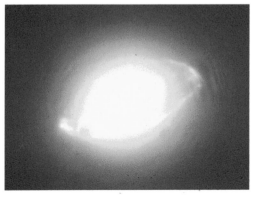

17 Auramine stain of *Isospora belli* in a stool specimen.

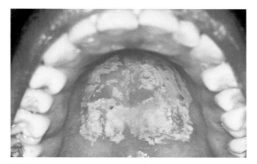

18 Pseudomembranous candidiasis on palate.

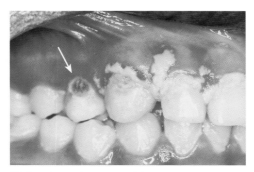

19 Pseudomembranous candidiasis on gingiva with caries lesion (arrowed).

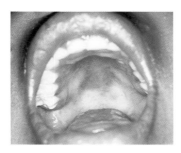

20 Erythematous candidiasis on palate.

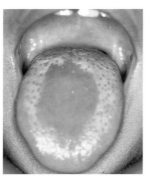

21 Median rhomboid glossitis.

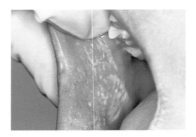

22 Hyperplastic candidiasis on buccal mucosa.

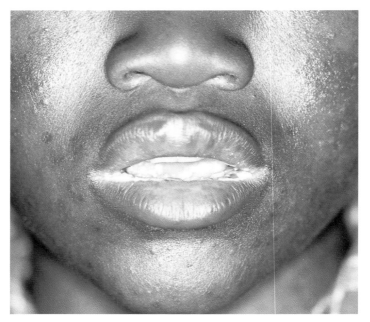

23 Angular cheilitis and pseudomembranous candidiasis.

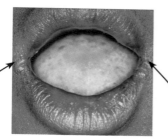

24 Angular cheilitis (arrowed).

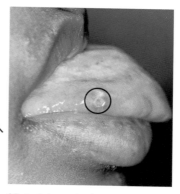

25 Early herpetic ulcer on the lateral border of the tongue (circled).

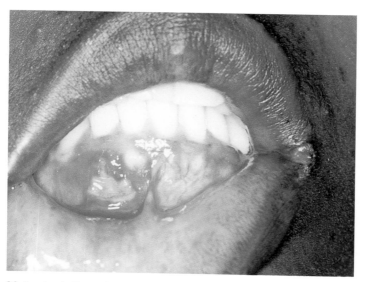

26 Angular cheilitis and aphthous ulcer on the lower gum margin.

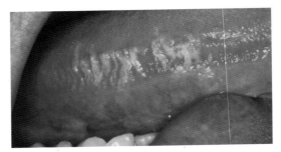

27 Oral hairy leukoplakia on the lateral border of the tongue.

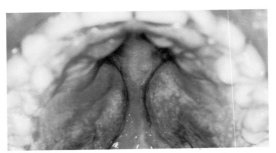

28 Florid Kaposi's sarcoma with haemorrhage on the palate.

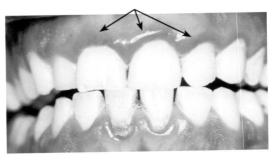

29 Linear gingival erythema (arrowed).

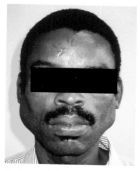

30 Parotid gland enlargement is a common feature of diffuse infiltrative lymphocytosis syndrome.

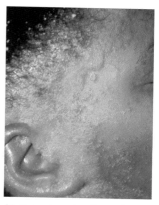

31 Extensive seborrhoeic dermatitis. Note angular configuration of lesions simulating a fungal infection.

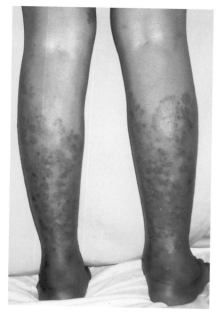

32 Fungal infection. The well-defined edge is characteristic.

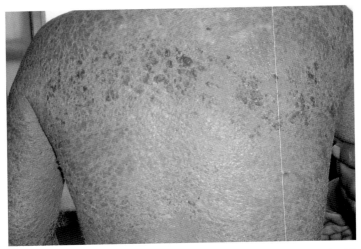

33 Widespread dermatitis on the back of a child. Unresponsive dermatitis should alert the practitioner to the possibility of associated HIV.

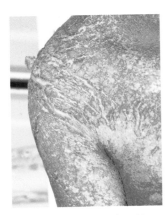

34 Crusted (Norwegian) scabies. There is thick scaling, with fissures at points of tension. Itching may be minimal or absent in this form of scabies.

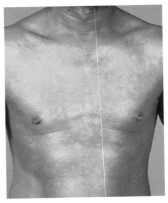

35 Diffuse maculopapular drug eruption due to a non-nucleoside reverse transcriptase inhibitor.

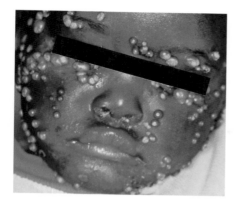

36 Molluscum contagiosum.

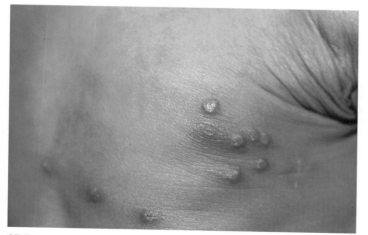

37 This crop of papules emerged suddenly with constitutional symptoms. Biopsy showed *Cryptococcus neoformans*.

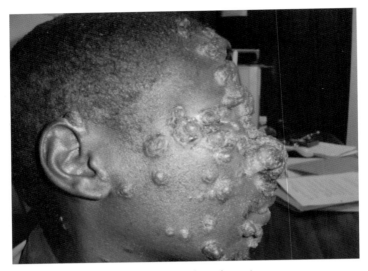

38 Cutaneous nodules and ulcers due to histoplasmosis.

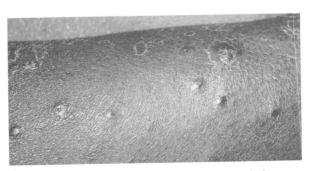

39 Pruritic papular eruption (PPE) of HIV also known as 'itchy bump disease' on a limb. Note active and healed lesions with post-inflammatory pigmentation.

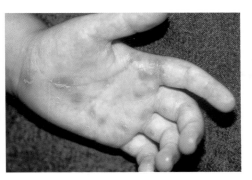

40 Keratotic scabies involving the anterior aspect of the wrist.

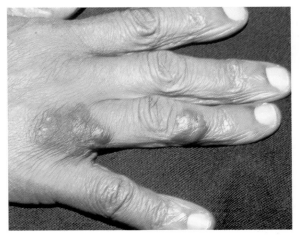

41 Kaposi's sarcoma.

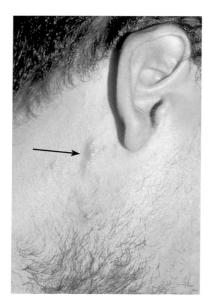

42 Kaposi's sarcoma may be very subtle in the early phase, with the lesion (arrowed) resembling a bruise or a callus.

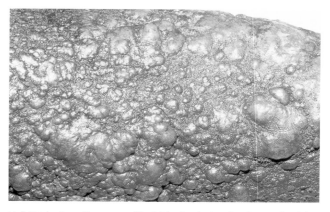

43 Extensive Kaposi's sarcoma of the thigh, showing lymphoedema and nodules.

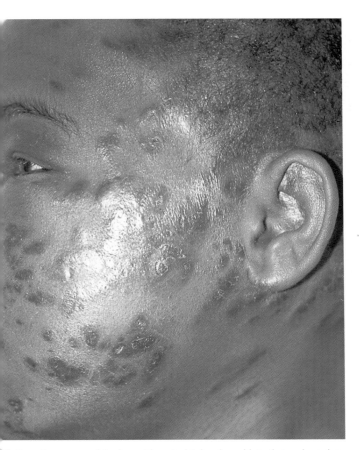

44 Kaposi's sarcoma of the face with periorbital oedema. Note that oedema due to Kaposi's sarcoma can present without visible lesions.

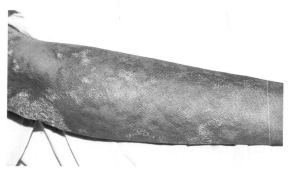

45 Lichenoid photo-aggravated drug reaction.

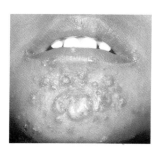

46
Primary impetigo of the chin. Note honey-coloured crusts.

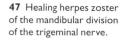

47 Healing herpes zoster of the mandibular division of the trigeminal nerve.

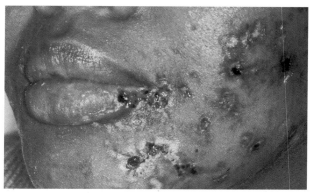

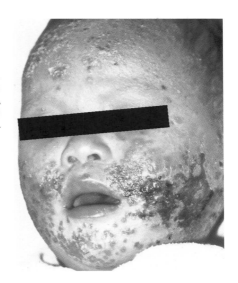

48 Herpes simplex virus infection. Note scattered vesicles, shallow erosions, and crusts on the face and forehead.

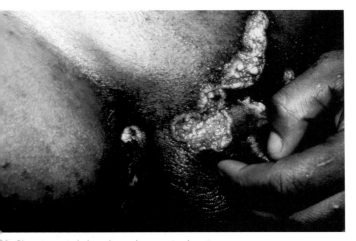

49 Chronic genital ulcer due to herpes simplex virus.

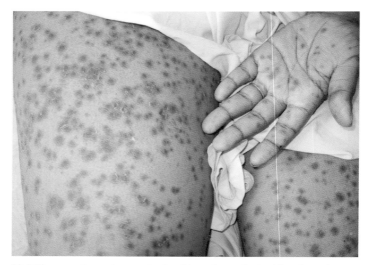

50 Diffuse maculopapular eruption involving palms and soles. *Histoplasmosis capsulatum* was detected on biopsy.

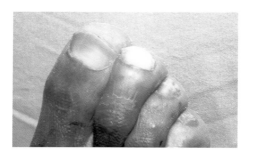

51 Proximal onychomycosis of the second toenail.

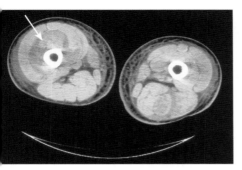

52 CT scan of bilateral thigh pyomyositis (arrowed).

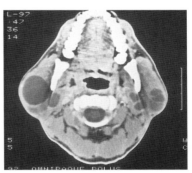

53 CT scan showing bilateral parotid gland cysts (arrowed).

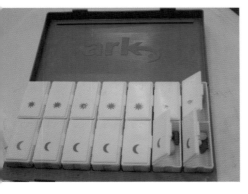

54 Pill box used to assist antiretroviral adherence.

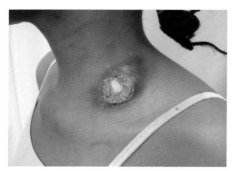

55 Paradoxical TB-IRIS lymphadenitis. The node enlarged and subsequently ruptured after patient started antiretrovirals while on TB treatment.

56 Paradoxical TB-IRIS. The patient developed recurrent cough and fever after starting antiretrovirals while on TB treatment. Chest radiograph shows worsening pulmonary infiltrate with cavitation.

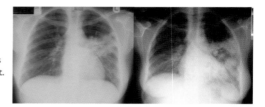

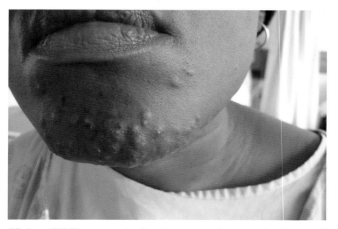

57 Acne IRIS. The patient developed an acne rash two weeks after switching to second line antiretrovirals following virological failure on first-line.

Treatment

- Treat the underlying cause (e.g. infection, hypoxia).
- Symptomatic treatment is with haloperidol (start with 0.5–1 mg bd) or atypical antpsychotic agents. Also lorazepam (1–2 mg 6–12 hourly) may help to control behavioural disturbance.
- Exclude underlying HIV-associated dementia.

HIV-associated dementia (HAD)

Epidemiology:

- 90% of AIDS patients have CNS changes post-mortem;
- 70–80% develop a cognitive disorder;
- 30% were thought to develop HAD. In an era of antiretrovirals, it has been recognised that many symptoms reverse, and this term may need better clinical clarity in future.

Mean survival after diagnosis of HAD is six months, in the absence of antiretroviral therapy. (See Chapter 35: Neurology, for neuropathology of HAD.)

Clinical presentation

- *Early minor cognitive and motor disorder*: asymptomatic HIV-positive patients may have very early CNS infection that is often discounted as 'stress'. Symptoms include cognitive slowing and memory deficits as well as motor slowing and subtle incoordination. Most will progress to HAD.
- *HIV-associated dementia (HAD)*: with worsening of symptoms, the clinical picture constitutes a dementia syndrome and is an AIDS-defining disorder. Clinical features are classified as *cognitive* (subcortical dementia, focal cognitive deficits, amnesia, mutism), *motor* (movement disorders) and *affective* (depression, apathy, agitation, disinhibition, mania) (see photo 12). Mild psychotic symptoms may progress to severe psychosis with manic and persecutory features, delusions and behavioural disturbance. Suicide is a serious risk, especially early in the course of HAD while insight remains intact. *Note: marked cognitive impairment is likely to adversely affect antiretroviral adherence.*

Core cognitive symptoms include:

- difficulty with switching tasks;
- decreased cognitive agility;

- difficulty with recall (worse than recognition);
- frontal-lobe symptoms;
- problem-solving difficulties

Treatment

Low doses of antipsychotic agents such as haloperidol or risperidone for psychotic and behavioural symptoms. Antiretrovirals have been shown to slow, arrest, or even reverse decline. Care must be taken before ascribing this diagnosis – it may be highly stigmatising. (Cognitive decline can be assessed using the HIV Dementia Scale.)

Other psychiatric problems and HIV/AIDS

Substance abuse

In South Africa, HIV transmission from sharing needles is uncommon. However, there is a high prevalence of other substance misuse in the general population, and this is a common comorbid problem. One should consider whether an HIV-positive patient's misuse of substances is in fact a form of self-medicating the stress, pain or depression associated with HIV.

Pain syndromes

Chronic pain (especially headache) is very common (experienced by up to 80% of patients at some stage). Pain is often severe (especially peripheral neuropathies) and frequently under-diagnosed, resulting in depression, self-medication with substances and an increased risk of suicide. The precise underlying cause may be difficult to determine. Adequate evaluation and treatment of pain is crucially important in maintaining quality of life. (See Chapter 56: Palliative care.)

Anxiety disorders

HIV infection is associated with increased risk for post-traumatic stress disorder (PTSD), obsessive complusive disorder (OCD), panic disorder and generalised anxiety disorder. A common time for anxiety symptoms is at testing and diagnosis.

Pregnancy and mental health

Pregnancy and the postpartum period are vulnerable periods for psychiatric problems, particularly affective and psychotic disorders. The combination of AIDS and pregnancy may be implicated in the exacerbation of these illnesses.

Children's mental health and AIDS

The mental health problems in children as a result of the AIDS epidemic are enormous and range from the loss of parents and siblings to the problems associated with being HIV-positive and having AIDS.

General principles of management

A thorough history, physical and mental state examination are essential in every HIV-positive patient presenting with psychiatric symptoms. Underlying medical causes of the psychiatric symptoms must be excluded and the clinical stage of HIV-infection must be determined. Appropriate investigations may include: CT scan of the brain; lumbar puncture; CD4 count and viral load; VDRL (to exclude neurosyphilis); FBC; U&E; liver functions. The clinician should consider the possible role of medications in precipitating psychiatric symptoms.

Important neuropsychiatric side-effects of drugs used in HIV treatment include:

- Efavirenz may cause vivid dreams, confusion, agitation, hallucinations, amnesia, anxiety, depression and suicidality, especially during the first two months of treatment. (Consider avoiding in patients with a psychiatric history.)
- Ritonavir + saquinavir combination may give neurological symptoms.
- INH can precipitate psychosis.

Some psychiatric medications may aggravate HIV-infection:

- Valproate   – plus ritonavir plus nevirapine may lead to hepato-toxicity.
- Carbamazepine – may aggravate leucopenia;
  - may decrease antiretroviral plasma levels.

Psychosocial treatment and rehabilitation

Psychosocial support for HIV-positive patients and their families is important to improve quality of life. Issues that require ongoing support include:

- education and information related to HIV;
- work discrimination;
- problems with accommodation; and
- dealing with the rejection of loved ones in the context of declining health. Psychosocial treatment strategies should be individualised and stage specific – being HIV-positive has markedly different implications from receiving a diagnosis of AIDS. Cognitive behavioural therapy (CBT), interpersonal and supportive therapies are useful for patients with adjustment disorders, and anxiety and mood disorders. Planning for wills, power of attorney, curatorship, and the care of dependants becomes important later in the course of the illness.

References and further reading

Bartlett, J.G., Treisman, G.J. and Angelino, A.F. 2004. *The Psychiatry of AIDS: A Guide to Diagnosis and Treatment*. The Johns Hopkins University Press.

Berger, J.R. and R.M. Levy. 1997. *AIDS and the Nervous System*. 2nd Edition. Lippincott-Raven Publishers.

McDaniel, J.S. et al. 2000. *Practice Guideline for the Treatment of Patients with HIV/AID* American Psychiatric Association. Available: http://www.psych.org

Saunders, J.N. 2001 *HIV and Mental Health*. In: B. Robertson, C. Allwood and C. Gagiano (Eds) *Textbook of Psychiatry for Southern Africa*. Cape Town: Oxford University Press.

Treisman, G.J. and A.I. Kaplin. 2002 'Neurologic and psychiatric complications of antiretroviral agents.' *AIDS*; 16:1201–1215.

Van Gorp, W.G. and S.L. Buckingham. 1998. *Practitioner's Guide to the Neuropsychiatry of HIV/AIDS*. The Guildford Press.

37 Ophthalmology

Ophthalmic manifestations of HIV infection are common and varied and occur in approximately 75% of all HIV-positive patients in the course of their disease. The ocular disease profile in patients with HIV/AIDS in Africa is dramatically different to that described in the developed world. Most notable is the comparative rarity of cytomegalovirus (CMV) retinitis in Africa (despite high CMV seroprevalence rates). Table 37.1 compares ophthalmic manifestations in the developing world with those in the developed world. Table 37.2 summarizes the relationship between CD4 counts and common HIV-associated disorders of the eye.

Table 37.1 Comparison of ophthalmic manifestations in the developed and developing world

Developed world	Developing world
HIV microvasculopathy	Herpes zoster ophthalmicus
CMV retinitis (15-30% of patients with AIDS)	HIV microvasculopathy
KS	Conjunctival neoplasia
	CMV retinitis (< 2% of patients with AIDS)

Table 37.2 CD4 counts and common HIV-associated disorders of the eye

<500 cells/µl	<250 cells/µl	<100 cells/µl
KS	Toxoplasmosis	HIV microvasculopathy
TB		Keratoconjunctivitis sicca
Syphilis		CMV retinitis
		Varicella-zoster retinitis

A symptom-based approach to HIV-associated eye disease is useful, and can be classified as:

- abnormal appearance on inspection or ophthalmoscopy;
- the painful red eye;
- painless loss of vision owing to retinal or optic nerve disease; and
- abnormal eye movements.

Abnormal appearance on inspection

The patient may present with any of the following diseases of the lids, external eye, and orbit:

- herpes zoster ophthalmicus;
- conjunctival neoplasia;
- molluscum contagiosum; and
- proptosis.

Herpes zoster ophthalmicus (HZO)

This is the most common ocular manifestation of HIV/AIDS in our setting. It usually occurs in the early stages of HIV disease and is associated with a higher rate of complications and recurrence than in HIV-negative patients.

Clinical features

The clinical features of HZO are:

- significant permanent lid damage with associated corneal damage, including:
  - ectropion (the lid margin turns away from the globe), and
  - entropion (the lid margin turns inward towards the globe);
- conjunctivitis, episcleritis, and scleritis (see the section on the painful red eye);
- keratitis in two-thirds of patients:
  - epithelial disease stains with fluorescein,
  - stromal and endothelial disease does not stain with flourescein – white/grey lesions are visible within the cornea;
- anterior uveitis (ranging from mild to very severe), which presents as a painful red eye with decreased vision, and occurs in up to 40% of patients;
- glaucoma in 10%-40% of patients with anterior uveitis;
- retinitis in approximately 15% of patients (see the section on painless loss of vision);
- oculomotor nerve palsy (other cranial nerves are more rarely involved); and
- post-herpetic neuralgia.

Primary care management

Treatment options include:

- systemic antivirals: aciclovir 800 mg five times daily for 10 days within 72 hours of the onset of the rash;
- chloramphenicol ointment as a lubricant and to prevent secondary infection of corneal lesions;
- potassium permanganate soaks 12 hourly followed by 1% silver sulfadiazine cream for skin lesions;
- analgesics (patients often require an opiate);
- antibiotics for added skin infection/cellulitis; and
- amitriptyline 25 mg at night for three months.

Refer all patients for ophthalmology review once acute skin lesions and swelling have subsided.

Criteria for same-day referral to an ophthalmologist

The criteria for same-day referral are:
- decreased visual acuity;
- Hutchinson's sign positive (skin lesions on the side of the tip of the nose) as this is associated with increased intraocular involvement; or
- corneal staining with fluorescein.

Conjunctival neoplasia

Squamous carcinoma of the conjunctiva

- In sub-Saharan Africa, 70%–80% of patients with squamous carcinoma of the conjunctiva are HIV-positive.
- It is associated with human papillomavirus-16.
- The tumour appears as a grey or white nodule that typically occurs medially between the upper and lower lids in the interpalpebral zone and has well-defined edges and surrounding hyperaemia. Most touch the corneal edge or grow onto the cornea. The surface of the lesion has a rough, foamy, or fungating appearance.
- Tumours are distinguishable from pterygium or pingueculum, which are covered with smooth, shiny, conjunctival epithelium.

Kaposi's sarcoma of the eyelid and conjunctiva

- The tumour can be flat or nodular. Conjunctival lesions range from bright red to purple, with surrounding dilated tortuous vessels. Lid lesions have the appearance of Kaposi's sarcoma of the skin elsewhere on the body.

- Differential diagnosis includes subconjunctival haemorrhage and haemangioma.

Refer all suspected malignancies to an ophthalmologist.

Molluscum contagiosum

Molluscum contagiosum occurs in the late stages of HIV disease. Lesions are larger than in HIV-negative patients, more numerous, and do not regress spontaneously.

See Chapter 40: Dermatology, for the management of molluscum contagiosum.

Proptosis

Orbital complications in AIDS patients are uncommon, but are associated with significant visual loss, morbidity, and mortality.

Causes of proptosis

The causes of proptosis are:
- neoplastic (malignant lymphoma);
- infective: fungal (aspergillus) and bacterial (usually secondary to sinusitis); and
- inflammatory (rare, usually due to orbital pseudotumour or myositis).

It is important to differentiate preseptal infection from orbital cellulitis: Open the eyelids and examine the eye. Table 37.3 shows the distinguishing findings on examination.

Table 37.3 Differentiating preseptal and orbital cellulitis

	Preseptal cellulitis	Orbital cellulitis
Conjunctival swelling/chemosis	Minimal	Significant
Eye movements	Normal	Limited
Proptosis	Absent	Present
Vision	Normal	May be decreased with afferent pupil defect*

* Afferent pupil defect: the pupil constricts to consensual light but not to direct light.

Refer patients with orbital disease to an ophthalmologist immediately.

Abnormal appearance on ophthalmoscopy

See also 'Painless visual loss', page 394.

Microangiopathy

Microangiopathy is the most common ocular manifestation of HIV disease in the developed world. The incidence in African patients is lower, as many patients die before they reach the degree of immunocompromise associated with HIV microvasculopathy. This is a benign condition and requires no treatment.

Clinical features

The clinical features of microangiopathy include:

- a CD4 count <100 cells/μl (if it is >100 cells/μl exclude other causes of retinopathy, such as diabetes, anaemia, and hypertension);
- cotton-wool spots (most frequent), microaneurysms, haemorrhages, and perivascular sheathing (see photo 13);
- changing signs that appear and disappear over a few weeks;
- signs that occur in both the retina (especially the posterior pole) and the conjunctiva; and
- no decrease in visual acuity.

Optic disc swelling

Papilloedema needs to be differentiated from optic nerve disease, and to be investigated appropriately. Table 37.4 summarizes the features, causes, and investigation of both.

Table 37.4 Differentiating papilloedema and optic nerve disease

	Papilloedema	Optic nerve disease
Clinical features	Usually bilateral Normal vision and normal pupil reflexes	Usually unilateral Decreased vision with afferent pupil defect
Causes	Mass lesions – CNS toxoplasmosis, lymphoma, or TB meningitis	Infective – toxoplasmosis, TB, cryptococcus, syphilis, herpes virus family Infiltrative – lymphoma
Investigation	Neuroimaging Perform LP unless contra-indicated by scan result	Refer the patient to an ophthalmologist

The painful red eye

All patients with a unilateral painful red eye, especially if this is associated with decreased vision, need to be referred to an ophthalmologist for assessment. Table 37.5 summarizes the clinical features and causes of the painful red eye.

Painless visual loss

The majority of the conditions listed in Table 37.6 present with painless loss of vision in a white, uninflamed eye. However, some of the causes of retinitis included in this section are sometimes associated with significant intraocular inflammation, and so present as a painful red eye. All patients presenting with loss of vision should undergo:

- an assessment of their visual acuity;
- an assessment of the red reflex;
- an external eye examination (zoster rash, conjunctival injection, corneal haze, flourescein staining of tear film);
- a swinging flashlight test for relative afferent pupil defect; and
- a fundoscopy examination through a dilated pupil.

Cytomegalovirus retinitis

CMV retinitis is the most common cause of visual loss, even in Africa, where the incidence is lower than in the developed world. It presents when the CD4 count ranges between 100 and 50 cells/µl. Bilateral disease is found at presentation in 20%–40% of patients.

Clinical features

The clinical features are:

- painless decrease in vision (lesions close to fovea or optic nerve) and floaters;
- relative afferent pupil defect if there is extensive retinal involvement;
- no vitreous haze – the fundus is clearly visible (this is important in the differential diagnosis);
- retinal whitening or opacification, with or without haemorrhages and with or without vascular sheathing 'frosted branch' angiitis (see photos 14 and 15);
- satellite lesions (small white lesions adjacent to the area of confluent retinitis); and
- optic nerve involvement in up to 5% of patients.

Table 37.5 Clinical features and causes of the painful red eye

Diagnosis	Clinical features	Common causes
Conjunctivitis*	Bilateral, injection increases further away from cornea Normal vision	Viral Bacterial
Episcleritis	Discomfort rather than pain Sectoral or focal conjunctival injection Normal vision	
Scleritis	Unilateral Severe pain (disturbs sleep) Sclera deep red or violaceous Vision may be abnormal or normal	
Keratitis	Stains with flourescein if there is an epithelial defect Corneal haze/whiteness if there is stromal keratitis Decreased corneal sensation in herpes simplex infection	Viral – herpes simplex, herpes zoster Bacterial Fungal Microsporidial
Uveitis	Photophobia Limbal flush (conjunctival injection around cornea) Irregular small pupil May see keratic precipitates on inflammation) close inspection with ophthalmoscope	Infective – herpes zoster, herpes simplex, syphilis, TB Drugs, e.g. cidofovir (severe pain) and rifabutin (marked iridocyclitis associated with retinitis) Immune recovery uveitis occurs in patients with pre-existing CMV retinitis commenced on antiretrovirals
Kerato-conjunctivitis sicca (KCS)†	Affects 25% of HIV patients Gritty 'foreign-body' sensation Burning or aching worsens in air-conditioned or dry environments Mild conjunctival injection with thin tear meniscus on close inspection Fine punctate staining of cornea with fluorescein	

Note: Refer conjunctivitis and KCS for ophthalmology assessment if the symptoms persist.
*Conjunctivitis should be treated with chloramphenicol eye drops.
†KCS should be treated with frequent application of lubricants.

Note that CMV encephalitis is commonly associated with optic nerve involvement.

Natural history

Untreated, CMV retinitis is relentlessly progressive and destroys the whole retina within six months. This progression is, however, slow compared with other causes of necrotizing retinitis in AIDS patients.

Treatment

Ideal therapy of CMV retinitis is systemic induction therapy followed by maintenance therapy with either intravenous ganciclovir or oral valganciclovir. In the South African public sector the main treatment modality is weekly intravitreal ganciclovir, which should be commenced by an ophthalmologist according to the following criteria:

- the patient should have a visual acuity 6/60 or better;
- there should be no CMV retinitis in the macula (the area between the temporal arcades); and
- there should be no optic nerve involvement.

Anti-CMV therapy can be discontinued when the CD4 count has increased to >100 cells/µl for six months on antiretroviral therapy. Initiation of antiretroviral therapy can result in a uveitis as a manifestation of the immune reconstitution inflammatory syndrome (refer to Chapter 50: Immune reconstitution inflammatory syndrome).

The patient should be counselled that the aim of treatment is to prevent further loss of vision (not to restore vision already lost), that treatment is lifelong, and that it involves weekly intravitreal injections. The ophthalmologist should explain the risks of intravitreal injections, namely endophthalmitis, retinal detachment, and vitreous haemorrhage.

Herpes zoster retinitis

This is the second most common cause of necrotizing retinitis and affects 1%–4 % of AIDS patients. It develops in approximately 15% of HIV-positive patients with HZO.

Table 37.6 Causes of painless loss of vision

Affected structure	Common causes
Retina Abnormality seen on dilated ophthalmoscopy If extensive, will have relative afferent pupil defect	Infective Viral: Herpes viruses (CMV, zoster, simplex) Bacterial: Toxoplasmosis, syphilis Neoplastic Large cell lymphoma Vascular Retinal artery occlusion Retinal vein occlusion
Optic nerve Optic disc may appear normal or abnormal Afferent pupil defect is present	Infective Papillitis or retrobulbar neuritis, HIV, syphilis, CMV, cryptococcosis, and TB. Neoplastic Lymphoma Vascular Constrictive optic neuropathy: Cryptococcal meningitis Anterior ischaemic optic neuropathy Other Toxic optic neuropathy: Ethambutol Compressive optic neuropathy: Orbital disease, intracranial mass lesion
Central visual pathways Normal ocular examination No afferent pupil defect May have visual field defect on confrontation Usually asymptomatic	Infective/neoplastic Mass lesion – lymphoma, tuberculoma Vascular Occipital infarction

Clinical features

Presentation is related to the level of immune compromise.

The features of acute retinal necrosis are:

- a CD4 count >50 cells/μl;
- retinitis in the peripheral retina (macula spared);
- prominent intraocular inflammation (hazy view of retina with red eye); and
- complications – optic nerve disease and retinal detachment are common.

The response to therapy is variable.

Features of progressive outer retinal necrosis (PORN) are:

- a CD4 count <50 cells/μl; and
- minimal intraocular inflammation.

As there is no vitritis, the view of the retina is good.

The visual prognosis is dismal, regardless of therapy. Features of PORN that differentiate it from CMV are: a lack of haemorrhages; rapid progression circumferentially then posteriorly to involve the macula; and the sparing of the retina just adjacent to the blood vessels (giving a 'cracked mud' appearance).

Treatment

The mainstay of therapy is intravenous aciclovir for a week, followed by four to six weeks of oral aciclovir.

Toxoplasmosis

Features of toxoplasmosis are:

- a CD4 count that is usually <100 cells/μl;
- retinitis that may be focal, multifocal, or diffuse, mimicking CMV retinitis (but with no retinal haemorrhages); and
- significant intraocular inflammation, giving vitritis and occasional anterior chamber activity on examination.

It is imperative to do neuroimaging (central nervous system toxoplasmosis is present in 30% of HIV-positive patients with retinal toxoplasmosis). The condition responds to treatment, and patients should be referred to an ophthalmologist.

Syphilis

Ocular syphilis is best conceptualized as neurosyphilis and may develop in people who have been adequately treated for primary or secondary syphilis. (See Chapter 25: Sexually transmitted infections.) Serum VDRL is often negative, while FTA is positive. Examination of the cerebrospinal fluid usually demonstrates a pleocytosis, but may be normal. All patients should be referred to an ophthalmologist for 10 days of intravenous penicillin.

Abnormal eye movements

Eye movement abnormalities in HIV-associated dementia

Patients with HIV-associated dementia have impaired anti-saccades. (See Chapter 35: Neurology.)

Decreased eye movement

Decreased eye movement is usually the result of mass lesion(s) or meningitis, and less commonly of brainstem viral infections, HIV encephalopathy, or cavernous sinus thrombosis.

References and further reading

Cunningham, E. T., and T.P. Jr. Margolis. 1998. 'Ocular manifestations of HIV infection'. *New England Journal of Medicine*; 339 (4):236–244.

Lewallen, S., and P. Courtright. 1997. 'HIV and AIDS and the eye in developing countries: A review'. *Archives of Ophthalmology*; 115 (10):1291–1295.

Martin, D.F. et al. 2002. ' A controlled trial of valganciclovir as induction therapy for cytomegalovirus retinitis.' *New England Journal of Medicine*; 346:1119–1126.

Gastroenterology and hepatology

Almost all HIV-infected patients have gastrointestinal tract (GIT) involvement during the course of their illness. The most common GIT symptoms are odynophagia, diarrhoea, weight loss, and medication intolerance.

Ascites, abdominal lymphadenopathy, and hepatosplenomegaly are frequent manifestations of tuberculosis (TB). This chapter deals with oesophageal disorders, diarrhoea, hepatobiliary disease, and weight loss. It also briefly touches on abdominal pain and perianal disease. Oral complications and nutrition are discussed in Chapter 39: Oral medicine and Chapter 23: Diet and nutrition respectively.

Oesophageal disorders

Odynophagia and dysphagia cause significant discomfort and, if severe enough, may lead to dehydration and loss of weight.

Oesophageal candidiasis

Oesophageal candidiasis is the commonest cause of odynophagia and dysphagia. Most cases (70%–80%) are accompanied by oral thrush. A history of retrosternal pain on swallowing in the presence of oral thrush is enough to make a presumptive diagnosis and start empiric treatment.

Management

The management of oesophageal candidiasis consists of the following:
- The standard treatment is fluconazole 100–200 mg daily for two weeks. Initial intravenous therapy can be given for patients unable to swallow. Symptomatic improvement occurs within a week in most patients.
- Itraconazole 200 mg daily is as effective as fluconazole. The oral solution has better bioavailability than the capsule.

Relapse occurs in about a third of patients. Prophylaxis is not generally recommended as it selects for azole resistant species, notably *Candida krusei*. This typically occurs in patients with advanced disease after prolonged azole exposure. It is important to send specimens for fungal culture and azole susceptibility if there is poor response to azole therapy. Amphotericin B 0.3–0.5 mg/kg/day IV is probably the best option for azole resistance, but some patients may respond to high-dose fluconazole (800 mg/day) or itraconazole. As with all opportunistic diseases, the best approach is immune reconstitution with antiretroviral therapy.

If symptoms fail to improve after a two-week course of treatment, the patient should undergo endoscopy to exclude other pathologies.

Cytomegalovirus oesophageal ulceration

Cytomegalovirus (CMV) ulcers may be small, or large and circumferential. Diagnosis is made on oesophageal biopsy. Treatment is with an induction course (two to three weeks) of intravenous ganciclovir or oral valganciclovir. The response is generally good. Relapses may occur, but maintenance therapy is not usually necessary. Antacids (notably sucralfate) and opiate analgesics are important for pain relief.

Aphthous ulcers

Aphthous ulcers may look similar to CMV ulcers macroscopically, and diagnosis is made after exclusion of CMV on biopsy. They are more common than CMV ulcers.

The treatment options for aphthous ulcers are:
- sucralfate and/or opiate analgesics;
- prednisone 0.5 mg/kg/day for two weeks (higher doses or a longer duration may be necessary, but should be avoided if possible);
- intralesional injections of steroids;
- thalidomide (not registered in South Africa)
- antiretroviral therapy, which is the best treatment.

Herpes simplex ulcers

This virus causes small, deep crops of ulcers. Diagnosis is made on biopsy. Aciclovir 400 mg eight hourly is effective treatment.

Other causes

Other HIV-associated causes of oesophageal disease are TB, Kaposi's sarcoma (KS), and lymphoma. Conditions unrelated to HIV, such as gastro-oesophageal reflux disease, are also common.

Diarrhoea in the HIV-infected patient

Between 40% and 90% of HIV-infected patients will present with diarrhoea at some stage of their illness, particularly in advanced disease. The approach to the patient with diarrhoea depends on the degree of immune suppression (e.g. a patient with a CD4 count of >200 cells/μl is unlikely to harbour opportunistic organisms) and the type of diarrhoeal illness. Table 38.1 lists common causes of diarrhoea specifically seen in immune-suppressed patients.

Table 38.1 Causes, presentation, diagnosis and treatment of HIV-related diarrhoea

Organism	Presentation	Diagnosis	Therapy
Coccidia:	Small bowel		
Cryptosporidium		Stool microscopy	Nil specific
Microsporidia spp.		Stool microscopy/biopsy	Albendazole* (4 weeks)
Isospora belli		Stool microscopy	Co-trimoxazole†
Cyclospora		Stool microscopy	Co-trimoxazole‡
Bacteria:	Large bowel		
Salmonella		Stool culture	Quinolone
Shigella		Stool culture	Quinolone
Campylobacter		Stool culture	Macrolide
C. difficile toxin		Stool toxin	Metronidazole
Mycobacteria:	Small bowel		Anti-TB therapy
Tuberculosis		Culture/biopsy/ultrasound	Clarithromycin &
MAC		Blood culture	ethambutol
Viral:			
CMV	Large bowel	Biopsy	Ganciclovir
HIV	Small bowel	Exclude other causes	Antiretrovirals

* Albendazole 400 mg twice daily 4wk.

† Co-trimoxazole 80/400 mg 4 tablets twice daily 2–4 wk., then 2 tablets as suppression.

‡ Co-trimoxazole 80/400 mg 2 tablets four times daily 10 d., then 2 tablets daily as suppression.

Diarrhoea is most commonly caused by infections, but drugs, notably the protease inhibitors, may be responsible. Malignancies like KS and lymphoma, and malabsorption related to pancreatic disease, may also present with diarrhoea.

Important factors are:

- access to safe water;
- travel history;
- the incidence of certain organisms or outbreaks in the community, e.g. cholera or amoebiasis;
- the duration of the diarrhoea;
- prior use of antibiotics;
- small bowel or large bowel diarrhoea;
- the degree of immune suppression.

Certain intestinal parasites are detected by specific stains, which may not be routinely performed; in particular *Cryptosporidium parvum*, *Cyclospora cayetanensis*, *Isospora belli*, and microsporidia. (See Table 38.2.)

Table 38.2 Commonly used stains for visualization of certain parasites

Cryptosporidium	Auramine, decolourized with acid alcohol Modified Ziehl-Neelsen stain (see photo 16) Sheather's sugar flotation
Isospora belli	Auramine decolourized with acid alcohol (see photo 17) Modified Ziehl-Neelsen stain
Microsporidium	Modified trichrome stain Calcufluor white
Cyclospora	Modified acid-fast stain

Some laboratories offer nucleic acid amplification tests for microsporidia. It is worthwhile liaising with the laboratory to determine which organisms are routinely looked for, and which organisms require additional investigations.

As a general rule, a maximum of three stool specimens should be sufficient to detect most parasitic infections. At least one specimen should also be cultured for the conventional bacterial causes, *Salmonella* spp., *Shigella* spp., or *Campylobacter* spp. If repeated stool samples are negative, endoscopy and small bowel biopsy should be considered.

Patients who develop diarrhoea while in hospital, or who have been on antibiotics, should have stool samples submitted for detection of *Clostridium difficile* toxin. (See Appendix 21.1)

Figure 38.1 is an algorithm for evaluating cases of diarrhoea more than two weeks in duration.

Figure 38.1 Algorithm for evaluating diarrhoea of >2 weeks' duration

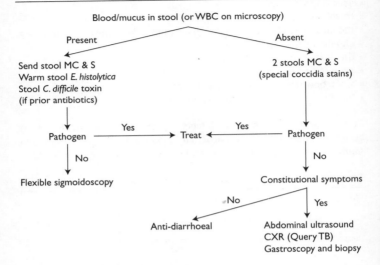

Small bowel diarrhoea

A patient with small bowel diarrhoea usually presents with large-volume watery stools, which are bland (i.e. absence of red or white blood cells). There may be associated malabsorption. The patient is often apyrexial. An acute illness in a patient with a well-preserved CD4 count should initially be treated symptomatically. Coccidian parasites are a likely cause of diarrhoea persisting for more than two weeks in patients with a CD4 count of less than 200 cells/μl. Special stains are required to diagnose the coccidian parasites, especially microsporidiosis, which is the most common cause of chronic diarrhoea in central Africa, but is less common in urban South Africa.

Large bowel diarrhoea

Tenesmus and frequent, low-volume stools with red and white cells or mucus suggest colitis. Acute illness is usually caused by conventional bacterial causes of dysentery. If a patient has an acute dysenteric-type illness (regardless of his or her HIV status or CD4 count):

- rehydrate;
- send blood and stool for microscopy and culture;
- commence an empiric course of a fluoroquinolone antibiotic.

CMV causes patchy mucosal ulceration of the colon and is typically seen with a CD4 count <100 cells/μl. Diagnosis is by biopsy of an ulcer, many of which are accessible by sigmoidsoscopy. Treatment is the same as that of CMV oesophageal ulceration.

HIV enteropathy

HIV can cause enteritis associated with malabsorption. This is a diagnosis of exclusion. Management is symptomatic and supportive, while awaiting immune restoration with antiretroviral treatment.

Antiretroviral-induced diarrhoea

Many of the antiretroviral drugs can cause diarrhoea, most notably the protease inhibitors. Diarrhoea may occasionally be severe, and adherence may be decreased. Substitution or symptomatic treatment (see below) should be considered.

Endoscopic procedures

For practical purposes, to speed up diagnosis, and because the differentiation between small and large bowel diarrhoea is sometimes not clear, gastroscopy (with duodenal aspirate and biopsy) and flexible sigmoidoscopy are often done at the same visit. A small number of right-sided colonic lesions will be missed on flexible sigmoidoscopy. If all tests are negative and there is a high index of suspicion, the patient should undergo colonoscopy. With intensive investigations, a causative organism may be found in up to 80% of patients.

Such intensive investigations are not always appropriate and efforts should be concentrated on performing the fewest invasive procedures necessary to find or exclude treatable organisms. Often chronic diarrhoea will resolve on antiretroviral therapy.

Management

Rehydration

Fluid and electrolyte replacement is essential in all forms of diarrhoea. Oral rehydration is preferable, and can be achieved using commercial formulations or a simple salt and water solution consisting of half a teaspoon of salt and eight teaspoons of sugar dissolved in a litre of boiled water. This can be given by nasogastric tube if necessary.

Dehydration with hypotension should be corrected with intravenous saline solution.

Symptomatic treatment

- Antidiarrhoeal agents should *never* be used in patients with colitis. Loperamide or codeine phosphate are often effective for small bowel diarrhoea. For protease inhibitor-induced diarrhoea loperamide, calcium carbonate and bulking agents have shown efficacy in small clinical trials.

Salmonella septicaemia

Non-typhoid salmonella species (e.g. *Salmonella typhimurium*) acquired from contaminated food cause recurrent severe septicaemia in AIDS patients. Infection presents with high fever and may be fatal if not promptly treated. Diarrhoea is absent in about half of the reported cases. A blood culture should be taken and antibiotics commenced (appropriate empiric choices would be a third-generation cephalosporin or a fluoroquinolone). The duration of antibiotic therapy should be four to six weeks to prevent relapse.

Atypical mycobacteria – *Mycobacterium avium* complex

Mycobacterium avium complex (MAC) infection is seen in severely immunocompromised patients (CD4 <100 cells/µl). The typical presentation is one of persistent fever of unknown origin with anaemia. GIT manifestations of wasting and diarrhoea may also occur.

The diagnosis is made on blood culture from a normally sterile site (e.g. blood, bone marrow, or biopsy). Stool culture is suggestive, but sputum culture often represents transient colonization, and only specimens that are repeatedly culture positive are clinically significant. A combination of ethambutol 15 mg/kg/day and clarithromycin 500 mg twice daily is effective long-term treatment. Rifabutin may be added in severe cases.

Weight loss and the HIV wasting syndrome

Weight loss and wasting contribute significantly not only to the morbidity and mortality of HIV and AIDS, but also to the stigma borne by patients, who sometimes go to great lengths to hide the wasting under many layers of clothing. Extreme wasting has given the name 'slim disease' to AIDS in Africa.

Many factors contribute to weight loss in HIV infection, and more than one factor is commonly present. Firstly, intake may be decreased due to anorexia (intercurrent infections, depression and adverse drug reactions are common causes), painful swallowing due to oropharyngeal or oesophageal disease, poverty (very common in the region), and drug or alcohol abuse. Secondly, the metabolic rate is raised early in the course of HIV infection, and increases further as the course of the illness progresses. Thirdly, malabsorption may occur due to infective diarrhoea or HIV-induced small bowel villus atrophy. Fourthly, the acute phase response induced by opportunistic diseases can cause profound weight loss. Finally, loss of subcutaneous fat (lipo-atrophy) may occur with the use of antiretrovirals, especially with stavudine.

When evaluating a patient with weight loss, consider the following:
- Take a careful dietary and substance abuse history.
- Determine the amount and pattern (rapidity) of weight loss. A history of weight loss of >2 kg or >5% of body weight in a month is probably due to an opportunistic disease. More gradual weight loss is usually the result of HIV wasting or malabsorption. Plotting serial weights on a graph is a useful clinical tool.
- The presence of fever or night sweats suggests an opportunistic disease, notably TB and malignancy (lymphomas and Kaposi's sarcoma are both associated with so-called 'B' symptoms).
- An elevated C reactive protein suggests that an opportunistic disease is the cause of wasting.

Wasting syndrome

This is an AIDS-defining illness and a diagnosis of exclusion.

Wasting syndrome is defined as: *An involuntary loss of weight of more than 10% of body weight, plus either chronic diarrhoea (two or more loose stools per day for more than 30 days) or fever, for more than 30 days in the absence of concurrent illness.* It is essential to exclude underlying opportunistic diseases, notably TB.

Treatment is with antiretrovirals together with nutritional supplementation. Anabolic steroids have no role in the routine management of wasting, but testosterone supplementation can be beneficial in men with low plasma testosterone concentrations.

Abdominal pain in the HIV-positive patient

In the immunosuppressed patient, abdominal pain is frequently a marker of OIs. If there is associated diarrhoea, investigations should proceed as above. In the absence of obvious localizing symptoms in the upper GIT, a chest radiograph and abdominal ultrasound may be helpful. Ascites, intra-abdominal and retroperitoneal lymphadenopathy, as well as splenic hypodensities are highly predictive of TB in a high-prevalence setting. Commencing antituberculous therapy while awaiting mycobacterial cultures is reasonable. Lymphoma and disseminated fungal infection should be considered if there is no response to TB treatment and cultures are negative.

Hepatobiliary disease

Hepatobiliary disease in HIV is commonly due to hepatic viruses, drug reactions, HIV itself, and opportunistic diseases. The differential diagnosis and management of hepatobiliary disease is complex.

Liver function tests

The two main patterns of liver enzyme elevations affect predominantly the hepatocyte transaminases (ALT is more useful to measure than AST) or the cannalicular enzymes (ALP and GGT). Cannalicular enzyme elevation suggests cholestasis or infiltration (with fat, granulomas or tumour), while transaminitis suggests hepatitis (viral or drug-induced). Mixed patterns are common. Minor abnormalities of liver enzymes (up to three times the upper limit of normal) are common, and should be investigated with hepatitis B and C serology and history of alcohol consumption.

Imaging

Abdominal ultrasonography will usually confirm or exclude biliary dilatation or the presence of gallstones, but definitive diagnosis of cholangiopathy sometimes requires an ERCP or MRI scan. Fatty infiltration may be seen on ultrasound, but a CT scan, if available, is more accurate.

If imaging shows an intrahepatic mass, a CT or ultrasound-guided biopsy can be undertaken.

Drug-induced hepatotoxicity

Most of the currently available classes of antiretrovirals have been associated with hepatotoxicity. Many of the drugs used to treat or prevent opportunistic infections may also be hepatotoxic. Many patients with suspected drug-induced hepatitis are on multiple drugs, making it difficult to ascribe the reaction to a particular drug. Diagnosis of drug-induced hepatitis is further complicated by co-existent chronic viral hepatitis, which is common in HIV infection (see below). Viral hepatitis increases the risk of drug-induced hepatotoxicity and flares of hepatitis due to IRIS are not uncommon.

In general drug-induced hepatotoxicity seen in HIV infection is thought to be idiosyncratic rather than dose-related. Several characteristic hepatotoxic reactions occur (Table 38.3).

Table 38.3 Patterns of hepatotoxicity from drugs commonly used in HIV medicine

Reaction	Examples
Hepatocellular	Pyrazinamide, rifampicin, isoniazid NNRTIs Protease inhibitors Azole antifungals
Hepatitis with systemic hypersensitivity	Nevirapine Co-trimoxazole Abacavir
Cholestasis	Macrolides
Steatosis	NRTIs Valproate
Unconjugated hyperbilirubinaemia	Some PIs (atazanavir and indinavir)

In general hepatocellular reactions and hepatitis develop within three months of starting the drug and settle within two weeks of discontinuing it. Steatosis and cholestatsis resolve much more slowly. Unconjugated hyperbilirubinaemia is a benign disorder, but can cause clinical jaundice. Steatosis (fatty liver) is generally mild with slight hepatomegaly, but may be severe in patients with symptomatic hyperlactataemia.

Management of suspected drug-induced hepatotoxicity is complex. Viral hepatitis should always be excluded. Three factors are important in decision-making: clinical features of hepatitis, the level of transaminase elevation (fivefold above upper limit of normal is significant), and the presence of other features of systemic hypersensitivity (rash, eosinophilia, fever, organ dysfunction). Drugs associated with hepatitis should be discontinued if the patient is symptomatic (either with systemic hypersensitivity or hepatitis) and liver function tests are deranged. Rechallenge should, in general, not be attempted (especially if there was systemic hypersensitivity). Rechallenge is reasonable with so-called biochemical hepatitis (i.e. asymptomatic) once the transaminases have improved; expert opinion should be sought.

Viral hepatitis

The course and prognosis of hepatitis A are not altered by concurrent HIV infection.

Hepatitis B virus

Poor cell-mediated immunity leads to increased hepatitis B virus (HBV) viral load and an increased incidence of chronic infection in the HIV-positive population. There is also more rapid progression to chronic liver disease. Hepatitis B vaccination should be offered if the hepatitis B surface antibody is negative, but responses are poor if the CD4 count is <200 cells/µl.

The use of antiretrovirals with activity against hepatitis B (lamivudine, emtricitabine and tenofovir) is recommended. Lamivudine (or the closely related emtricitabine) suppresses hepatitis B viral load and improves outcome in cirrhosis, but resistance develops after two years of therapy in about half. Therefore tenofovir should be combined with lamivudine or emtricitabine, as this delays the emergence of resistance. Three problems may occur when using antiretrovirals in hepatitis B co-infected patients:

- increased risk of drug hepatotoxicity;
- hepatitis B IRIS, which presents as a hepatitis flare within three months of commencing antiretroviral thearpy (this is difficult to distinguish from drug-induced hepatitis – the re-appearance of anti-core IgM is a clue);
- hepatitis B flares, often severe, may occur when antiretrovirals with hepatitis B activity are discontinued.

Hepatitis C virus

Hepatitis C infection is found mainly in haemophiliacs and intravenous drug-users, and is thus not a common co-infection in our region. As with hepatitis B, co-infection with HIV results in more rapid progression of liver disease, higher hepatitis C viral loads, hepatitis C IRIS, and increased risk of drug hepatotoxicity. Some hepatitis C genotypes can be cured with prolonged courses of ribavirin plus pegylated interferon-α, but this is currently prohibitively expensive.

Opportunistic diseases and the liver

Sepsis is associated with a variety of liver function test abnormalities, typically cannalicular enzymes are more elevated than transaminases and conjugated hyperbilirubinaemia may occur. A similar pattern is seen with granulomatous infiltration, usually due to TB in the region. Hepatic involvement occurs with a wide variety of opportunistic diseases, illustrating the potential value of liver biopsy in fever of unknown origin. However, the diagnosis can usually be made using less invasive tests.

Disease of the biliary tree

Disease of the biliary tree commonly presents with elevated cannalicular enzymes, conjugated hyperbilirubinaemia, and right upper-quadrant pain.

Acalculous cholecystitis

Acalculous cholecystitis is associated with late-stage disease and typically presents as acute or chronic cholangitis in the absence of gallstones. It may be caused by non-opportunistic Gram negative bacilli or opportunistic infections, (e.g. CMV, microsporidiosis, *Isospora belli*, or cryptosporidiosis). The ultrasound may be normal, but usually shows a thickened and dilated gall bladder. There may be associated cholangiopathy. Surgery may be necessary.

AIDS cholangiopathy

This disease is similar to sclerosing cholangitis. Most patients with cholangiopathy have advanced HIV infection. The pathogenesis is unclear, but in some cases opportunistic pathogens have been implicated, (e.g. CMV, *Cryptosporidium*, or *Microsporidium*). Often no organism is identified.

An ultrasound will show dilated ducts in about 80% of patients. However, the gold standard is ERCP, which outlines the biliary system. Duodenal biopsies can be taken at the same time to isolate the causative organism. The main aim of management is to improve symptoms, especially relief from pain. Specific pathogens should be treated, but the response is usually poor. Intercurrent cholangitis can be treated with broad spectrum antibiotics. If papillary stenosis is present, an endoscopic sphincterotomy relieves obstruction. There is no treatment for intrahepatic disease.

Perianal disease

Anorectal disease is seen most frequently in men who have sex with men (MSM). The commonest cause is herpes simplex virus (type II, often recurrent). Other sexually transmitted infections, notably *Neisseria gonorrhoea*, *Chlamydia trachomatis*, and human papillomavirus (HPV) also occur commonly. Anal warts are frequently large and difficult to manage. Rectal discharge, perianal abscesses, fistulae, ulceration, and proctitis may be found. TB is an occasional cause of chronic perianal disease. Rectovaginal fistulae are particularly difficult to manage. Chronic diarrhoea may lead to excoriations. Anorectal carcinoma is more common in MSM. Initial examination of MSM should include proctoscopy to exclude tumours, warts, and proctitis. A pus swab should be taken if a discharge is present. All patients with symptoms and no obvious diagnosis should undergo sigmoidoscopy.

References and further reading

Corcoran, C., and S. Grinspoon. 1999. 'Drug therapy for wasting with the Acquired Immunodeficiency Syndrome'. *New England Journal of Medicine*; 340 (22):1740–1750.

Gordon, M.A., Banda, H.T., Gondwe, M. et al. 2002. 'Non-typhoidal salmonella bacteraemia among HIV-infected Malawian adults: high mortality and frequent recrudescence.' *AIDS*; 16:1633–1641.

Sharpstone, D., and B. Gazzard. 1996. 'Gastrointestinal manifestations of HIV infection'. *Lancet*; 348 (9024):379–383.

Southern African HIV Clinicians Society. 2011. 'Management oh HIV-Hepatitis B co-infection.' *SA Journal of HIV Medicine*; 12:27–33.

Vincent Soriano, V., Puoti, M., Bonacini, M., Brook, G., Cargnel, A., Rockstroh, .J, Thio, C., Benhamou, Y. 2005. 'Care of patients with chronic hepatitis B and HIV co-infection: recommendations from an HIV–HBV International Panel.' *AIDS*; 19:221–240.

Paediatric oral medicine

Several studies have emphasized the prognostic significance of oral candidiasis and hairy leukoplakia as predictors of immunosuppression and AIDS-defining conditions in adults. Similar studies documenting the prognostic implications of oral lesions in HIV-seropositive children have emerged recently. Cervical lymphadenopathy and oral candidiasis are the most prevalent head and neck manifestations. Both of these lesions are associated with a decline in the number of CD4 T-cells and an increase in IgG. There is also a significant relationship between oral candidiasis and declining CD4 T-cell and neutrophil counts in HIV-infected children.

Oral manifestations should be considered the earliest clinical sign of HIV infection and a good indicator of progression in children. Oral lesions can be asymptomatic or can present with pain, discomfort, and eating restrictions. Oral examination is quick and inexpensive. Early detection of HIV-related oral lesions can be used to:

- diagnose HIV infection;
- elucidate progression of the disease;
- predict immune status;
- provide a basis for more aggressive and appropriate treatment of HIV and considerably improve well-being.

Oral candidiasis

Oral thrush occurs in healthy infants in the first six months of life. However, the lesions are often mild, readily amenable to treatment, may regress spontaneously, and are rarely seen beyond infancy in the absence of predisposing factors. Candidiasis is the most frequently occurring oral manifestation in HIV-infected children. It is often recurrent, persists for long periods of time, and is often resistant to conventional antifungal therapy. The clinical presentation is variable. Lesions are often characteristic of the pseudomembranous and erythematous types, can be widespread, and occur anywhere in the oropharynx.

Median rhomboid glossitis, a red, smooth, depapillated patch on the middle of the tongue, is a variant of erythematous candidiasis. Tenderness, or a burning sensation, may be experienced. Angular cheilitis presents with fissures or linear ulcers at the corners of the mouth, with varying degrees of inflammatory erythema. Hyperkeratosis and hyperpigmentation may occur peripheral to the fissure. Concurrent intraoral candidal involvement is a common clinical finding. These lesions are usually tender and slow to heal because of repeated opening of the mouth.

Management

Candidiasis should be treated promptly and thoroughly with topical antifungal agents. If compliance is good, most regimens will effectively clear oral lesions. However, there may be non-adherence due to the unpleasant taste of some preparations and the quantity of tablets that need to be dissolved in the mouth. Oral suspensions that have a high sucrose content contribute to tooth decay and topical fluoride should be used if given for long periods.

- Treat with nystatin oral suspension 100 000 IU/mL 2.5 mL five times daily.
- Systemic therapy with ketoconazole (3 mg/kg/day) once a day for seven days, or fluconazole (3-6 mg/kg/day) once a day for seven days is used for lesions that do not respond to topical agents and for oesophageal candidiasis.

Herpes simplex virus infections

Herpetic stomatitis caused by the herpes simplex virus 1 (HSV-1) is commonly seen in HIV-infected children and often recurs (two or more episodes in one year). The primary lesions of HSV infections in children may manifest as gingivostomatitis. Recurrent lesions are seen as vesicles on the vermilion border, which rupture to form ulcers on the lips, or appear as clusters of small, painful ulcers on the palate and gingiva. They are extremely painful. Primary HSV lesions may also be seen in healthy children aged between two and six years. However, in healthy children, HSV lesions resolve within 10–14 days and may only require symptomatic treatment. In HIV-infected children, these lesions are chronic, recurrent, and may progress rapidly and become widespread.

Patients may exhibit fever, malaise, swollen and tender lymph nodes, and intraoral and perioral lesions on the gingiva, hard palate, and vermilion border of the lips, but any mucosal surface may be involved. Initially presenting as vesicles, these lesions rupture and coalesce to become painful, irregular ulcers.

As immunosuppression increases, an increase in severity and frequency of orolabial lesions occurs. Recurrent cases are characterized by extensive lesions and marked crust formation on the vermilion border of the lips.

Management

- Early diagnosis and treatment of lesions is important, as lesions may affect nutrition and hydration.
- Most herpetic lesions, even in HIV-infected children, are self limiting.
- Lesions can be treated with aciclovir (40–80 mg/kg/dose eight hourly, maximum 1 g/day). Viruses may occasionally become resistant. Antibiotics may be necessary to treat superinfection.

Recurrent aphthous ulcers

Recurrent aphthous ulcers appear to be more common among HIV-infected children. They occur in several different clinical forms, based on the size, number, and duration of the lesions:

- Minor recurrent aphthous ulcers are small, <5 mm in diameter, covered with a pseudomembrane, and surrounded by an erythematous halo.
- In major recurrent aphthous ulcers, the lesions are much larger, sometimes 1-2 cm in diameter, and may persist for weeks at a time.
- Herpetiform lesions appear as clusters or crops of tiny, recurrent aphthous ulcers, which may coalesce.

All lesions are painful and may interfere with mastication and swallowing. They tend to occur on the soft palate, buccal mucosa, tonsillar area, and tongue. A prompt response to steroids confirms the diagnosis.

Management

The severity and location of recurrent aphthous ulcers will dictate appropriate treatment:

- Topical steroid therapy is usually the first choice. Triamcinolone acetonide 0.1% ointment eight hourly may reduce inflammation and accelerate healing.
- Paracetamol and 2% viscous lidocaine gel will reduce pain. A 0.2% chlorhexidine digluconate mouth rinse two to four times daily or 1% topical povidone-iodine mouthwash may also be useful. Reinforce good oral hygiene.
- Topical beclomethasone spray, benzydamine hydrochloride spray, or betamethasone tablets (used as a mouthwash by dissolving a 0.5 mg

tablet in 15 mL of water and keeping in the mouth for three minutes before spitting out) are all often effective for large, persistent ulcers.
- For long-standing, intractable ulcers, systemic steroids such as prednisolone may be used, but it is important to exclude cytomegalovirus, as steroids may exacerbate this condition.

Gingival and periodontal lesions

Gingival and periodontal lesions include linear gingival erythema (LGE), necrotizing ulcerative gingivitis (NUG) and necrotizing ulcerative periodontitis (NUP), and acute necrotizing ulcerative gingivitis (ANUG):
- LGE is the most common form of HIV-associated periodontal disease in HIV-infected children. It presents as an intensely erythematous, linear band involving the labial margin and attached gingiva and may be accompanied by petechiae-like or diffuse red lesions. The amount of erythema is disproportionate to the amount of plaque present.
- NUG and NUP may also been seen. In NUG, there is destruction of one or more papillae, accompanied by necrosis, ulceration and/or sloughing. Destruction is limited to the marginal tissues.
- In ANUG, the gingival tissues are very red and swollen, with yellowish-grey necrotic tissue that bleeds easily. Severe pain and halitosis also occur.

Management

Management centres on the following:
- Encourage thorough oral hygiene, including plaque removal, scaling, and root planing.
- Irrigate with 1% povidone-iodine solution for acute disease.
- Mouth rinses of 0.2% chlorhexidine gluconate are an adjunct therapy to good oral hygiene. Therapeutic responses may vary, and relapses are common.
- Patients with pain and severe acute lesions should receive antibiotics:
  o amoxicillin 30–40 mg/kg/day oral 8 hourly for five days; *or*
  o for penicillin-allergic patients, erythromycin 20–40 mg/kg/day oral 8 hourly before meals, for five days;
  o metronidazole 7.5 mg/kg/dose oral 8 hourly for five days.
- For refractory cases, clindamycin for 7–14 days, or co-amoxiclav for five days.

Parotid enlargement

Parotid enlargement is a distinct feature of HIV infection in children. It is reported in 10-30% of children with symptomatic HIV infection and is a predictor of long-term survival. Typically, the parotid glands are diffusely swollen and warm without inflammation or tenderness. The swelling is chronic with unilateral or bilateral involvement, occasionally accompanied by xerostomia (a dry mouth). It may be accompanied by pain and associated with lymphocytic interstitial pneumonitis and diffuse lymphadenopathy, which probably represents a lymphoproliferative stage of HIV infection in children.

Xerostomia is far more common in HIV-infected children than in adults. It may present not only as a result of HIV infection, but also as a result of some medications. It may occur with or without parotid swelling.

Management

No definitive treatment is indicated for HIV-related salivary gland disease, but efforts should be made to relieve the symptoms of xerostomia with salivary substitutes containing methylcellulose, or with artificial saliva containing a mucin base, and sugarless chewing gum to stimulate salivary flow. Glycerine may be useful.

For parotid abscess, the treatment of choice is co-amoxiclav or clinda-mycin for patients with a penicillin allergy. Children with decreased salivary flow and xerostomia should maintain thorough oral hygiene and use topical fluorides (varnishes, gels, rinses) to prevent xerostomia-induced dental caries. Dietary control is essential to limit the intake of sugar and sugary foods.

Molluscum contagiosum

Molluscum contagiosum is a virally induced lesion of the skin, mucous membranes, and, rarely, the oral cavity. (See Chapter 40: Dermatology.)

Adult oral medicine

The oral manifestations of HIV infection include fungal, viral, and bacterial infections, as well as opportunistic cancers. These conditions are often asymptomatic, but can cause pain, discomfort, and eating restrictions. Oral lesions such as candidiasis and herpetic ulceration are among the first signs of HIV infection.

Early detection of oral lesions can:

- indicate HIV infection;
- predict immune status, allowing timely therapeutic interventions; and
- indicate the response to antiretroviral therapy.

The treatment and management of oral HIV lesions can considerably improve well-being. Oral examination is quick, inexpensive, and ideal for use in screening for HIV infection in the primary health care setting. Diagnosis of oral mucosal disease predicts HIV infection, and it may be useful in antenatal screening so that appropriate drug management can be instituted to reduce vertical transmission.

Oral candidiasis

The clinical presentation of oral candidiasis is variable. It can manifest as creamy white pseudomembranous plaques, erythematous patches, non-scrapable hyperplastic plaques, or as angular cheilitis. Early presentations of these manifestations are usually asymptomatic.

- Pseudomembranous candidiasis is the most common oral lesion. It presents as creamy white or yellow, loosely adherent plaques anywhere in the mouth that can be wiped off to reveal an erythematous surface, with or without bleeding. (See photos 18 and 19.)
- Erythematous candidiasis presents as multiple, flat, diffuse or discrete, red, non-removable plaques. It is usually found on the palate, tongue, and occasionally the buccal and labial mucosa. (See photo 20.) A variant of erythematous candidiasis is median rhomboid glossitis – a red, smooth, depapilated area on the middle of the tongue. (See photo 21.)
- Hyperplastic candidiasis is usually seen on the buccal mucosa as diffuse, white, adherent lesions. (See photo 22.) Hyperplastic candidiasis needs to be distinguished from oral hairy leukoplakia.
- Angular cheilitis appears as fissures or linear ulcers at the corners of the mouth, with varying degrees of inflammatory erythema. Hyperkeratosis may be present, peripheral to the fissure. Concurrent with angular cheilitis, intraoral candidal involvement is a common clinical finding. These lesions are usually tender and slow to heal because of repeated opening of the mouth. (See photos 23 and 24.)

Once colonization and superinfection by *Candida* spp. is established, concomitant mucosal infections caused by bacteria and herpes simplex virus (HSV) may facilitate deeper penetration into submucosal tissue.

Candidiasis may be accompanied by pain and altered taste sensation, both of which interfere with nutrition and hydration, and may be exacerbated by decreased salivary production.

Management

Early treatment of candidiasis is warranted, not only because of discomfort, but also because infection may spread to the pharynx and oesophagus. Either topical or systemic antifungal agents may be used. Topical treatments include:

- 0.5% gentian violet aqueous solution painted in the mouth three times daily; and
- nystatin suspension 100 000 IU/mL rinse and swallow 2.5 mL five times daily.

In severe cases, or if the above treatment fails:

- apply 2% miconazole oral gel two to three times daily for 10 days; and
- suck amphotericin B lozenges 10 mg six hourly for 10 days.

Oral candidiasis in HIV patients usually responds to initial topical therapy, but recurrences are common and if there is no response in one to two weeks, systemic agents for treatment may be required:

- ketoconazole 200–400 mg, once a day for seven days;
- fluconazole 50–100 mg, once a day for seven days; or
- itraconazole 200 mg, once a day for seven days.

Angular cheilitis is best managed with topical nystatin cream or miconazole gel.

Comments

Different manifestations of candidiasis may occur simultaneously, but all must be treated promptly and vigorously, especially if there is oesophageal involvement.

Owing to the high sugar content of some formulations, fluoride mouth-wash should be used daily.

- 0.2% chlorhexidine gluconate mouth rinse, two to four times daily, may also be useful.
- Chlorhexidine should not be used at the same time as either nystatin or amphotericin B.

Local contributory factors such as continuous denture wear, poor denture hygiene, and xerostomia (dry mouth) should be minimized. Patients must be advised to remove dentures when using medication and not to sleep with their dentures in overnight. Dentures should be disinfected in a proprietary denture cleaning solution.

Oral ulceration

Herpes simplex virus

Herpetic stomatitis caused by HSV type I or II is commonly seen and has a tendency to recur.

Initial vesicles soon rupture to become painful, irregular ulcers. Lesions may be found on the gums, hard palate, vermilion border of the lips, and adjacent facial skin. (See photo 25.) Chronic, recurrent (two or more episodes in one year) ulcerations can progress rapidly to cause extensive mucocutaneous involvement that may persist for several weeks and extend to the oesophagus.

Aphthous ulcers

Aphthous ulcers can be small or large, single or multiple, and occur anywhere in the mouth. These painful ulcers are well-circumscribed lesions with a whitish covering surrounded by a reddish halo, usually limited to the mucosa of the soft palate, buccal mucosa, tongue, and tonsillar area. (See photo 26.)

Aphthous ulcers are deeper than herpetic ulcers and have a well-defined edge, unlike herpetic ulcers, which are shallower, with an irregular border. Preceding vesiculation is characteristic of herpetic lesions. Severe recurrent aphthous ulcers may occur in the mouth, oropharynx, and oesophagus. Large lesions are progressive, chronic, and heal slowly. They often interfere with speech and swallowing, and may contribute to inadequate oral intake and rapid weight loss.

Management of oral ulcerations

Early diagnosis and treatment of severe, long-standing and painful lesions is important because they may interfere with nutrition and hydration:

- Adequate pain control is essential. Use paracetamol or paracetamol-codeine with topical 2% viscous lidocaine gel.
- Herpes simplex lesions often heal spontaneously, but some patients have prolonged bouts with frequent recurrences that are accompanied

by severe pain and local tissue destruction. A 0.5% gentian violet aqueous solution painted in the mouth three times daily or 1% topical povidone-iodine may be useful for small ulcers. Aciclovir 400 mg eight hourly for five days will effectively treat large ulcers.

Aphthous ulcers respond to topical steroids such as triamcinolone aceto-nide 0.1% in sodium carboxymethylcellulose base (Kenalog in Orabase®) given eight hourly. A 0.2% chlorhexidine digluconate mouth rinse two to four times daily or 1% topical povidone-iodine may also be useful. For large, persistent ulcers, try:

- beclomethasone spray (one to two puffs twice daily onto ulcer);
- benzydamine mouthwash; or
- betamethasone 0.5 mg tablets dissolved in 15 mL water and used as a mouthwash for three minutes daily.

For long-standing, intractable ulcers, systemic steroids such as predni-solone may be used, but it is important to exclude cytomegalovirus (CMV) and herpes, as steroids may exacerbate these ulcers.

Comments

- Herpes viruses may occasionally become resistant to aciclovir.
- Patients should be advised to avoid acidic foods and drinks and a fluid diet should be prescribed.
- Chlorhexidine should not be used at the same time as topical steroids or antifungals.
- Patients with ulcers that are refractory to treatment should be referred for biopsy to exclude malignancy or CMV.

Oral hairy leukoplakia

Oral hairy leukoplakia (OHL) is a benign and usually asymptomatic lesion. It usually presents as white, vertical corrugations on the lateral borders of the tongue, unilaterally or bilaterally, which cannot be rubbed off. (See photo 27.) It can cause discomfort. Studies have shown that it is associated with intraepithelial proliferation of Epstein-Barr virus (EBV) and that multiple strains of the virus are often present in OHL tissues.

Management

Effective treatment is not available. Specific treatment is rarely indicated, but for patients with discomfort, aciclovir 800 mg three to five times daily for 10 days may be used. Antiretroviral therapy may clear the lesions but none of the treatments eliminate the underlying EBV infection. Despite the benign nature of the lesion, its presence indicates immunosuppression and the patient should commence co-trimoxazole prophylaxis.

Kaposi's sarcoma

Kaposi's sarcoma (KS) is a multifocal neoplastic proliferation of endothelial cells. It presents as one or more reddish or slightly bluish swellings, with or without ulcerations. Kaposi's sarcoma-associated herpesvirus or human herpesvirus-8 has been identified in all forms of KS. (See also Chapter 40: Dermatology.) Oral lesions of KS occur commonly on the hard palate, adjacent to the gingival ridge. (See photo 28.) Intraoral lesions are initially asymptomatic but, as they progress, patients may have pain associated with ulceration, bleeding, or superinfection. Lesions on the palate are associated with pulmonary KS. Nearly two-thirds of patients with oral KS have pain, discomfort, or dysphagia, or complain of poor aesthetics and require treatment. A biopsy is essential for a definitive diagnosis.

Management

Treatment decisions are made on the basis of the extent of the disease. For isolated oral lesions, local therapy may include laser or surgical excision, radiotherapy, or intralesional chemotherapeutic injections. Intralesional injections of vinblastine can cause lesions to regress. However, in some patients vinblastine produces pain and they may require repeated visits before a response is achieved. Systemic chemotherapy is usually indicated for patients with widespread progressive disease. (See also Chapter 41: Oncology.)

Non-Hodgkin's lymphoma

Non-Hodgkin's lymphoma (NHL) is the second most common malignant condition associated with HIV infection. Lymphomas present as a focal soft swelling that may be red and inflamed. These lesions are painful and may progress rapidly. Suspected lesions should be biopsied for histological diagnosis.

Management

Treatment requires systemic combination chemotherapy, and radiotherapy on occasion. Large exophytic or pedunculated lesions can be surgically removed, providing pain relief and reducing interference with chewing and speaking. Because of their size and location, some lesions may be hard to access. In such cases, radiotherapy is the treatment of choice. Treatment is almost always palliative and not curative.

Comments

Physicians need to encourage good oral hygiene, plaque control, and frequent professional cleaning for patients with KS and lymphomas, because lesions might become infected in advanced stages. Patients require on-going oral health care to help prevent and manage the specific oral complications of mucositis and xerostomia, and the increased risks of bacterial or fungal superinfection that are associated with both chemotherapy and radiotherapy. Benzydamine hydrochloride mouth rinse may provide relief and is recommended mainly when there are obstructive symptoms. The immune reconstitution associated with antiretroviral therapy may cause lesions to regress.

Gingival and periodontal lesions

A number of specific periodontal changes have been associated with HIV infection:

- Linear gingival erythema is characterized by a profound erythema of the free gingival margin. (See photo 29.)
- In necrotizing ulcerative gingivitis, there is destruction of one or more interdental papillae with bleeding, ulceration, necrosis, and sloughing. Tissue destruction is limited to the gingival tissues and does not involve alveolar bone.
- Necrotizing ulcerative periodontitis is characterized by advanced necrotic destruction of the periodontium. There is rapid loss of the periodontal attachment, destruction or sequestration of bone, and teeth may become loose. It is accompanied by severe pain and halitosis.

Management

Dental treatment is based on plaque reduction and thorough debridement:

- Patients should be encouraged to brush and floss meticulously to achieve a maximum level of oral health.
- Dental referral is necessary for a multistep regimen of professional scaling, local debridement with subgingival irrigation, local and systemic antimicrobial therapy, immediate follow-up care, and regular long-term maintenance.

- Intervention usually involves intensive curettage and debridement of all involved tissues.
- A regimen of topical antiseptic agents, such as 1% povidone-iodine solution and 0.2% chlorhexidine gluconate mouth rinse two to four times daily is often initiated as an adjunct therapy. This regimen should be continued until all the diseased hard and soft tissues are removed and the patient is no longer symptomatic.

In severe cases, topical antimicrobial therapy should be supplemented by a short course of systemic antimicrobial therapy, usually metronidazole 400 mg 8 hourly for five days. Alternatives are:
- clindamycin 300 mg eight hourly for 7–14 days; or
- co-amoxiclav 375 mg eight hourly for five days.

Comments

- Recurrences are common and result in delayed healing and continued destruction of soft tissues and bones.
- The importance of strict, regular oral hygiene measures including brushing, flossing, and using mouth rinses cannot be overemphasized.
- Mobile teeth may need to be splinted or extracted.
- Bony sequestrations should be removed under antibiotic cover.

Salivary gland disease

Several salivary gland disorders are found in patients who are HIV-positive. Parotid gland enlargement often accompanies a syndrome of persistent generalized lymphadenopathy caused by lymphoid proliferation in response to HIV infection (see photo 30). It may manifest as unilateral or bilateral non-tender gland enlargement with xerostomia. Recurrent bacterial parotitis may occur.

Management

No definitive treatment is indicated for HIV-related salivary gland disease if there is no super-added infection, but efforts should be made to relieve the symptoms of xerostomia. Note the following points:
- Oral broad-spectrum antibiotics should be used in the treatment of suspected bacterial salivary gland infection.
- Treat dry mouth with salivary substitutes containing methylcellulose, or artificial saliva that has a mucin base, as well as sugarless chewing gum to stimulate salivary flow. Glycerine may be useful.

- Encourage thorough oral hygiene and the daily use of topical fluoride varnishes, gels, or rinses to maintain optimal oral hygiene and prevent xerostomia-induced dental caries.
- Dietary control is essential to limit the intake of sugar and sugary foods.

References and further reading

Common oral lesions in children and adults with HIV/AIDS. Available: http:// www.oralhivlesions.com.

Department of Community Dentistry. 2001. *Common oral lesions in children and adults with HIV. Visual reference for health care workers.* University of Stellenbosch.

Lifson, A. R. 1995. 'Oral lesions and the epidemiology of HIV'. In *Oral manifestations of HIV infection,* ed. J. S. Greenspan and D. Greenspan. Chicago: Quintessence Publishing.

Ramos-Gomez, R.J. 1997. 'Oral aspects of HIV infection in children'. *Oral Diseases.*; (3) Suppl. 1:531–535.

Dermatology

Skin lesions are frequently seen in people with HIV/AIDS and are often a presenting sign of the disease or its complications. Certain skin conditions, such as herpes zoster and Kaposi's sarcoma (KS), may help in the clinical staging of HIV. In addition, skin disorders may offer useful clues to the presence of major systemic opportunistic infections and, being easily accessible to biopsy, may enable the clinician to identify an organism rapidly. Skin disorders frequently cause the patient great discomfort, yet, when correctly diagnosed, may be easily treated. Shortly after the initiation of antiretroviral therapy dermatological conditions may flare. This is known as the immune reconstitution inflammatory syndrome (refer to Chapter 50: Immune reconsititution inflammatory syndrome). As in other settings, differential diagnosis is based largely on the characteristic morphology of the lesion, together with the anatomical distribution.

This chapter will cover both paediatric and adult skin manifestations of HIV infection.

Common presentations include the following:

- scaly rashes;
- non-itchy papules and nodules;
- itchy papules and nodules;
- purple-brown lesions;
- blisters, erosions, and crusts;
- ulcers;
- pigmentary changes; and
- nail disorders.

Scaly rashes

Note whether the rash is generalized or confined to key regions such as body folds or sun-exposed areas. Itching may indicate inflammation. A history of drug use or previous eczema or psoriasis may be helpful.

Seborrhoeic eczema/dermatitis

This occurs in the axillae, groin, neck, and scalp, with weeping and redness. Scaly, erythematous or yellowish patches typically involve the scalp, face, chest, back, axillae, or pubic area. These lesions can be confused with dermatophyte infection, lupus erythematosus, or psoriasis. Crusting may indicate secondary infection. The rash may spread to involve the face and trunk. (See photo 31.)

Management

- Use a potent topical steroid (e.g. betamethasone valerate 0.1%). In hairy areas and body folds use creams or lotions rather than ointments. On the face, use hydrocortisone 1% cream or lotion.
- Treat secondary infections with flucloxacillin.
- Wean the patient onto a steroid cream of lower potency as soon as possible after the initial response.
- Use 'anti-dandruff' shampoo, such as selenium sulphide, cetrimide, or povidone-iodine.
- If there is no response, give a trial of an azole antifungal agent, either topically or orally.

Fungal infection (tinea)

Dermatophytes infect keratinized skin, hair, and nails. Superficial fungal infection can have an atypical clinical presentation or may be extensive, recurrent, and difficult to treat. Infection may occur at any site, often at multiple sites and caused by multiple organisms. Lesions have an active, well-defined edge and asymmetrical distribution, e.g. scaling of one hand suggests fungal infection, but this is not invariable. Facial involvement can mimic seborrhoeic dermatitis. Lesions may be psoriasiform and palmoplantar lesions are commonly hyperkeratotic. (See photo 32.)

Tinea capitis is common in children and can display the following patterns:

- grey patches of scaling with hair loss;
- a seborrhoeic dermatitis-like picture;
- an alopecia areata-like picture;
- an abscess-like (kerion) picture; and
- patches of hair loss with pustulation and crusting.

Secondary impetigo is common in all forms. Impetigo of the scalp should always prompt a search for tinea capitis, scabies, and lice infestations.

Management

- Use clotrimazole cream for localized infection.

- Use oral griseofulvin for extensive disease, or if the nails are involved. This is usually well tolerated but may be replaced by itraconazole or terbinafine in people who are allergic to griseofulvin, or if the infection is refractory.
- If the infection does not respond, reconsider the diagnosis and examine skin scrapings (with KOH 20%) microscopically for hyphae, or send scrapings to the laboratory for fungal culture.

Worsening of pre-existing dermatosis

Atopic eczema, contact eczema, and psoriasis may all flare up during the course of HIV infection and may be the presenting illness. A flexural or generalized, itchy, lichenified rash suggests eczema (particularly if there is asthma or hay fever in the patient or family). (See photo 33.)

Psoriasis may present shortly after HIV seroconversion. Advanced HIV disease may exacerbate mild, pre-existing psoriasis and make it resistant to therapy. Individuals typically develop discrete, red, scaly plaques, or a more diffuse hyperkeratotic dermatitis with palmoplantar keratoderma. Psoriasis may present with the typical plaque form of variable extent or may be erythrodermic (i.e. the whole surface area is involved). Psoriatic arthropathy can be severe. (See also Chapter 42: Rheumatology.)

Management

Use a potent steroid ointment and moisturisers for eczema and erythrodermic psoriasis. Treat any secondary bacterial infection. When prescribing systemic therapy for psoriasis, note that methotrexate is generally contraindicated in immunosuppressed individuals, but could be considered if the patient is taking antiretroviral therapy or if the CD4 count can be monitored regularly. Acitretin may be used in severe psoriasis. These agents should usually only be prescribed by a dermatologist.

Photosensitive dermatoses

Photosensitive dermatoses may result from eczema, drug reactions, or pellagra. People with AIDS may show marked photosensitivity, sometimes with increased pigmentation or dramatic loss of pigment. Look for 'flaky paint' and the sharp definition of pellagra. Take a history of drugs, soaps, creams, and spray exposure.

Management

- Use a moderate potency steroid ointment.
- Stop the patient from using the suspected drug.
- Treat pellagra with niacin supplementation.

Dry skin or ichthyosis

Acquired ichthyosis occurs commonly in patients with advanced HIV disease. The condition involves the trunk and limbs and is characterized by dry, scaly skin, which may resemble fish scales or give a sensation of dryness of the skin. The condition is very common, and associated pruritus may be severe.

Management

- Use moisturizers, such as emulsifying ointment, Cetomacrogol ointment or Vaseline®.
- It is important to give an adequate supply (500 g) each month.
- Avoid excessive use of soaps; aqueous cream may be used as a substitute.

Crusted ('Norwegian') scabies

Patients present with extensive, thick scales that may cover the whole body. The scales are parchment-like, inflexible, and crack at the flexures. The rash may not be itchy. (See photo 34.)

Management

Crusted scabies is highly contagious – treat all close contacts and family members:

- Use moisturizer (Vaseline®) or a keratolytic (salicylic acid 5%) to soften the scale.
- Apply benzyl benzoate to the whole body excluding the head for 24 hours and repeat after 72 hours.
- The patient may also use sulphur ointment 5–10% three times per day for three days.

Drug hypersensitivity syndrome

The patient's whole skin is inflamed and scaly, the face is swollen, and there may be fever and lymphadenopathy, with an associated hepatitis and eosinophilia. This reaction tends to occur four to six weeks after starting, or restarting, a drug. It is seen most frequently, but not exclusively, with anticonvulsant agents (carbamazepine and phenytoin), co-trimoxazole, anti-tuberculous agents, and the non-nucleoside reverse transcriptase inhibitors (NNRTIs). (See photo 35.)

Management

- Stop the patient from using the suspected drug. Use sodium valproate if he or she requires an anticonvulsant.
- Monitor liver function.
- Patients may use topical steroid ointment if there is no evidence of secondary skin infection.
- Desensitization can be attempted, with careful monitoring for skin and liver toxicity, if fever and hepatotoxicity were not a feature of the initial reaction.

(See also Appendix 40.1.)

Non-itchy papules and nodules

Papular eruptions may be easily recognizable, (e.g. warts), but may be difficult to identify clinically and a biopsy may be needed to detect infectious agents. (See Appendix 21.1.) If the papules appear in a crop, if there are vesicles or crusted areas, and if the patient is systemically ill, a systemic infection should be suspected and a skin biopsy performed.

Molluscum contagiosum

Lesions are of variable size and are smooth papules, showing characteristic central umbilication (dimpling). This infection is common on the face, particularly in young children, and shows a tendency to spread slowly to adjacent skin. In immunocompetent individuals it is usually self limiting. In severely immunosuppressed individuals these lesions may be extensive and very disfiguring. (See photo 36.)

Management

Management is difficult in the immunosuppressed patient:
- Use local destructive treatment, such as potassium hydroxide, silver nitrate, trichloroacetic acid, or liquid nitrogen. Patients usually require repeated applications.

- imiquimod cream might be helpful, but is expensive and may cause marked skin irritation.

Molluscum-like papules due to other organisms

The variable morphology and cropping of these lesions, coupled with systemic illness, should alert the clinician to the possibility of other infections, such as cryptococcosis or histoplasmosis. (See photo 37 and photo 38.)

Management

When in doubt, do a biopsy, sending the specimen for fungal culture and histology.

Warts

Warts are usually easy to identify, but may be very persistent, large, and troublesome, particularly in the anogenital area. This condition is common in babies and young children.

Management

- Apply podophyllin 25% to anogenital warts weekly if the patient is not pregnant. Wash off after four hours to prevent severe irritation.
- Apply 80% trichloroacetic acid in water, weekly.
- Cautery, liquid nitrogen, or laser therapy may be used, but lesions frequently recur.
- Imiquimod cream is helpful, but is expensive, and may cause marked local skin irritation.

Bacillary angiomatosis

These lesions are vascular papules and nodules that result from infection with *Bartonella* spp. They range from a single nodule to a widespread eruption and are usually red to purple, sometimes with erosions or crusting. Clinically, this condition is easy to confuse with KS, but is much less common, does not produce plaques or lymphoedema, and may be self limiting. Co-trimoxazole may prevent bacillary angiomatosis.

Management

- Do a biopsy for histological diagnosis if the patient has a sudden eruption of vascular papules.

- Prescribe erythromycin 500 mg six hourly, or doxycycline 100 mg 12 hourly, for four weeks.

Skin nodules

Skin nodules of recent onset have many causes that are frequently difficult to establish without a biopsy. If the lesion is growing, a deep skin infection (such as tuberculosis (TB), bacillary angiomatosis, atypical mycobacterium, or yeast) or a neoplasm should be considered likely.

Management

- Do a biopsy.
- If the histology shows a granulomatous pattern, culture for mycobacteria and fungi.

Itchy papules

Itchy papules are among the commonest skin problems in people in Africa with HIV/AIDS and may occur at all stages of the disease, sometimes improving with the development of profound immunosuppression.

'Itchy bump disease', or pruritic papular eruption of HIV

Pruritic papular eruption of HIV could be a group of disorders, some follicular and others severe forms of papular urticaria (insect bite allergy). This skin eruption appears to be particularly common in Africa. The patient usually complains of severe itch and demonstrates scattered papules, particularly on the limbs and trunk. Lesions are often in different stages of evolution, including early blisters, inflamed papules, and old inactive lesions. Post-inflammatory pigmentation is usually prominent. Other skin lesions, such as scabies and KS, may co-exist. (See photo 39.)

Management

- Give a potent topical steroid ointment.
- Treat secondary bacterial infection, if present.
- Give a sedating antihistamine, such as promethazine 25 mg, at night.

Scabies

Scabies is easy to confuse with 'itchy bump disease', or may co-exist with it. Small papules in the web spaces, on the wrists, and around the umbilicus and axillae suggest this diagnosis.

In early HIV infection, scabies has a classic presentation with erythematous pruritic papules and burrows on the finger webs, wrists, and anogenital region. In babies, lesions are often widespread, affecting the palms, soles, and scalp. These areas are not commonly affected in adults. Specific lesions (burrows) occurring on normal skin, or surmounting a red papule, are often obscured by secondary pyoderma or primary irritation dermatitis because of inappropriate treatment. Lesions may be accompanied by erythema, urticaria, or dermatitis caused by hypersensitivity to parasitic antigens. In exceptional cases, a multitude of greyish lines, representing burrows, may be present.

With progressive immunodeficiency, individuals may develop either a diffuse papular eruption or hyperkeratotic, yellowish plaques on the scalp, face, hands, back, and trunk (keratotic scabies), see photo 40. Pruritus is minimal or absent. Infesting mites may number in the millions, making this condition highly contagious. Excoriations may be prone to secondary infection. Other members of the household may be affected. The crusted form is sometimes seen (see 'Scaly rashes').

Diagnosis is confirmed by identifying mites, eggs, eggshells, or faecal pellets in lesional skin scrapings or skin biopsy.

Management

- Apply benzyl benzoate lotion to the whole body for 24 hours and repeat once after 72 hours. Treat all members of the household, even those who are not itching.
- In patients younger than six months, sulphur ointment applied three times per day for three days is the treatment of choice. Recurrence of keratotic scabies is common due to the large number of infesting organisms; ivermectin may become the treatment of choice.

Folliculitis

Several forms of follicular disease are seen in HIV-infected individuals, including the worsening or explosive onset of acne. An itchy monomorphic eruption (i.e. many similar follicular papules) may be infective, caused by bacteria or yeasts, or may be sterile in the case of eosinophilic or neutrophilic folliculitis.

Eosinophilic folliculitis (EF) is a chronic and extremely pruritic dermatosis, characterized clinically by multiple, reddish, oedematous papules
arising on the face, neck, upper trunk, and extremities. Pustules are
occasionally seen. Excoriations and post-inflammatory hyperpigmentation occur commonly, secondary to chronic scratching. In infants, EF
should be distinguished from EF of infancy and erythema toxicum
neonatorum, as neither is associated with HIV disease. A skin biopsy is
usually required to confirm the diagnosis and shows a perivascular and
perifollicular mononuclear cell infiltrate with numerous eosinophils.

Management

- Try simple remedies such as calamine lotion or benzoyl peroxide
  cream and oral antibiotics.
- Topical steroids are generally not effective.
- If the condition is severe, consider taking a biopsy for histology and
  culture, or referring to a specialist.

Purple-brown skin lesions

Kaposi's sarcoma

KS presents with multifocal vascular plaques or nodules in the skin
and viscera. The nodules are purple-to-brown, may grow, and have a
firm consistency. (See photo 41.) Lesions can occur in any location,
but are usually multiple and occur frequently on the face, oral mucous
membranes, and lower extremities. Early lesions of KS may be very subtle,
suggesting a bruise or a callus. (See photo 42.) Purple nodules on the
buccal mucosa, and particularly the hard palate, may help to confirm
the diagnosis and indicate visceral involvement. The lesions are usually
painless, but considerable pain can be experienced if oedema is present,
owing to lymphatic involvement. (See photo 43.) Lymphoedema may
involve the face, the clinical picture mimicking nephrotic syndrome.
(See photo 44.) In the disseminated form of KS the lymph nodes,
lung, and gastrointestinal tract can be involved. Bilateral lower-lobe
infiltration and pleural effusions are common in pulmonary KS. KS
follows a variable clinical course, ranging from indolent skin plaques to
aggressive malignancy with early visceral involvement, but ultimately it is
a progressive disease in all its forms. KS can occur at any CD4 count, but is
more aggressive at low counts.

Management

Without antiretroviral therapy, the disease is progressive. Management consists of:

- radiotherapy to relieve local obstructive symptoms on the palate or in the throat (if in doubt, discuss the problem with an oncologist); and
- cryotherapy with liquid nitrogen for small facial lesions.

(See Chapter 41: Oncology.)

Drug reaction

Lesions vary, depending on the type of reaction (for instance lichenoid, photosensitive, or fixed drug eruptions). Lichenoid reactions are characterized by itchy, violaceous, or brown papules and plaques and may be seen on sun-exposed areas. (See photo 45.) The lesions are often followed by areas of post-inflammatory hyperpigmentation or hypopigmentation. A history of repeated episodes at the same sites and the presence of round areas of persistent hyperpigmention suggest a fixed drug reaction.

Management

- Stop the patient from using the suspected drug.
- Treat the skin with a moderate-potency steroid ointment, if it is inflamed.

(See Appendix 40.1.)

Skin blisters, erosions, or crusts

Blisters, erosions, and crusts are often seen at different stages of the same process and may be seen together in the same person. In the immunosuppressed patient these lesions are most commonly due to infection with viruses, bacteria, or yeasts. The distribution of the lesions and the presence of fever or other systemic illness may alert the clinician to the diagnosis.

Bacterial infections

Bacterial infection is the most frequent cause of crusted skin lesions or pustules and should always be considered in this clinical setting. Although *Streptococcus pyogenes* and *Staphylococcus aureus* are the commonest pathogens in the skin, a variety of other bacterial infections may occur. *Pseudomonas aeruginosa* may produce severe otitis externa, folliculitis, or destructive skin ulcers.

Cutaneous infections are associated with advancing immunodeficiency. Impetigo, ecthyma, folliculitis, furunculosis, abscesses, or cellulitis are common:

- Impetigo presents with chronic, crusted erosions of the head or neck, or atypical bullous lesions of the axillae or groin (see photo 46).
- Folliculitis is often pruritic and accompanied by eczematization.
- Furunculosis refers to chronic, recurrent episodes of pyogenic folliculitis. Hidradenitis suppurativa can be especially troublesome and requires surgical excision of the involved skin.
- Ecthyma presents with crusted ulcers, usually on the limbs, as a consequence of bacterial infection of the dermis, and sometimes the subcutaneous fat. It heals with scarring and is refractory to treatment.

S. *aureus* may also cause secondary infection of atopic dermatitis, scabies, herpetic ulcers, or KS. Infection of indwelling venous catheters is common and has significant morbidity. Unusual clinical patterns of infection may occur, such as botryomycosis, which is a chronic suppurative infection with grains in the purulent material, and atypical plaque-like lesions of the scalp, axillae, and groin.

If lesions are atypical, or do not respond to the usual antibiotics, a sample should be sent for culture.

Management

- If the lesion is localized, wash it well and give the patient an antibacterial cream such as povidone-iodine.
- If the lesions are more extensive, wash them well and give the patient an oral antibiotic (e.g. flucloxacillin).
- Eradicating the organism from the nares with topical mupirocin or chlorhexidine gluconate solution can prevent recurrent staphylococcal infections.

Varicella-zoster virus

Chickenpox, a varicella-zoster virus (VZV) infection in immunocompetent children is characterized by a vesicular eruption (dewdrops on a rose petal) on the face, trunk, and proximal extremities. In immunocompromised patients the rash may be more widespread, with a high frequency of visceral complications and a mortality rate as high as 20%, if untreated.

Children with low CD4 counts exhibit extensive mucocutaneous disease with persistent new vesicle formation. Necrotizing and haemorrhagic lesions are not uncommon. The interval between primary VZV infection and reactivated VZV disease (herpes zoster) may be reduced to weeks or months instead of decades.

Herpes zoster infection (shingles) is easy to identify and typically presents as a unilateral, painful, vesicular, erosive dermatomal eruption, which resolves uneventfully. (See photo 47.) With increasing immunodeficiency it can be multidermatomal (usually contiguous), disseminated, or recurrent, followed by post-herpetic neuralgia and scarring. Lesions that persist for months after primary infection, reactivation, or disseminated VZV infection may appear as painful hyperkeratotic, ulcerated, or crusted nodules. Zoster infection is a common presenting condition in the early stages of HIV infection and, when occurring in patients under the age of 40 years, strongly suggests underlying HIV infection. A recurrence of zoster infection is common in the first weeks after starting antiretroviral therapy.

Management

- Prescribe a regular dosage of a good analgesic (e.g. paracetamol-codeine six hourly). Stronger opiate analgesics are often necessary in acute zoster virus infection, but should be avoided in patients with post-herpetic neuralgia.
- Apply a soothing antibacterial cream, such as silver sulfadiazine or povidone-iodine.
- Give aciclovir 800 mg five hourly or valaciclovir 1 g, eight hourly, for seven days (preferably within the first 72 hours).
- If the pain is not controlled, either during the attack or after the lesions heal, give amitriptyline at night.

Herpes simplex

Herpes simplex virus (HSV) infection is usually localized and starts with a group of vesicles on an inflamed base, followed by erosions, crusting, and eventual healing. (See photo 48.) Periungual lesions (herpetic whitlow) and herpetic folliculitis on the face are frequently misdiagnosed as bacterial infections. In early HIV disease, HSV has a classic presentation with grouped vesicles or erosions that heal in one to two weeks without treatment. In immunosuppressed individuals the virus may cause a disseminated eruption (haemorrhagic vesicles or bullae) or a persistent destructive ulcer. (See photo 49.) Prolonged treatment may be required.

These ulcers occur most commonly in body folds, particularly in the anogenital area, but may also appear on other skin surfaces. HSV can also infect the mucosa, producing proctitis, glossitis, oesophagitis, or severe gingivostomatitis (which is seen mainly in children). HSV ulceration lasting for >4 weeks is an AIDS-defining condition.

In atypical cases, a positive Tzanck smear is helpful but cannot distinguish between herpes simplex and varicella-zoster infection. Specific diagnosis requires fluorescent antibody staining, polymerase chain reaction testing, or culture.

Management

- Apply antibacterial cream.
- If the lesions are extensive, if the eye is involved, or if there is persistent ulceration, give aciclovir 400 mg eight hourly for at least five days. Children should be given aciclovir 80 mg/kg/day in three divided doses; or >2-years-old – adult dose, <2-years-old – half the adult dose.
- Long-term, low-dose prophylaxis with aciclovir 400 mg 12 hourly may be needed in people with recurring ulcers.

Yeast infections

Candidiasis is extremely common in HIV infection and may produce a range of mucosal lesions. These often spread to the oesophagus and may also involve the body folds and nails. Other yeast infections present with a variety of skin lesions. These include solitary gelatinous nodules and widespread molluscum-like papules or vesicles with crusts and erosions. Infections of *Cryptococcus* and *Histoplasma* species are commonly seen in immunosuppressed people and both may present in this way. (See photo 50.) The patient may be unwell, with fever, weight loss, meningitis, or pneumonia, but this is not invariable.

Management

If you suspect a yeast infection, take two skin biopsies (for histology and for culture). The material may appear gelatinous. Direct microscopy on a stained smear may help the clinician to diagnose yeast infection rapidly. Systemic therapy is always necessary.

Drug reaction

Erosions and blisters develop in many drug reactions, notably bullous fixed-drug eruption, erythema multiforme, and toxic epidermal necrolysis

(TEN). TEN produces large areas of dusky skin necrosis, followed by the stripping of sheets of skin as with a burn. Fixed-drug eruption is characterized by the recurrence of lesions at previous sites of inflammation and marked post-inflammatory pigmentation (usually in round spots). Erythema multiforme is usually easy to recognize because of the presence of 'target' lesions. There may also be mucosal erosions involving the eyes, mouth, and genitalia.

Management

- Stop the patient from using the suspected drug.
- If the eyes are involved, or there is extensive skin involvement (i.e. more than 10% of body surface area), refer the patient to a specialist unit if possible.
- If the mouth is ulcerated, use regular mouthwash and analgesics and encourage the patient to take oral fluids.
- Do not treat the reaction with systemic steroids.

(See Appendix 40.1.)

Skin and mucosal ulcers

Ecthyma

Ecthyma is the commonest form of skin ulcer and is usually caused by S. *aureus* infection. Other organisms, such as *Pseudomonas aeruginosa* or *Cryptococcus neoformans*, may produce a similar picture.

Management

- Clean the ulcer with fresh, running water or potassium permanganate solution.
- Apply antibacterial cream.
- If there is no response, consider an unusual organism and send material for culture.

Herpes simplex

HSV is the usual cause of shallow, persistent, painful ulcers, particularly in the anogenital area. A herpetic ulcer lasting more than four weeks is considered to be AIDS defining. (See also note under 'Skin blisters, erosions, or crusts, page 435.)

Other infections, including TB, occasionally cause very similar ulcers and should be considered if there is no response to treatment.

Nodulo-ulcerative syphilis

Syphilis may present with multiple ulcers and ulcerated nodules, involving both the skin and mucosa. This form of syphilis is more common in immunosuppressed patients.

Management

- Confirm the diagnosis with syphilis serology.
- Give the patient procaine penicillin daily 2.4 million units IM daily and probenecid 500 mg six hourly for 10 days. (The patient may need a longer course if the response is slow.)

Changes in pigmentation

Increased or decreased pigmentation

Changes in pigmentation are frequently seen after inflammatory skin diseases, particularly in people with dark skin. It is common in drug-induced photosensitivity states (when the changes may appear explosively in the patient with HIV infection), in fixed drug eruption, and in the itchy papular eruption of HIV.

Both HIV infection and treatment with zidovudine or hydroxyurea are associated with Addisonian type hyperpigmentation of skin and mucous membranes. True Addisonian pigmentation may develop secondary to opportunistic infection of the adrenal glands – TB and cytomegalovirus are the usual causes.

Nail abnormalities

Blue nails

Blue nails appear to be a feature of HIV infection and may be of diagnostic value. The cause of the discolouration is unknown.

White discolouration of the nails

White discolouration of the nails suggests a fungal infection (onycho-mycosis) and, especially when in the proximal part of the nail plate, suggests immunosuppression. (See photo 51.)

Management

- Send a specimen of the affected white nail for fungal culture if possible. (The material should be taken from under the nail plate.)
- Treat with a systemic antifungal if the infection is troublesome. If griseofulvin is the only available oral antifungal, treatment will be required for six to18 months. Liver enzymes should be monitored monthly. Itraconazole may be preferable and can be given as monthly pulses (200 mg twice daily for one week per month, for two months for fingernails and for three months for toenails), but is more expensive.
- Consider the possibility of psoriatic nail dystrophy if the culture is negative. (There is no satisfactory treatment for this condition.)

Hair changes

In advanced HIV infection the hair characteristically becomes sparse and fine. Excessive elongation of the eyelashes is also a recognized feature.

Oral lesions

See Chapter 39: Oral medicine.

References and further reading

Bason, M. M. et al. 1993. 'Pruritic papular eruption of HIV-disease'. *International Journal of Dermatology*; 32:784-789.

Berger, T. G. and A. Dhar. 1994. 'Lichenoid photoeruptions in human immunodeficiency virus infection'. *Archives of Dermatology*; 130:609–613.

Porras, B., et al. 1998. 'Update on cutaneous manifestations of HIV infection'. *The Medical Clinics of North America*; 82:1033–1080.

Resneck, J.S. et al. 2004. 'Etiology of pruritic papular eruption with HIV infection in Uganda.' *Journal of the American Medical Association*; 292:2614–2621.

Saxe, N. S. et al. 1997. *Handbook of Dermatology for Primary Care*. Cape Town: Oxford University Press Southern Africa.

Smith, K. J. et al. 1994. 'Cutaneous findings in HIV-1-positive patients: A 42-month prospective study'. *Journal of the American Academy of Dermatology*; 31:746-754.

Appendix 40.1 Common cutaneous drug reactions

Drug reaction	Skin lesions	Other features	Common causes	Treatment
Urticaria	Itchy weals Change rapidly	May be airway obstruction	Penicillin Other drugs Foods Stings	Antihistamines
Erythema multiforme	Target lesions Mucosal ulcers	Eyes may be involved	Sulphonamides Non-steroidals Laxatives	Supportive Eye and mouth care
Toxic epidermal necrolysis	Sheets of necrotic epidermis	Fluid loss Shock Bronchial slough	Anticonvulsants Sulphonamides	High-care Monitor fluid and electrolytes Sepsis control
Lichenoid rash	Purple/brown papules on face & arms	Changes in pigmentation may persist	Anti-tuberculous drugs Thiazides Chloroquine	Sun protection Topical steroids
Fixed-drug eruption	Round Eroded Recurs at same site Leaves pigmentation		Laxatives Analgesics Non-steroidals Sulphonamides	Symptomatic
Drug hyper-sensitivity syndrome	Swollen face Diffuse, inflamed, scaly rash	Adenopathy Hepatitis Fever Eosinophilia	Anticonvulsants Anti-tuberculous agents Sulphonamides NNRTIs	Monitor liver functions Emollients Consider topical steroids

HIV-infected individuals are at far greater risk of developing cancer than the general population. Chemotherapy should be limited to patients on antiretroviral therapy or ideally those with CD4 counts >200 cells/µl; in some cases, rapid successive initiation of both therapies can be considered. In the patient with advanced HIV and cancer, palliative care is a priority.

Common HIV-associated malignancies

AIDS-defining cancers include:
- Kaposi's sarcoma (KS);
- non-Hodgkin's lymphoma (NHL); and
- invasive cervical cancer (see Chapter 26: Gynaecology).

Other cancers associated with HIV include:
- Hodgkin's lymphoma;
- anal carcinoma;
- glioma;
- leiomyosarcoma in children with HIV; and
- squamous carcinoma of the conjunctiva.

In addition, there is accumulating evidence for a host of other 'non-AIDS' cancers being linked to HIV, as patients live much longer on antiretrovirals.

Kaposi's sarcoma

KS is a spindle cell tumour, presumably of endothelial cell lineage, and is associated with human herpesvirus-8 (HHV-8) infection. It is an opportunistic neoplasm and is AIDS defining. Because HHV-8 is largely sexually transmitted, KS is uncommon in children, or people infected with HIV by blood products.

Clinical features

See Chapter 40: Dermatology, for a clinical description of KS.

Staging

Because the disease is multicentric, the standard tumour-node-metastases staging system that is used for solid tumours is not useful for classifying KS. The AIDS Clinical Trial Group Staging System given in Table 41.1 provides an alternative.

Table 41.1 AIDS Clinical Trial Group Staging System for epidemic Kaposi's sarcoma

	Good risk	Poor risk
Tumour	Confined to skin	Oedema Ulcers Oral and visceral involvement
Immune status	CD4 >200 cells/µl	CD4 < 200 cells/µl
Systemic illness	No B-symptoms or OIs	Prior OIs B-symptoms* Performance status <70† Other HIV-related illness

Source: Adapted from von Roenn, J. H. 1998. Reprinted with permission.
Copyright 1998 by the American Society of Clinical Oncology.
B-symptoms: fever, night sweats, and >10% loss of body weight.
† Karnofsky score (see Appendix 19.1).

Treatment

An optimal and/or standard therapy for AIDS-related KS has not been defined. Because palliation of KS-related symptoms is the primary goal of treatment, assessment of the therapeutic benefit of an agent should include:

- assessment of the agent's toxicity;
- objective tumour regression achieved;
- relief of tumour-related symptoms; and
- prevention of new disease.

Optimal antiretroviral therapy, with maximal viral suppression and prevention of other opportunistic infections (OIs), is an essential part of the treatment of KS and can lead to complete remission, even without other therapy.

Local treatment

Local treatment has an important palliative role. Individual cutaneous or oral lesions respond to:
- radiation therapy;
- intralesional chemotherapy; and/or
- cryotherapy.

In general, the smaller the lesion, the better the response will be. For modalities other than radiation therapy, repeated treatments may lead to some shrinkage of the lesions, but a complete response is uncommon, and tumour regrowth is frequently seen over a four to six month period. The most effective local treatment, radiation therapy, provides response rates of 80%–90%. It may provide effective palliation of painful, bulky, obstructive, and cosmetically disturbing lesions. Generally, the highest possible dose over a more protracted course will result in the longest duration of benefit.

Systemic treatment

Systemic therapy is generally indicated for KS patients who are on antiretroviral therapy, and can take the form of biological treatment or chemotherapy.

Biological therapy should be considered when a patient only has slowly growing skin lesions or mucocutaneous lesions. Interferon-α (IFN-α) has antiviral, anti-angiogenic, immune modulating, and antiproliferative properties. It is now considered first-line therapy for patients with cutaneous KS. Subcutaneous, intralesional, or intravenous therapy all resulted in remissions in 20%–60% of patients studied. Results are similar to the results achieved with single-agent chemotherapy. Response can take up to four months and is more effective with higher CD4 counts and the use of antiretroviral therapy. IFN-α can cause myelosuppression and hepatotoxicity and patients should be monitored carefully, especially if they are also taking antiretrovirals. (See Chapter 44: Adult antiretroviral therapy and Chapter 45: Paediatric antiretroviral therapy.)

Chemotherapy is indicated for patients with symptomatic visceral disease, pulmonary KS, symptomatic or rapidly progressive mucocutaneous lesions, and patients with lymphoedema.

Outcome

HIV-associated KS is generally associated with lower response rates and a shorter duration of responses. In spite of the significantly improved survival rates for patients with AIDS, the survival of patients with advanced KS has remained poor, even with the use of antiretroviral therapy.

Lymphoid neoplasms

HIV-positive patients have an increased incidence of high-grade non-Hodgkin's lymphoma, including primary B-cell lymphoma of the brain. Apart from the brain, extra-nodal sites include the liver, skin, gastrointestinal tract, bone marrow, and mucous membranes. Although most AIDS lymphomas are of B-cell origin, there is an increasing number of case reports of T-cell tumours. Generally, these lymphomas have an aggressive course, with relatively poor responses to chemotherapy, and are associated with high mortality rates. In HIV-positive patients, Hodgkin's disease (usually the lymphocytic depleted and mixed cellular types) follows an atypical aggressive clinical course, with involvement of multiple extra-nodal sites.

Central nervous system (CNS) lymphomas in HIV-infected patients are intracranial, intraparenchymal tumours that are multifocal and have indistinct borders. They are generally high-grade: mostly large-cell immunoblastic and small-cell non-cleaved lymphomas. Most tumours are of B-cell origin. The differential diagnosis of a parenchymal brain lesion in a patient with HIV infection includes toxoplasmosis and tuberculoma. Malignant cells were found in about 25% of patients in whom it was considered safe to perform a lumbar puncture, and Epstein-Barr virus polymerase chain reaction testing is sensitive and also specific for the diagnosis. The prognosis for CNS lymphoma is extremely poor.

Treatment

To date the treatment of AIDS lymphoma has largely involved modifications of conventional therapy involving cytotoxic agents. The morbidity and mortality associated with such treatments are increased in AIDS lymphoma patients, but dose reduction has been associated with improved outcome in AIDS lymphoma, even when tumour control was diminished. Median survival times for AIDS lymphoma are <18 months in most series.

Initially, oncologists treating AIDS lymphoma used complex regimens. However, patients tolerated chemotherapy poorly. Complete responses occurred in a minority of AIDS lymphoma patients and were usually of short duration. In order to improve patient tolerance, oncologists began to explore the role of low-dose chemotherapy. This resulted in a better quality of life, with fewer treatment-related complications. The anti-B cell monoclonal antibody rituximab has shown promising results when added to standard chemotherapy.

When treating AIDS lymphoma patients with both chemotherapy and antiretroviral therapy, it is important to consider the advantages and disadvantages of both these combination treatments. Overlapping toxicities and pharmacokinetic interactions may affect the therapeutic efficacy of the various drugs. Increased toxicity may lead to delay of chemotherapy and/or dose reductions that could compromise the potential cure of the lymphoma. Ideally, all patients receiving chemotherapy should also receive antiretroviral therapy, as immune reconstitution can be associated with an anti-tumour effect. Note, however, that chemotherapy can deplete the CD4 count by up to 50%.

As 15%–20% of patients with AIDS lymphoma have CNS involvement at presentation, CNS prophylaxis with intrathecal chemotherapy (methotrexate or cytarabine) is standard practice in AIDS lymphoma patients. To date, the studies regarding immune depletion, chemotherapy dose intensity, scheduling, and the role of antiretrovirals during chemotherapy on treatment outcome, have failed to yield precise conclusions that can easily be applied to standard clinical practice guidelines.

Other malignancies

It is best to refer AIDS patients with secondary neoplasms, whether they are AIDS-defining cancers or tumours in immune-compromised patients, to a team experienced in the complicated treatment options for such patients. Optimal antiretroviral therapy, with maximal viral suppression, and the prevention and treatment of OIs, should be an integral part of the AIDS malignancy treatment plan.

References and further reading

Antman, K. and Y. Chang. 2000 'Kaposi's sarcoma.' *New England Journal of Medicine*; 324 (14):1027–1036.

Boue, F. et al. 2006. 'Phase II trial of CHOP plus rituximab in patients with HIV-associated non-Hodgkin's lymphoma.' *Journal of Clinical Oncology*; 24 (25):4123–4128.

Little, R. F. et al. 2000. 'Systemic chemotherapy for HIV-associated lymphoma in the era of highly active anti-retroviral therapy'. *Current Opinion in Oncology*; 12 (5):445–449.

Spano J.P. et al. 2008. AIDS-related malignancies: State of the art and therapeutic challenges. *Journal of Clinical Oncology* (in press).

Rheumatology

A wide spectrum of musculoskeletal conditions is associated with HIV infection. Principles to remember when evaluating an HIV-infected patient with a rheumatological syndrome include the following:

- Musculoskeletal syndromes and HIV infection may be unrelated.
- HIV infection may alter the clinical picture of these syndromes, which may be more severe or more subtle in presentation.
- The stage of the patient's HIV disease is important in determining aetiology. Infectious complications are more common with lower CD4 counts, and account for the majority of serious clinical musculoskeletal conditions prior to the initiation of antiretroviral therapy.
- Diagnosis is the same in HIV-negative and HIV-positive patients.
- Immunosuppressive therapy should be used with caution in HIV-positive patients. Antiretroviral therapy is often very effective in the treatment of musculoskeletal conditions, and has a profound impact on decreasing the incidence of psoriatic arthritis and reactive arthritis, as well as other syndromes.

Common, benign conditions

HIV-associated arthralgia

Arthralgia is the commonest rheumatic manifestation associated with HIV infection. This can occur at any stage of HIV infection, and is generally mild to moderate in intensity, intermittent, and oligoarticular. Arthralgia usually involves large joints such as shoulders, elbows, and knees, but can affect small joints. It is uncommon for polyarthralgia to progress to inflammatory joint disease and the most appropriate treatments are non-narcotic analgesia and reassurance. Pyrazinamide commonly causes arthralgia.

Painful articular syndrome

This self-limiting syndrome is characterized by idiopathic, severe, oligo-articular pain, usually in the knee, elbow or shoulder. It usually occurs in the later stages of the HIV infection. Examination shows no evidence of synovitis and the intense pain usually lasts <24 hours. The treatment is symptomatic and patients may require short-term use of narcotics.

Myalgia and fibromyalgia

Myalgias have been reported in up to a third of HIV-positive out-patients. They are common in the first few weeks after starting zidovudine. Fibromyalgia syndrome (FMS) can also complicate HIV infection. The treatment of HIV-associated FMS is similar to that of non-HIV-associated FMS and includes non-narcotic analgesics, low-dose tricyclic antidepressants, and reassurance.

HIV infection and arthritis

The following types of arthritis may occur:
- HIV-associated reactive arthritis (Reiter's syndrome variant);
- psoriatic arthritis; and
- HIV-associated arthritis (which may be due to the virus directly involving joint synovium).

Reactive arthritis

Reactive arthritis (for example secondary to *Chlamydia* infection) is the most common arthritis seen in patients with HIV infection. It is not more common in HIV-infected individuals, but is more severe.

Patients develop asymmetric oligoarthritis, predominantly of the lower extremities, which is usually accompanied by dactylitis (sausaging of toes or fingers). Erosive polyarthritis, severe enthesopathy, and poor response to treatment may be seen in about two-thirds of patients. The remaining third exhibit a mild and self-limiting course. Classic Reiter's syndrome (urethritis, conjunctivitis, and arthritis) may occur as part of the spectrum of reactive arthritis.

Treatment of reactive arthritis

- The first-line treatment is with non-steroidal anti-inflammatory drugs.
- Chloroquine or sulfasalazine may be used as disease-modifying agents. Methotrexate should be used with caution.
- Low-dose oral steroids (e.g. 5–10 mg of prednisone) may be necessary in refractory cases.

Psoriatic arthritis

Psoriasis and psoriatic arthritis occur with greatly increased prevalence in HIV-infected individuals. New onset or exacerbation of underlying psoriasis in high-risk individuals should alert clinicians to the possible presence of underlying HIV infection.

Psoriatic arthritis tends to occur late in the course of HIV infection. The foot and ankle are the most common sites of inflammation in HIV-infected patients with psoriatic-like arthritis. Erosive changes and crippling deformities may occur. Enthesopathy can be a major cause of disability. From a clinical point of view, psoriatic arthritis and Reiter's syndrome with keratoderma blennorrhagica may be indistinguishable.

Treatment

Low-dose methotrexate (12.5–25 mg once a week), used under specialist supervision, has led to rapid (<4 weeks) improvement in the joint symptoms and skin lesions seen in severe inflammatory arthritis:

- Methotrexate can be given until the skin and joint disease is under control, then slowly tapered by 2.5 mg per month, aiming for a maintenance dose of 12.5 mg per week.
- Folic acid 5 mg daily should be given and full blood count, differential, and liver functions should be checked frequently.
- Patients must be monitored closely for progressive immunodeficiency and OIs. Methotrexate should be avoided if the CD4 count is <200 cells/μl.
- Antiretrovirals may ameliorate symptoms in the longer term, but may paradoxically worsen the condition in the short term (see immune reconstitution inflammatory syndrome below).

Intra-articular steroid injections may provide substantial relief to individual arthritic joints. Systemic glucocorticoid use is generally discouraged.

HIV-associated arthritis

HIV-associated arthritis tends to be oligoarticular and occurs predominantly in the lower extremities. It tends to have a self-limiting course, lasting <6 weeks. Radiographs of the affected joints generally show no erosive changes. Patients also lack the extra-articular clinical manifestations associated with Reiter's syndrome.

More recently, an HIV-associated polyarthritis has been described that resembles rheumatoid arthritis (RA) in distribution and course of illness.

The rheumatoid factor may be positive or negative. Synovitis abates with a progressive decline in the CD4 count, but joint destruction continues.

Treatment of HIV-associated arthritis

- Disease-modifying agents are seldom needed in the oligoarticular presentation, owing to the self-limiting nature of the illness.
- Methotrexate may need to be used to control joint disease in the RA-like variety.

Table 42.1 contrasts the features of HIV-associated arthritis with those of reactive arthritis.

Table 42.1 Contrasting features of HIV-associated arthritis and reactive arthritis

Feature	HIV-associated arthritis	HIV-associated reactive arthritis
Joint involvement	Highly variable (mono/polyarthritis)	Asymmetric oligo/polyarthritis
Mucocutaneous involvement	Absent	Occurs
Enthesopathy	Absent	Frequent
Synovial fluid cultures	Negative	Negative
Microorganisms in synovial membranes	HIV-1 virus	Chlamydia*
HLA-B27 association†	Absent	70–90% ‡
Course	Usually self-limited	Chronic/relapsing

*Demonstrated in non-HIV-associated reactive arthritis.
†HLA is human leukocyte antigen.
‡The B27 association in black patients is substantially less.

HIV-associated muscle disease

The spectrum of muscle involvement in patients with HIV infection ranges from uncomplicated myalgias, fibromyalgia, or asymptomatic creatine kinase (CK) elevation, to disabling and life-threatening HIV-associated polymyositis or pyomyositis.

The spectrum of muscle involvement in HIV-infected individuals includes:

- asymptomatic sporadic CK elevation;
- myalgia/fibromyalgia (see 'Myalgia and fibromyalgia' above);
- HIV-associated polymyositis;
- zidovudine-associated myopathy; and
- pyomyositis.

HIV-associated polymyositis

HIV-associated polymyositis is rare, tends to occur in early infection, and is characterized by proximal muscle weakness. The presentation, diagnosis, and treatment of HIV-associated polymyositis are similar to those in HIV-negative individuals, and should be managed by a specialist rheumatologist.

Zidovudine-associated myopathy

Zidovudine-associated myopathy is rare, and is characterized by the gradual onset of myalgias, muscle tenderness, and proximal muscle weakness. It tends to be dose related, and associated with chronic zidovudine usage. Zidovudine myopathy is difficult to distinguish from HIV-associated polymyositis, both clinically and on EMG and biopsy. A muscle biopsy is seldom indicated, but mitochondrial myopathy-like changes may be seen.

The symptoms tend to improve as the drug is discontinued, with CK returning to normal within four weeks and muscle strength returning within eight weeks.

Pyomyositis

Pyogenic infection (usually staphylococcal) of muscle is more common in HIV-infected individuals, and tends to occur in advanced infection. *The typical presentation is acute, with severe muscle pain, usually without obvious erythema or fluctuation.* CK levels are elevated. Ultrasound is much less sensitive than CT or MRI in demonstrating the infected muscle. Open drainage or debridement, together with antibiotics, is curative. (See photo 52.)

Diffuse infiltrative lymphocytosis syndrome

Diffuse infiltrative lymphocytosis syndrome (DILS) is a Sjögrens-like syndrome, with salivary gland enlargement and peripheral CD8 lymphocytosis. In HIV-positive individuals it is often accompanied by sicca symptoms and extraglandular features. DILS usually presents with painless parotid enlargement, owing to benign lympho-epithelial cysts. The parotidomegaly is often massive. (See photo 53.) Co-existing sub-mandibular and lacrimal gland enlargement are common. Sicca symptoms (xerostomia and xerophthalmia) occur in over 60% of patients.

Extraglandular features of diffuse infiltrative lymphocytosis syndrome

The extraglandular features of DILS are:

- pulmonary:
  - lymphocytic interstitial pneumonitis;
- neurologic:
  - VIIth nerve palsy,
  - aseptic lymphocytic meningitis,
  - peripheral neuropathy;
- gastrointestinal:
  - lymphocytic hepatitis;
- renal:
  - renal tubular acidosis,
  - interstitial nephritis; and
- musculoskeletal:
  - peripheral arthritis,
  - polymyositis.

Treatment

See Chapter 39: Oral medicine, for the treatment of xerostomia. Corticosteroids are helpful for both glandular and extraglandular features, but should only be considered if there are significant symptoms. Parotidomegaly may respond to radiotherapy. Antiretrovirals are effective in treating the glandular swelling and sicca symptoms associated with DILS, as well as the complications, such as neuropathy.

Other autoimmune disease

A variety of vasculitic syndromes has been reported in association with HIV. Of interest is a rapidly progressive focal necrotizing vasculitis of the aorta and large arteries that is similar to Takayasu's arteritis. Isolated central nervous system (CNS) vasculitis can present with organic brain syndromes and neurologic deficits.

Rheumatoid arthritis and systemic lupus erythematosus appear to improve in the face of CD4 lymphocyte depletion associated with HIV.

Autoantibodies tend to occur, in low titre, in HIV-positive individuals, including antinuclear antibodies, rheumatoid factor, and anti-neutrophil cytoplasmic antibodies. These are rarely of clinical significance.

Musculoskeletal infections in HIV

Typical musculoskeletal infections encountered in HIV-positive patients include:

- osteoarticular tuberculosis (TB);
- septic arthritis;
- osteomyelitis;
- cellulitis;
- septic tenosynovitis;
- bursitis;
- soft-tissue abscesses; and
- pyomyositis (see above).

Osteoarticular tuberculosis (TB)

The presentation of osteoarticular TB is similar to that of TB in HIV-negative patients, but disseminated TB is more common.

Septic arthritis and acute osteomyelitis

The presentation of septic arthritis and osteomyelitis is similar to that occurring in HIV-negative patients. *Staphylococcus aureus* is the agent most commonly isolated.

Other musculoskeletal complications

Cellulitis, septic tenosynovitis and bursitis, and soft-tissue abscesses may also occur. Gram-positive microorganisms, particularly *Staphylococcus aureus* and *Streptococcus pyogenes*, are the most common aetiologic agents. Bacillary angiomatosis secondary to *Bartonella henselae* may give destructive osseous lesions along with skin and lymphatic involvement. Lymphoma in advanced AIDS cases may present with extensive bone involvement.

Children

The most common musculoskeletal syndromes in children include bone and joint infection caused by pyogenic organisms. Polyarthritis, with and without psoriasis, may occur. Human leukocyte antigen B27 status should be checked. Management should take place in consultation with a paediatric rheumatologist, but is similar to that of adults.

Immune reconstitution inflammatory syndromes (IRIS)

Some patients experience paradoxical worsening of symptoms and signs pertaining to a condition in the weeks and months after the initiation of antiretrovirals. While this was initially recognized with OIs, they have been increasingly described with other conditions, including rheumatoid arthritis, SLE, sarcoid, psoriasis, Reiter's, Grave's Disease and other auto-immune thyroid conditions. The pathogenesis of IRIS is complex, and treatment generally involves continuing antiretroviral therapy while addressing the underlying condition conventionally. Occasionally, the underlying disease process may be unrecognised (referred to as 'occult' IRIS) and the diagnosis only confirmed when antiretrovirals are started.

Acute HIV

An assortment of symptoms that may resemble aspects of rheumatological conditions occur during acute HIV, almost always before the development of antibody responses (the 'window period'), meaning that the diagnosis is often missed. Arthralgias, oral ulcers, fevers, myalgias, pharyngitis, rash and headaches occur in association with a variety of other symptoms, especially diarrhoea. Diagnosis is made on PCR testing or serial ELISA testing.

References and further reading

Adebajo, A., and P. Davis. 1994. 'Rheumatic disease in African blacks.' *Seminars in Arthritis and Rheumatism*; 24 (2):139–153.

HIV Insite. Rheumatologic and musculoskeletal manifestations of HIV. Available: http:hivinsite.ucsf.edu/.

Reveille, J. D. 2000. 'The changing spectrum of rheumatic disease in Human Immunodeficiency Virus infection.' *Seminars in Arthritis and Rheumatism* 30 (3):147–166.

PART 5

Antiretroviral drug management

43 Antiretroviral drug classes 459

44 Adult antiretroviral therapy 465

45 Paediatric antiretroviral therapy 474

46 Prevention of mother-to-child transmission of HIV 498

47 Antiretroviral drug resistance 508

48 Adherence to antiretroviral therapy 512

49 Drug-drug interactions 520

50 Immune reconstitution inflammatory syndrome 526

51 Principles of managing adverse drug reactions 531

52 Occupational post-exposure prophylaxis 543

43 Antiretroviral drug classes

Antiretroviral drug resistance is discussed in Chapter 47, drug interactions in Chapter 49, and the management of adverse drug reactions in Chapter 51.

Figure 43.1 The replication cycle of HIV, with the sites of action of antiretroviral drug classes numbered (described below)

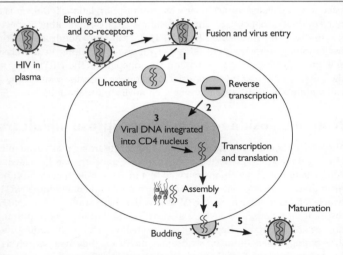

1 There are two classes of entry inhibitors: fusion inhibitors (e.g. enfuvirtide) and chemokine receptor antagonists (e.g. maraviroc).
2 There are two classes of reverse transcriptase inhibitors: nucleosides (e.g. zidovudine) and non-nucleosides (e.g. nevirapine).
3 Integrase inhibitors (e.g. raltegravir).
4 Protease inhibitors (e.g. saquinavir).
5 Maturation inhibitors (still investigational).

Four classes of antiretrovirals are currently available in southern Africa: nucleoside/nucleotide reverse transcriptase inhibitors (NRTIs), non-nucleoside reverse transcriptase inhibitors (NNRTIs), protease inhibitors (PIs), and integrase inhibitors. Currently available entry inhibitors are either very expensive (enfuvirtide) or require expensive tests to determine chemokine receptor tropism (maraviroc), so they are unlikely to be used in our region.

Nucleoside reverse transcriptase inhibitors

NRTIs resemble the natural nucleotide building blocks of DNA and block the conversion of viral RNA into proviral DNA. NRTIs are pro-drugs that need to be activated intracellularly by tri-phosphorylation. Tenofovir is a nucleotide RTI that contains one phosphate group, but in other respects it is similar to the rest of the NRTIs. NRTIs impair mitochondrial function by inhibiting mitochondrial DNA polymerase-γ, resulting in the class side effects of hyperlactataemia and steatohepatitis. The NRTIs vary in their ability to impair mitochondrial function: didanosine > stavudine > zidovudine > lamivudine = abacavir = tenofovir = emtricitabine.

Non-nucleoside reverse transcriptase inhibitors

Three NNRTIs, efavirenz, nevirapine, and etravirine are currently available. NNRTIs do not bind at the active site of reverse transcriptase, but cause a conformational change in the enzyme that inhibits it. Both efavirenz and nevirapine have long half-lives. Etravirine is a second generation NNRTI, which retains activity against HIV strains that have some of the NNRTI resistant mutations. The NNRTIs are involved in a number of important drug interactions (see Chapter 49). Hypersensitivity rashes (including life-threatening Stevens-Johnson syndrome and Toxic Epidermal Necrolysis) are common in the first six weeks of therapy, but are more severe with nevirapine. Hepatitis is also more severe with nevirapine, and, unlike efavirenz, the hepatitis is often accompanied by a rash; therefore it is essential to check liver function tests in patients developing rashes on nevirapine. Rash-associated hepatitis from nevirapine is more common in patients with higher baseline CD4 counts (>250 cells/μl in women and >400 cells/μl in men), and the drug is best avoided in this setting. Transient neuropsychiatric symptoms (e.g. insomnia, vivid dreams, dizziness) occur commonly with efavirenz. Efavirenz should be avoided in the first trimester as it is reported to be teratogenic, associated with craniofacial and neural tube defects.

Table 43.1 Nucleoside reverse transcriptase inhibitors currently available in southern Africa: dosing and common or severe adverse drug reactions

Generic name	Dosage	Adverse drug reactions
Zidovudine (AZT)	300 mg 12 hourly	Anaemia, elevated red cell MCV, neutropaenia, nausea, headache, myalgia, myopathy (rare), hyperlactataemia/steatohepatitis (medium potential), lipoatrophy
Didanosine (ddI)	400 mg daily (250 mg daily if <60 kg) (take on empty stomach)	Peripheral neuropathy, pancreatitis, nausea, diarrhoea, hyperlactataemia/steatohepatitis (high potential)
Lamivudine (3TC)	150 mg 12 hourly or 300 mg daily	Hyperlactataemia/steatohepatitis (low potential), may precipitate severe hepatitis B flare if discontinued, red cell aplasia (rare)
Stavudine (d4T)	30 mg 12 hourly (note – higher doses for >60 kg no longer recommended due to toxicity)	Peripheral neuropathy, elevated red cell MCV, hypertriglyceridaemia, lipoatrophy, hyperlactataemia/steatohepatitis (high potential)
Abacavir (ABC)	300 mg 12 hourly or 600 mg daily	Systemic hypersensitivity reaction, hyperlactataemia/steatohepatitis (low potential)
Tenofovir (TDF)	300 mg daily	Renal failure, decreased bone mineral density, hyperlactataemia/steatohepatitis (low potential), may precipitate severe hepatitis B flare if discontinued
Emtricitabine (FTC)	200 mg daily (co-formulated with TDF)	Headache, nausea, hyperpigmentation, hyperlactataemia/steatohepatitis (low potential), may precipitate severe hepatitis B flare if discontinued

Table 43.2 Non-nucleoside reverse transcriptase inhibitors currently available in southern Africa: dosing and common or severe adverse drug reactions

Generic name	Dosage	Adverse drug reactions
Nevirapine	200 mg daily for 14 days then 200 mg 12 hourly	Rash, hepatitis
Efavirenz	600 mg at night	Rash, neuropsychiatric symptoms, hepatitis, dyslipidaemia
Etravirine	200 mg 12 hourly	Rash, hepatitis

Protease inhibitors

Protease inhibitors (PIs) interfere with HIV protease, which cleaves transcribed viral polyproteins into functional proteins. Inhibition of protease results in the release of immature non-infectious viral particles. PIs are involved in many drug interactions (see Chapter 49). Small doses of ritonavir markedly increase the plasma concentrations and prolong the half-lives of most PIs. This is known as ritonavir boosting and has become the standard of care for administering these agents (see Chapter 44). Gastrointestinal intolerance (nausea, vomiting and/or diarrhoea) are common side effects of protease inhibitors. Insulin resistance and dyslipidaemia are class side effects, but the individual drugs differ in their propensity to cause this (see Table 43.3). There is an increased risk of myocardial infarction in patients on PIs, probably because of these metabolic side effects.

Table 43.3 Protease inhibitors currently available in southern Africa: dosing and common or severe adverse drug reactions

Generic name	Dosage	Adverse drug reactions
Indinavir	800 mg 8 hourly (on an empty stomach) or 800mg 12 hourly with 100 mg ritonavir 12 hourly (no food restrictions)	Kidney stones, unconjugated hyperbilirubinaemia, GI upset, hair loss, insulin resistance, dyslipidaemia
Ritonavir	600 mg 12 hourly	Poorly tolerated and rarely used as sole PI. GI disturbances, hepatitis, taste perversion, insulin resistance, dyslipidaemia
Saquinavir	1000/100 bd or 2000/100 daily (only if PI naïve)	GI upset (mild), headache, hepatitis, insulin resistance/dyslipidaemia
Atazanavir	400 mg daily (only if PI naïve) or 300 mg with ritonavir 100 mg daily	Unconjugated hyperbilirubinaemia, GI upset, dyslipidaemia (low potential)
Lopinavir/ Ritonavir	400/100 mg 12 hourly or 800/200 mg daily (only if PI naïve)	GI upset, hepatitis, dyslipidaemia
Darunavir	600 mg 12 hourly with 100 mg ritonavir 12 hourly	Rash, GI upset, hepatitis, dyslipidaemia

Integrase inhibitors

Raltegravir is the only member of this class currently available. The mechanism of action is inhibition of the HIV integrase enzyme, which is responsible for inserting proviral DNA into the genome of the CD4+ cell. Raltegravir is generally well tolerated, with headache and insomnia being the two commonest adverse drug reactions. It may be used in salvage therapy, provided it is combined with an active protease inhibitor, or in initial therapy.

Constructing a combination antiretroviral regimen

The best-studied regimens consist of two NRTIs together with either a NNRTI or a PI.

Several factors need to be considered when selecting the dual NRTI combination. First, some combinations (AZT and d4T; TDF and ddI) cannot be used because of adverse drug interactions (see Chapter 51). Second, several NRTIs (3TC, FTC and TDF) are active against hepatitis B. Discontinuing these agents can cause severe flares of hepatitis B. It is preferable to combine TDF with either FTC or 3TC when treating HIV in patients co-infected with hepatitis B in order to delay the emergence of hepatitis B resistant mutations. Hepatitis B is a common infection in our region and it is advisable to always screen for it in patients starting anti-retroviral therapy. FTC and 3TC share the same HIV-resistant mutation and can be used interchangeably. Third, it is prudent to avoid NRTIs in patients with co-morbidities that are also adverse drug reactions of the NRTI (e.g. anaemia and AZT, renal failure and TDF). Fourth, if the NNRTI or protease inhibitor selected is to be administered once daily, then NRTIs that can also be dosed once daily should be chosen (ABC, 3TC, FTC, TDF). Finally, d4T and ddI are associated with higher risk of toxicity and should generally be avoided. Several fixed-dose combination dual NRTI formulations (some of which also contain NNRTIs) exist that can reduce the patient's pill burden. It is essential to have a complete history of previous NRTI exposure in order to select combinations that are less likely to have cross-resistance (although mutations conferring resistance to all NRTIs may occur – see Chapter 47).

Selecting an NNRTI or a PI as the third agent in a regimen depends on whether it is the initial or subsequent regimen. NNRTIs are best used in initial regimens, except in children who have been exposed to single dose nevirapine for prevention of mother-to-child transmission because they will often have NNRTI resistance.

Alternative combination antiretroviral regimens to the conventional dual NRTI plus NNRTI or PI have been studied, and doubtless more will be studied with the newer classes of antiretrovirals now available. Triple NRTI combinations are inferior to conventional regimens, especially if the viral load is >100 000 copies/ml, but may be considered in exceptional circumstances. PIs and NNRTIs can be combined (with a dose increase required for some PIs due to the induction of metabolism by the NNRTI) if there is resistance to all NRTIs or if a severe NRTI class side-effect has occurred such as lactic acidosis.

References and recommended reading

Current versions of adult antiretroviral guidelines can be downloaded from the following websites:
Southern Africa: http://www.sahivsoc.org/
United Kingdom: http://www.bhiva.org/
USA: http://www.aidsinfo.nih.gov/guidelines/
WHO: http://www.who.int/hiv/pub/guidelines/en/
The DAD study group. 2007. 'Class of antiretroviral drugs and the risk of myocardial infarction'. *New England Journal of Medicine*, 356:1723–1735.

Adult antiretroviral therapy

Other important chapters on antiretroviral therapy are: antiretroviral drug classes (Chapter 43), adherence (Chapter 48), resistance (Chapter 47), managing adverse drug reactions (Chapter 51), drug interactions (Chapter 49), and the immune reconstitution inflammatory syndrome (Chapter 50).

Goals of antiretroviral therapy

Antiretroviral therapy reduces the HIV viral load in the blood (ideally to below the detectable limit of the assay). This allows gradual recovery of the immune system and consequently results in a reduction of HIV-related illnesses. HIV-associated morbidity and mortality are dramatically reduced. It is difficult to estimate the survival benefit from combination antiretroviral therapy because treatment is evolving. Recent estimates suggest a survival benefit of as much as 30 years.

There is a downside to these benefits. Antiretroviral therapy is complex, typically requiring the use of at least three drugs in combination in order to keep the viral load suppressed. Adverse drug reactions caused by antiretrovirals are fairly frequent. Furthermore, high levels of adherence are necessary to avoid the risk of inducing viral resistance (see Chapter 48). Antiretroviral therapy suppresses but does not cure HIV, so therapy is lifelong. It was thought that antiretroviral therapy could be discontinued in patients with high CD4 counts and recommenced if the CD4 counts fell. However, this strategy, known as structured treatment interruption, has been shown to be associated with an increased risk of death, often due to vascular disease, even in patients with high CD4 counts.

When to start antiretroviral therapy

Clinical stage and CD4 count

The optimal time to start combination antiretroviral therapy is controversial. Current recommendations are based on either the CD4 count or the clinical status of the patient. Cohort studies suggest that patients should not start therapy too early (CD4 count >350 cells/µl) in the course of the infection as there is very little risk of disease progression at this stage. It is clear that outcomes on combination antiretroviral therapy are worse in patients with CD4 counts <200 cells/μl because they remain at risk of AIDS events, often for many months, and they experience more adverse drug reactions, and immune reconstitution inflammatory syndrome events (see Chapter 50). Thus, current evidence supports starting antiretroviral therapy when the CD4 count is between 200–350 cells/μl. However, it is important to note that many patients do well despite starting antiretroviral therapy with very low CD4 counts; it is never too late to start antiretroviral therapy. It is also clear that patients with AIDS-defining illnesses or other severe HIV-related morbidity should start antiretrovirals irrespective of the CD4 count.

The current Southern African HIV Clinicians Society and WHO guidelines recommend starting antiretroviral therapy when *either*:

- the CD4 count is <350 cells/μl (this should be confirmed with a second CD4 count within three months as CD4 counts vary considerably) *or*
- the patient has WHO Stage 3 or 4 disease.

The current South African public sector guidelines are similar, but do not include WHO stage 3 as a criterion for starting ART.

Major opportunistic infections, notably TB, should be identified and treatment started before starting antiretroviral therapy. The immune reconstitution inflammatory syndrome is much more likely to occur if antiretroviral therapy is started before the opportunistic infection is brought under control. With TB this risk is highest when antiretroviral therapy is started within the first eight weeks of antitubercular therapy. However, randomised controlled trials have shown that patients with advanced disease need to start antiretroviral therapy at around two weeks. See Chapter 49 for appropriate antiretroviral regimens to use in combination with rifampicin.

Table 44.1 Guidelines for when to initiate antiretroviral therapy in patients being treated for tuberculosis (TB)

CD4 count	Duration of TB therapy
<50	Start antiretroviral therapy after 2 weeks
50–350	Start antiretroviral therapy after 8 weeks
>350	Defer antiretroviral therapy*

*Current South African guidelines – WHO and the Southern African HIV Clinicians Society recommend treating all patients with TB irrespective of CD4 count

Guidelines of when to start also need to be flexible. There are a number of severe conditions that may present with CD4 counts >350 cells/µl but that are not WHO stage 3 or 4 illnesses. Examples of conditions that fall into this category are listed in Table 44.2.

Table 44.2 Examples of severe conditions in which antiretroviral therapy initiation should be considered irrespective of the CD4 count

Multidrug-resistant TB
Non-AIDS malignancies
Severe manifestations of the diffuse infiltrative lymphocytosis syndrome (e.g. polymyositis, lymphocytic interstitial pneumonitis)
Severe manifestations of primary HIV infection
Chronic liver disease due to hepatitis B (using antiretrovirals active against both infections)

Social and psychological stage

Psychosocial readiness for antiretroviral therapy is at least as important as meeting medical criteria in deciding when to initiate such therapy. It is essential that patients are ready to commit to lifelong antiretroviral therapy before starting treatment. They need to be educated about the risks and benefits of antiretroviral therapy. They must have insight into the progression of HIV disease and understand the importance of monitoring antiretroviral therapy efficacy and toxicity. Patients need to understand the importance of high levels of adherence. Substance abuse and depression should be actively excluded and, if present, managed.

First-line antiretroviral regimens

The first regimen has the best chance of sustained success. Standardized antiretroviral regimens, similar to the drug regimens used in TB management programmes, have been used with success in resource-limited settings. However, there are frequently compelling reasons to select or to avoid certain antiretrovirals in individual patients.

Conventional combination antiretroviral therapy consists of two nucleoside reverse transcriptase inhibitors (NRTIs) together with either a non-nucleoside reverse transcriptase inhibitor (NNRTI) or a protease inhibitor (PI). The principles involved in selecting an appropriate dual NRTI combination for individuals are covered in Chapter 43: Antiretroviral drug classes.

Table 44.3 Advantages and disadvantages of appropriate dual NRTI combinations for initial therapy

Dual NRTI	Advantages	Disadvantages
Tenofovir + lamivudine/ emtricitabine	Once daily Low potential for mitochondrial toxicity Effective for hepatitis B	Need to monitor renal function
Zidovudine + lamivudine	Long track record, including pregnancy	Need to monitor full blood count
Abacavir + lamivudine	Once daily Low potential for mitochondrial toxicity	Expensive Shared resistance pathway
Stavudine + lamivudine	Cheap	High potential for mitochondrial toxicity

NNRTIs are at least as effective as protease inhibitors (when combined with two NRTIs) in clinical trials. There are several compelling reasons for preferring NNRTIs to protease inhibitors in first-line therapy:

- cheaper;
- lower pill burden;
- no increased risk of vascular disease (unlike the protease inhibitors, which are associated with a 16% increased relative risk of myocardial infarction per year of use);
- lower genetic barrier to resistance (therefore less robust in second line antiretroviral therapy where there may be some mutations compromising the NRTIs).

Efavirenz should be avoided in pregnant women in the first trimester and in patients with uncontrolled depression or psychosis. Nevirapine should be avoided with co-existing liver disease, and in patients with higher CD4 counts (>250 cells/μl in women and >400 cells/μl in men) because of the increased risk of rash-associated hepatitis.

Second-line antiretroviral regimens

The most likely causes of resistance after failing first line NNRTI-based therapy (see the definition of failure below) are mutations conferring high level resistance to the NNRTIs (there is cross resistance between efavirenz and nevirapine) and/or high level resistance to lamivudine (or the similar NRTI emtricitabine). If the patient continues to take the failing antiretroviral regimen for years, NRTI mutations slowly accumulate that may affect the entire class.

The definition of virological failure requires a confirmed increase in viral load. In other words the viral load must be repeated at least a month apart. It is essential to assess adherence and enhance adherence support if the viral load increases on therapy. Transient minor increases in viral load up to 1000 copies/mL are known as "blips". Blips are of no significance and do not cause resistance. The simplest definition of virologic failure in patients who were suppressed is a confirmed viral load increase above an arbitrary value, typically 1000 or 5000 copies/mL. A more aggressive definition is any sustained viral load increase above the level of detection of the assay. There is no hard evidence to back either approach. The Southern African HIV Clinicians Society recommendation is to consider switching antiretroviral therapy with a confirmed viral load increase of >1000 copies/mL.

When selecting a second-line antiretroviral regimen two NRTIs should be used, one of which is new, together with a third drug from a new drug class. Lamivudine (or emtricitabine) should be used in the second-line regimen even if either was used in the initial regimen, despite the fact that a mutation conferring high level resistance to both drugs is likely to be present because this resistance mutation partially cripples HIV and increases viral susceptibility to tenofovir, zidovudine and stavudine (see Chapter 47).

A ritonavir boosted PI is recommended in second-line antiretroviral therapy. Ritonavir boosted PIs have a relatively high genetic barrier to resistance and the second-line regimen may be effective even if there are some mutations which limit the efficacy of the NRTIs.

Table 44.4 Advantages and disadvantages of appropriate ritonavir boosted protease inhibitors for second-line therapy

Protease inhibitor	Advantages	Disadvantages
Lopinavir + ritonavir	High genetic barrier to resistance Fixed dose combination	High potential for dyslipidaemia
Atazanavir + ritonavir	Low potential for dyslipidaemia Once daily dosing*	Moderate genetic barrier to resistance Unconjugated hyperbilirubinaemia is common
Saquinavir + ritonavir	Low potential for dyslipidaemia	Moderate genetic barrier to resistance
Indinavir + ritonavir	Long track record	Poorly tolerated due to nephrolithiasis Insulin resistance and hair loss

*Once daily dosing is also possible with boosted lopinavir and saquinavir

Monitoring antiretroviral efficacy

Viral loads

The key determinant of long-term antiretroviral success is the suppression of the viral load below the limit of detection of the assay. Virological failure is therefore the most important criterion for switching antiretroviral regimens. An early viral load at about four to eight weeks after initiating antiretroviral therapy is helpful because there should be at least a tenfold reduction in viral load at this stage. Viral suppression should occur by six months. If this does not occur, then in nearly all cases the explanation will be poor adherence (see Chapter 48). If the viral load is undetectable this test should be repeated approximately every six months.

CD4 counts

With effective antiretroviral therapy, CD4 counts should rise approximately 100 cells/μl in the first year and about 50–80 cells/μl per year thereafter. However, the CD4 response is very variable. About 10-20% of patients fail to have a CD4 response despite virological suppression. There is no point in changing the antiretroviral regimen in this setting.

In many resource-limited countries viral load monitoring is not available and decisions to switch to second line antiretroviral therapy are made on the basis of CD4 responses. The WHO has suggested the following CD4 criteria for switching antiretrovirals:

- CD4 count below 100 cells/μl after six months of antiretroviral therapy;
- return to the pre-therapy CD4 baseline;
- 50% decline from the on-treatment peak CD4 value.

Switching antiretroviral therapy on the basis of CD4 count responses will result in unnecessary changes in patients who have poor CD4 responses, and failing antiretroviral therapy will be continued (with the risk of accumulating more resistance mutations) in many patients.

Once CD4 counts have increased to >200 cells/μl prophylaxis against opportunistic infections can safely be discontinued. CD4 counts should be monitored six-monthly.

Safety monitoring

Most safety monitoring of antiretroviral therapy is done by clinical assessment. Routine laboratory monitoring is required for only a few antiretrovirals:

- Zidovudine: full blood counts should be monitored to detect anaemia and neutropenia. Most haematological toxicity occurs within six months, so routine monitoring after this period is of questionable value.
- Nevirapine: liver transaminases (it is cost effective to monitor only the ALT) should be monitored for the first three months. Hepatitis beyond this period is very unusual and clinical monitoring should be enough.
- Protease inhibitors: fasting lipogram should be done after three months and annually thereafter.
- Tenofovir: creatinine should be monitored closely for three months, then six monthly.

Managing toxicity

This is covered in Chapter 51.

Salvage therapy

Salvage antiretroviral therapy is defined as therapy in patients who have failed an NNRTI regimen and a PI regimen. These patients are difficult to manage, because their adherence is often sub-optimal and they frequently have resistance mutations, limiting treatment options. Achieving viral suppression is unlikely unless at least two drugs are used to which the patient's HIV is susceptible. Until recently viral suppression could only be achieved in a minority of salvage patients, but recent results from clinical trials of potent new drugs (notably the integrase inhibitor raltegravir, the second generation NNRTI etravirine and the PI darunavir that is active against many HIV isolates resistant to all available protease inhibitors) indicate that virological suppression is a realistic goal.

Selection of a salvage antiretroviral regimen should be done in consultation with an HIV expert. A thorough antiretroviral history with reasons for switching and viral load results is critically important. It is essential to assess adherence to and tolerability of prior antiretroviral regimens, which are often the underlying reasons for failure. A viral resistance genotype test (see Chapter 47) is very useful in selecting salvage antiretroviral therapy. Studies of patients failing second line regimens show that only about 5% of failing patients have resistance mutations to protease inhibitors - they are failing because of poor adherence. However, resistance tests are very expensive and will often not detect resistance to antiretrovirals from previous regimens that are archived and will reappear on re-exposure. Continuing antiretroviral therapy in patients who are failing virologically, with documented resistance to the NRTIs and PIs they are taking, still experience a clinical benefit. The CD4 count continues to climb with failing antiretroviral therapy until the viral load exceeds 10 000 copies/mL. The main explanation for benefit, despite resistance, is that resistant HIV is less fit than the wild type. Note that NNRTI resistance does not impair viral fitness and this class should not be used in salvage therapy. Eventually CD4 counts decline when failing antiretroviral therapy is continued and there is an increased risk of death. The problem with continuing failing antiretroviral therapy while waiting for new drugs is the accumulation of more resistant mutations, which may impair newer drugs. Nevertheless, the clinical benefits are important and discontinuing antiretroviral therapy is associated with an increased risk of death, even with high CD4 counts.

Thus, in our region where newer antiretrovirals take a long time to become available, or are unlikely to become available due to expense, continuing a failing protease inhibitor-based regimen is sometimes the only option. Lamivudine (or emtricitabine) should be continued in salvage antiretroviral therapy because it does result in a modest viral load response despite the presence of resistance.

References and further reading

Current versions of adult antiretroviral guidelines can be downloaded from the following websites:

Southern Africa: http://www.sahivsoc.org/

United Kingdom: http://www.bhiva.org/

USA: http://www.aidsinfo.nih.gov/guidelines/

WHO: http://www.who.int/hiv/pub/guidelines/en/

Imaz, A. et al. 2011. 'Antiretroviral salvage therapy for multiclass drug-resistant HIV-1-infected patients: from clinical trials to daily clinical practice.' *AIDS Reviews*, 13:180-93.

The DAD study group. 2007. 'Class of antiretroviral drugs and the risk of myocardial infarction.' *New England Journal of Medicine*, 356:1723–1735.

The PLATO Collaboration. 2004. 'Predictors of trend in CD4-positive T-cell count and mortality among HIV-1-infected individuals with virological failure to all three antiretroviral-drug classes.' *The Lancet*, 364:51–62.

45 Paediatric antiretroviral therapy

(See also Chapter 44: Adult antiretroviral therapy.)

The goals of antiretroviral therapy are to:
- prevent severe immunodeficiency or end organ dysfunction such as growth failure and neurological disease;
- halt and reverse the progression of HIV infection;
- restore normal growth and development;
- normalize quality of life.

As infants survive into adulthood, a long-term strategy to preserve antiretroviral options is essential.

How does antiretroviral therapy in children differ from adults?

The liver and renal function are immature in neonates but undergo rapid maturation in the first few months of life. Hepatic function becomes 'super-efficient' exceeding adult levels until four to five years, explaining the rapid clearance and need for higher relative dosages for drugs such as nelfinavir in this age group. Neonates have diminished clearance so require reduced dosages of zidovudine and lamivudine. Premature infants have immature absorption, diminished clearance and also more immature enzyme systems and therefore require alternative dosing strategies. Premature infants experience different adverse events. More research is urgently needed for this group.

Frequent dosage adjustments need to be made for growth. Infants and children depend on their caregivers for adherence to medication. Occasionally infants or children may refuse to take medications, mainly because of poor palatability.

When to start antiretroviral therapy in children

The CHER trial, evaluating antiretroviral initiation at a median of seven weeks of age versus deferred therapy in infants with a median CD4 of 35%, showed a 76% decrease in early mortality for early therapy.

This study therefore established early diagnosis with rapid access to treatment as the gold standard. However, despite early therapy young infants still experienced significant morbidity and mortality with mortality declining in both arms in the second six months of life. In the screening phase of the study, 20% of infants already had extreme CD4 depletion (CD4 <25%). The results of the CHER study and various cohort studies indicate that high CD4 values do not preclude rapid and unexpected clinical deterioration and death.

The PREDICT study conducted in Thailand and Cambodia randomized children from between the ages of one and 12 to immediate therapy or deferral until immune suppression. There were no differences between the arms, but this study enrolled few children under three years of age. The neurocognitive outcomes were identical, but significantly lower than matched uninfected controls.

Guidelines for starting antiretroviral therapy

Initially, in 2008, the WHO recommended antiretroviral therapy for all infants below a year of age and then revised this recommendation to include the first two years of life, as progression in the second year of life is still unacceptably rapid. The South African guidelines of 2010 still recommend early antiretroviral therapy regardless of CD4 in the first year of life. We recommend early initiation for all infants under two years of age.

Above two years of age, clinical monitoring (three to six monthly), traditional CD4 criteria and WHO staging criteria can be used.

The CD4 assay is the most useful for prognosis of disease progression in children. The CD4 count and percent provides important information about rate of progression. Total lymphocyte counts are not very useful in adults or children and should only be used where CD4 is not available at all.

Viral load is less predictive of progression and more expensive but is useful to confirm a positive HIV DNA PCR at baseline and as a measure of adherence later on.

Recommendations for infants ≤24 months of age

Initiate antiretroviral therapy as soon as possible (ideally within one to two weeks of diagnosis).

For infants and children over two years of age

WHO stage Stages 3 and 4 disease *or* CD4 criteria in Table 45.1.

In newly diagnosed infants and children, especially those with failure to thrive, always consider tuberculosis (TB) and other reversible causes. If TB is clinically suspected (see Chapter 16: Paediatric tuberculosis) or diagnosed on microbiological evidence, first initiate treatment for TB prior to starting antiretroviral therapy to avoid problems with adherence, drug interactions, and immune reconstitution inflammatory syndrome (IRIS). Antiretroviral therapy should be started within approximately two weeks of starting anti-TB therapy (see TB and antiretroviral section below). The full blood count (FBC) and transaminases are useful at base-line for toxicity monitoring, and monitoring weight-for-age is invaluable. In very young and ill infants, one need not wait for two weeks.

What treatment do you start?

The principles of antiretroviral therapy are the same as in adults; a mini-mum of three drugs must be used. Quadruple therapy, although not adequately assessed, has been successfully used in infants under three months of age. Do not use quadruple therapy without expert consulta-tion. In addition, data also indicate that in some situations specific drugs may be used once daily. These are important data as simplification of regi-mens are essential for sustained adherence. The validation of simplified weight based dosing charts and the development of fixed drug formula-tions remain a priority. New drugs and classes are under investigation and offer hope for new strategies for failing children and those newly initiating therapy.

Failed PMTCT leads to transmitted resistance. Nevirapine exposure leads to resistance to nevirapine, efavirenz and potentially etravirine (the newest non-nucleoside reverse transcriptase inhibitor).

Where infants become infected despite the mother taking combina-tion antiretroviral therapy or second line therapy, resistance tests should be done if the circumstances and the timing allow. AZT can still be used but 3TC may be lost, if the mother received these as part of dual therapy. Where triple therapy has been given to the mother during pregnancy, attempt to select different classes of drugs for the infant.

Table 45.1 Recommendations for initiating ART in infants and children (revised in 2010)

Age	Infants and children <24 months[a]	24 months through 59 months	Five years or older
% CD4+	All[c]	<25%	NA
Absolute CD4[b]		≤750 mm³ [d]	≤350 mm³ As in adults

[a] Absolute CD4 count is more reliable than CD4% for determining prognosis, but because of natural decrease with age, is harder to use than percentage. All HIV-infected infants should receive ART due to the rapid rate of disease progression.

[b] [40, 42–43]

[c] Countries with reliable and affordable access to CD4 and VL monitoring may choose to use immunological and/or virological thresholds for initiation of ART in children aged 12–23 months.

[d] In children with absolute lymphopaenia, the CD4 percentage may be falsely elevated.

Table 45.2 lists the antiretrovirals registered in South Africa.

Table 45.2 Antiretroviral therapy registered in South Africa

Generic name/other comments Strength	Dosage	Major toxicities
Nucleoside reverse transcriptase inhibitors (NRTIs)		
Zidovudine (AZT) Double dose Syrup: 10 mg/ml (180 mg/m² 6 hourly) Capsules: 100 mg	180–240 mg/m² 12 hourly (all ages) from 4 wks Neonates: 2 mg/kg 6 hourly Premature: 1.5 mg/kg 12 hourly for 2 weeks, then 2 mg/kg 8 hourly IV: 120 mg/m² 6 hourly or 20 mg/m²/hr.	Neutropaenia; anaemia; headaches; myopathy (rare)
Lamivudine (3TC) Well tolerated Store at room temperature (use within 1 month of opening) Syrup: 10 mg/ml Tablets: 150 mg (can be broken)	4 mg/kg 12 hourly once weight >11 kg, can combine into single daily dose (8 mg/kg/day) Neonates <30 days: 2 mg/kg 12 hourly; >50 kg: 150 mg 12 hourly (can use Combivir® AZT 300 mg & 3TC 150 mg)	Headache; abdominal pain; pancreatitis; peripheral neuropathy; neuropaenia (all rare)

Didanosine (ddI) Can be combined for single daily dose, on empty stomach, 1 hour before or 2 hours after food. Solution: 10 mg/ml (must be refrigerated – stable for 30 days) Tablets: 25, 50, 100, 150 & 200 mg Tablets can be dissolved in water. To obtain sufficient antacid buffer use 2 tablets; if cost is a consideration, give 1 tablet with 10 ml antacid as ddI is inactivated by stomach acid	Oral solution: 2 weeks to <3 months: 50 mg/m^2 12 hourly >3 to 8 months: 100 mg/m^2 12 hourly After 8 months: 90–150 mg/m^2 12 hourly (max – 200mg/dose 12 hourly) Tablet or enteric coated: 20–25kg: 200mg X1 daily 25–<60kg: 250 mg X1 daily ≥60kg: 400mg X1 daily	Pancreatitis; peripheral neuropathy (dose related and rare) Diarrhoea; abdominal pain
Stavudine (d4T) Solution: 1 mg/ml Large volume of suspension must be refrigerated, stable for 30 days Capsules: 20, 30 & 40 mg Well tolerated and can be opened up	1 mg/kg 12 hourly 30–60 kg: 30 mg 12 hourly	Headache; GI upset; peripheral neuropathy & pancreatitis (both rare) Long term use causes lipoatrophy
Abacavir (ABC) Solution: 20 mg/ml Tablet: 300 mg	8 mg/kg 12 hourly if >3 months of age Can give X1 daily at 16–20 mg/kg/day to max of 600mg if clinically stable and undetectable VL once body weight >11 kg	Screen for HLA-B*5701 prior to initiation. 1–3% develop hypersensitivity – fever, malaise, mucositis with/without rashes, usually in first 6 weeks. Stop drug – do not re-challenge. (See later)
Tenofovir (TDF) 300 mg tablets Awaiting paediatric formulations Baseline and yearly DXA Creatinine clearance after 3 months and then yearly Serum phosphate at 3 months and then yearly	8 mg/kg/day (maximum 300 mg)	Renal dysfunction Osteopenia Do not use with ddI

Non-nucleoside reverse transcriptase inhibitors

Nevirapine (NVP) Rifampicin reduces levels Can give with food Store at room temperature Solution: 10 mg/ml Tablet: 200 mg	Start at 200 mg/m^2 daily for 14 days, then, if no rash, increase to 200 mg/m^2 12 hourly (maximum daily dosage: 400 mg) <2 months of age: 120 mg/m^2 for daily and 12 hourly dosages	Rash most common in first 2 weeks. Do not increase dosage until rash resolves. Monitoring ALT necessary in first 3 months, then less frequently
Efavirenz (EFV) Take at night to decrease CNS side effects Avoid taking with high fat meal Capsules: 50 & 200 mg Can open capsule & give with stewed apple & other food and drinks Do not use <3 years of age	15 mg/kg daily Or 10–15 kg: 200 mg 15–20 kg: 250 mg 20–25 kg: 300 mg 25–33 kg: 350 mg 33–40 kg: 400 mg >40 kg: 600 mg daily	Sleepiness; abnormal dreams; skin rash Limited pharmacokinetic data in children <3 years – avoid in children of this age

Protease inhibitors

Nelfinavir (NFV) Take with food to increase absorption Tablet: 250 mg Crush tablets Powder formulation not recommended	<10 kg: 75 mg/kg twice daily 10–19.9 kg: 60 mg/kg twice daily Adolescent: 1250 mg twice daily	Vomiting; rash; abnormal lipids Unboosted PI – not recommended
Indinavir (IDV) Take fasting or with low fat snack Drink lots of water daily Avoid Coke® Capsules (hard gel): 200 mg	33 mg/kg 8 hourly	Nausea; hyper-bilirubinaemia; abnormal lipids. Avoid in neonates/ Unboosted PI – not recommended
Ritonavir (RTV) To improve tolerability, coat mouth with peanut butter prior to medication Suspension: 80 mg/ml Capsules: 100 mg	>3 months : start at 250 mg/m^2 12 hourly; increase over 5 days to 400 mg/m^2 12 hourly	Nausea; vomiting; abdominal pain (severe); increase in liver enzymes; abnormal lipids

*Lopinavir/Ritonavir (LPCV/r) *Kaletra*® Take with a meal to increase absorption Solution tastes bitter Solution: 80/20 mg/ml Aluvia Tablets: 200/50 mg or 100/25 Aluvia® Do not break or crush tablets	230/57.5 mg/m^2 12 hourly 300/75 mg/m^2 12 hourly if used with nevirapine or efavirenz or if PI experienced	Nausea; abnormal lipids
Darunavir (DRV) *Prezista*® Not for children <3y of age 75mg, 150mg, 400mg & 600mg tablets 2nd or 3rd line option	≥20 to <30 kg: 375 mg + Ritonavir 50 mg ≥30 to <40kg: 450 mg + Ritonavir 60mg >40kg: 600mg + Ritonavir 100 mg (Can use ritonavir 100 mg for all weight bands if more tolerable) Twice daily with food >18y and if no Darunavir mutations, give once daily at 800 mg with 100 mg Ritonavir	Caution if sulpha allergies
Atazanavir (ATZ) *Reyataz*® Capsules –100 mg, 150 mg, 200 mg & 300 mg	≥6y to <18 y of age 15 to <25 kg: 150 mg + Ritonavir 80 mg 25 to <32 kg: 200 mg + Ritonavir 100 mg 32 to <39 kg: 250mg + Ritonavir 100 mg ≥ 39kg: 300 mg + Ritonavir 100 mg Once daily with food	Not for neonates as associated with unconjugated hyperbilirubinemia & kernicterus Caution with hepatic impairment Needs low gastric Ph for absorption – needs 12hr gap if using Omepazole Not recommended without ritonavir boosting in children

*For 'super-boosted' Kaletra®, add 0.75 ml Ritonavir for each ml of Kaletra®

Evidence from the P1060 trial suggests that first line therapy using LPV/r in infants is more potent than a NVP-containing regimen regardless of exposure through MTCT and should remain the first-line treatment of choice for children under three years of age. Data from the Neverest study supports a switch strategy; if a child is confirmed to be virally suppressed on LPV/r after at least a year of treatment, a switch to NNRTI-based therapy is possible, provided that VL monitoring is done at least six to eight weeks after switching and six-monthly for a year afterwards. This may be particularly helpful where children can neither tolerate LPV/r liquid (Kaletra®) nor swallow Aluvia® tablets. However, if a prolonged course of nevirapine has been used to prevent breastfeeding related HIV transmission, this strategy should best be avoided.

Choices for first-line treatment include:

- two NRTIs (ABC + lamivudine [3TC]; stavudine (d4T) + 3TC; ABC + AZT;) plus one PI (Lopinavir/ritonavir); or
- two NRTIs plus efavirenz or nevirapine.

South African Guidelines currently recommend:

- ABC + 3TC + Lopinavir/ritonavir (LPV/r) for infants <3 years;
- ABC+ 3TC + efavirenz (EFV) children >3 years.

d4T and AZT are available for substitution should toxicity occur.

The combination of d4T and AZT is contraindicated as both are thymidine derivatives. d4T combined with ddI is implicated in lactic acidosis and should be avoided.

Data from the PENTA group support ABC and 3TC as the most durable first-line NRTI combination for children. Using d4T in first-line and zidovudine in second-line therapy exposes children to failure, because thymidine-associated mutations accumulate with both drugs. Also, d4T is implicated in lipoatrophy (loss of subcutaneous fat), which can affect between 30 and 40% of children on long-term use.

Specific issues associated with paediatric formulations:

- Zidovudine (AZT), lamivudine (3TC), nevirapine (NVP) (10 mg/ml), and abacavir (ABC) (20 mg/ml) are available in pleasant-tasting formulations, in reasonable concentrations to permit relatively low volumes. None have food restrictions.
- Stavudine liquid formulation requires refrigeration. Stavudine capsules can be opened and the powder mixed with water or milk. For a child weighing 15 kg, a single 30 mg capsule may be opened and dissolved in 30 ml of water with 15 ml being given as a single dose. The

other 15 ml may be refrigerated and given in the evening or discarded if it is not possible to store safely.

- Didanosine (ddI) is reconstituted at 10 mg/ml. It can be given once daily although twice daily is preferable. (An extended release formulation has been developed for once daily use. A disadvantage is the need to administer 30 minutes before, or one hour after, meals. The liquid formulation, once reconstituted, requires refrigeration and is only stable for 30 days. It must be reconstituted in a 500 ml bottle and antacid added. Many prefer the dispersible/chewable tablets, dissolved in 30 ml water or clear apple juice. Dosage should *always* comprise at least *two* tablets to ensure adequate buffering (ddI is broken down at acidic pH). Didanosine cannot be given at the same time as PIs and must be at least *two* hours apart.

- Tenofovir (TDF) has recently been approved by the FDA for children above two years of age. It should be reserved for teenagers but may have a place in younger children – get expert advice.

- Protease inhibitors (PIs) are usually taken with food. Lopinavir-ritonavir is poorly palatable. Coating the mouth with peanut butter (anecdotally, Nutella™ is more effective) pre- and post-dosing improves palatability. Giving the child a frozen ice-lolly can also help before the dose is given.

- Efavirenz is given as a daily dose. Currently, it is only locally available in capsule form (a syrup is available but not registered in South Africa). Because of limited pharmacokinetic data, efavirenz is not given to children below three years of age (and weighing <10 kg). The capsule can be opened and sprinkled on food.

- Only two protease inhibitors and one NNRTI are currently available in liquid formulation. The protease inhibitors are poorly palatable.

Paediatric dosages

Remember to increase the dosage as the child gains weight. The more successful the therapy, the more the weight gain, and the more frequently you need to adjust the dosage. Recalculate the dosage at every patient consultation.

For zidovudine, didanosine, and nevirapine, dosage is ideally calculated by body surface area (BSA). This is calculated from a formula

$$BSA = \sqrt{\frac{ht \times wt}{3\,600\,(m^2)}},$$

or read from a nomogram. In both cases, weight in kilograms and height in centimetres are necessary.

More recently, weight-band dosing has been introduced to simplify treatment. This approach is based on modeling known pharmacokinetic data and is yet to be scientifically validated. Studies are in progress.

(See the weight-based dosing table recommended by the Paediatric Group of the Southern African HIV Clinicians Society in Appendix 45.2.)

The ideal paediatric antiretroviral formulation:

- is a pleasant-tasting soluble or chewable tablet;
- can be given in low volume if liquid;
- is uninfluenced by the need for concomitant food;
- can be given once or twice per day;
- is non-toxic; and
- does not require refrigeration.

There are currently no chewable or small tablets for infants and children available in South Africa. Generic chewable fixed-dose combinations (FDCs containing nevirapine are registered in South Africa). The WHO is developing a harmonized strategy for the pharmaceutical industry to develop simpler solid formulations for children.

Children >10 kg can often swallow tablets or capsules and efforts should be made to teach them to do so as soon as possible. Introduce children to tablets by asking them to swallow small sweets (candies), starting with a small size and then moving on to those of similar size to the capsules prescribed. The reward for swallowing a sweet is then to give one for enjoyment.

Advantages of solid formulations include:

- easier to transport;
- easier to store (e.g. stavudine solution, but not capsules, requires re-frigeration);
- adherence may be improved;
- administration is simplified and the need to draw up exact amounts of liquid in a syringe is eliminated.

How to promote adherence to therapy

Long-term adherence in children is a major challenge. The goal should be 100% adherence. Rapport with health care providers plays an important role in improving adherence. Spending time educating the parent or caregiver prior to prescribing therapy is essential. This process may take as long as two to three weeks. However, this should not become a barrier to children accessing antiretroviral therapy. If transport is too expensive, ways of expediting this process should be sought:

- Go through the child's daily routine and determine who will take responsibility for the medication. Identify a single caregiver. Ensure adequate communication between multiple caregivers, often best accomplished by bringing role players together for a counseling session.
- Use medications that can be given once or twice daily.
- Ensure that adequate supplies are available over weekends and during holidays.
- Help the parents to plan ahead.
- Get the child and caregiver to fill in a diary card.
- One person should take primary responsibility but needs a treatment supporter, who should come to the clinic for adherence training. Disclosure by the mother to trustworthy family and friends is fundamental for a successful outcome but is not mandatory.
- Ask the parents to bring the medication along when you are seeing the child, and check that they are giving it correctly.
- Work with the pharmacist, nursing colleagues and adherence counselors to promote adherence.
- Remember to continue adherence support on a long-term basis as motivation may wane over time.
- If medicine requires refrigeration, make sure that a refrigerator is not only available, but in good working order and actually in use.

It is difficult to assess accurately the best methods of promoting adherence and a combination of different techniques, e.g. diary cards, pill counts, viral load monitoring are all helpful. Most important is the relationship developed between the patient, their caregiver and the staff with whom they interact at the health care services. The power of this important relationship in nurturing the trust of the family and ensuring clear understanding of what the patient is to expect with the medication will positively impact on adherence.

Resistance testing

Resistance testing is recommended for all infants failing MTCT if the mother has been exposed to antiretroviral therapy. If affordable, resistance testing should be performed with any regimen failure (while still on the failing regimen) in order to build up a profile on individual patients over time. Resistance testing may be limited by affordability.

Complications of therapy

Immune reconstitution inflammatory syndrome (IRIS)

This occurs from two weeks after starting therapy and is most common in the first three months. It occurs most commonly with a rapid CD4 response from a low initial level. It may be difficult to differentiate from recurrence of an opportunistic infection already present at the start of antiretroviral therapy. Systemic steroids may be useful and antiretrovirals should be continued. The exception is for intracranial pathology where IRIS is associated with mass effects and raised intracranial therapy (consult an expert). In South Africa, BCG adenitis and clinical tuberculosis occur commonly. Most opportunistic infections can present as IRIS.

Adverse drug reactions

Most side-effects of antiretrovirals are mild and usually disappear with persistence of treatment. The side-effect profile is similar in children to adults although children are thought to tolerate treatment better. Please refer to Table 45.3 for drug specific side-effects. Adverse events can be graded, providing a guide to responding to the event.

Table 45.3 Grading the severity of paediatric adverse reactions (DAIDS)

Laboratory Test Abnormalities				
Item	Grade 1 toxicity	Grade 2 toxicity	Grade 3 toxicity	Grade 4 toxicity
Haemoglobin 22–35 days	9.5–10.5	8–9.4 g/dL	7.0–7.9 g/dL	<7 g/dL
Haemoglobin 36–56 days	8.5–9.4 g/dL	7.0–8.4 g/dL	6.0–6.9 g/dL	<6 g/dL
Haemoglobin >56 days.	8.5–10 g/dL	7.5–8.4 g/dL	6.5–7.4 g/dL	<6.5 g/dl
Absolute neutrophil count (>7 days)	1–1.3 ×10⁹/L	0.75–0.99 ×10⁹/L	0.5–0.79 × 10⁹/L	<0.5 × 10⁹/L
ALT (SGPT)	1.1–4.9 × upper normal limit	5.0–9.9 × upper normal limit	10.0–15.0 × upper normal limit	>15 × upper normal limit

Triglycerides	–	1.54–8.46 mmol/L	8.47–13.55 mmol/L	>13.56 mmol//L
Cholesterol	–	4.43–12.92 mmol/L	12.93–19.4 mmol/L	>19.4 mmol/L

Clinical Adverse Events

Item	Grade 1 toxicity	Grade 2 toxicity	Grade 3 toxicity	Grade 4 toxicity
Peripheral neuropathy	Diagnosis of peripheral neuropathy is difficult in children. Screen motor function against milestones and refer to specialist if peripheral neuropathy is suspected.			
Skin rash / dermatitis		Diffuse maculo-papular rash OR dry desquamation	Vesiculation OR ulcers	Exfoliative dermatitis OR Stevens-Johnson syndrome OR erythema multiforme OR moist desquamation

Adverse reactions can be graded according to the International Maternal Paediatric and Adolescence Clinical Trial Group (IMPAACT) grading.

Action on grading

- Grades 1 and 2: patient remains on therapy. Repeat the test. Reassess clinically within two weeks.
- Grade 3: test should be repeated within one week and if still Grade 3, stop *all* antiretroviral drugs and seek expert medical advice.
- Grade 4: Stop all drugs immediately and seek specialist advice. If most likely caused by a NNRTI, continue NRTIs for 7–14 days. If the patient restarts therapy after the event has resolved, and the same grade 4 event recurs, appropriate changes or withdrawal of antiretroviral therapy may need to be made.

Some class-specific adverse events which are particularly harmful and/or life threatening

Lactic acidosis

All nucleoside analogues have been associated with lactic acidosis, a rare, but potentially life-threatening metabolic complication of treatment. The pathogenesis involves drug-induced mitochondrial damage. Initial symptoms are variable; cases have occurred as early as one month and as late as 20 months after starting therapy. It is usually associated with ddI plus d4T, although either alone has been implicated. There are no good screening tests to detect lactic acidosis and a high index of clinical suspicion should be maintained.

Clinical features:
- generalized fatigue, weakness;
- gastrointestinal symptoms (nausea, vomiting, diarrhoea, abdominal pain, hepatomegaly, anorexia, and/or sudden unexplained weight loss);
- respiratory symptoms (tachypnoea and dyspnoea);
- neurological symptoms (including motor weakness);
- loss of weight.

Laboratory abnormalities:
- hyperlactataemia (>2 mmol/L);
- increased anion gap $[(Na + K) - (Cl + HCO3)$; normal <15];
- elevated aminotransferases, CPK, LDH, lipase, and amylase;
- microvesicular steatosis – liver histology.

Management:
NB: *Discuss with a treatment expert.*

Antiretroviral therapy should be discontinued in patients with symptoms associated with lactic acidosis that continue or worsen.
- Therapy is primarily supportive (fluid, bicarbonate administration and respiratory support).
- Administration of riboflavin, thiamine and/or L-carnitine may have benefit (case reports).

Hepatotoxicity

Hepatotoxicity may occur mainly in the first eight weeks after starting therapy with nevirapine (efavirenz and PI's may also be implicated). In the initial phases of NVP therapy ALT should be monitored frequently. The patient may present with nausea, vomiting, right upper quadrant tenderness, and jaundice if severe. Always exclude hepatitis A and B infection.

Management:
Grade the level of toxicity. Antiretrovirals should be stopped if the toxicity is grade 3 or 4.

NB: *Skin rash associated with nevirapine toxicity may occur in association with liver dysfunction. Always check liver function tests if skin rash occurs (see above).*

Lipodystrophy/lipoatrophy syndrome

HIV-associated lipodystrophy includes fat loss and/or fat accumulation in distinct regions of the body: increased fat around abdomen, buffalo hump, breast hypertrophy, and fat loss from limbs, buttocks and face.

Other manifestations: insulin resistance, hyperglycaemia, hypertriglyceridaemia, hypercholestrolaemia and low HDL levels. These individuals are at risk of type 2 diabetes mellitus and coronary artery disease.

Association with antiretrovirals usually occurs in patients who have been on long-term therapy. Lipodystrophy is more common in individuals taking stavudine or protease inhibitors.

Management:
There are no established methods for treating lipodystrophy. Encourage exercise to reduce fat accumulation. Some patients improve if switched from a protease inhibitor to an NNRTI.

Lipoatrophy may improve if d4T or AZT is replaced with abacavir. Only switch if the viral load is undetectable.

Statins and/or fibrates are effective at lowering cholesterol and triglyceride levels (beware of drug interactions). Insulin resistance can be improved with anti-diabetic agents.

Abacavir hypersensitivity

This can occur in children. Approximately 8% of Caucasian patients receiving abacavir develop a hypersensitivity reaction (HSR), which rarely is fatal. The symptoms or signs are of multi-organ/body involvement. The hypersensitivity reaction is genetically linked to HLA-B*5701, a rare allele in Africans.

Symptoms usually appear within the first six weeks of abacavir (median time to onset is 11 days) and most often include fever, rash, gastrointestinal symptoms (nausea, vomiting, diarrhoea, or abdominal pain), and lethargy or malaise. Respiratory symptoms (dyspnoea, sore throat, cough), musculoskeletal symptoms (myalgia, rarely myolysis, arthralgia), headache, paraesthesia and oedema also occur. It has been confused with pneumonia, bronchitis, pharyngitis and flu-like illness. Renal failure and anaphylaxis have also been reported. Physical findings include lymphadenopathy and occasionally, mucous membrane lesions (conjunctivitis and/or mouth ulceration) and hypotension. The rash is often maculopapular or urticarial, but may be absent.

Laboratory abnormalities include lymphopenia, elevated liver enzymes, creatinine, and creatine phosphokinase.

Symptoms worsen with continued therapy and usually resolve upon discontinuation of abacavir. Restarting abacavir following a HSR results in a prompt return of symptoms, usually within hours. This recurrence may be life-threatening. Abacavir must not be re-introduced.

Note:

- If there is a need to discontinue antiretroviral therapy, stop *all* antiretrovirals rather than continuing with one or two agents alone. When stopping a NNRTI-containing regimen, attempt to continue the NRTIs for another seven days (for example, if NNRTI-related hepatotoxicity suspected).
- Adverse events should be recorded and reported regularly to the National HIV and AIDS Cluster. Serious adverse events (SAEs) should be reported within 48–72 hours (Grade 4 or death) to the Medicines Control Council. Adverse event forms (on yellow paper) will be made available at all centres.
- After the patient has recovered from the adverse event it may be possible to start a different regimen. Decide in consultation with a treatment expert.

Safe monitoring of therapy

CD4 counts and viral load should be monitored six monthly in the first year after starting treatment. If the patient is stable annual VL and CD4 testing can occur. More frequent monitoring is required if there is reason to suspect treatment failure e.g. change in caregiver, other psychosocial stressors, poor growth or clinical deterioration. Monitor growth and use weight-for-age and height-for-age percentile charts as an adjunct to monitoring. (See Chapter 44: Adult antiretroviral therapy.)

Changing therapy

WHO definition of treatment failure:

- Immunological failure is recognized as developing or returning to the following age-related immunological thresholds after at least 24 weeks on ART, in a fully treatment-adherent child, as:
  - CD4 count of <200 cells/mm^3 or %CD4+ <10% for a child more than two years to less than five years of age;
  - CD4 count of <100 cells/mm^3 for a child 5 years of age or older.
- Clinical failure is recognized as appearance or reappearance of stage 3 or stage 4 events after at least 24 weeks on ART in a fully treatment-adherent child. Virological failure is recognized as a persistent VL above 1000 RNA copies/ml, after at least 24 weeks on ART, in a fully adherent child.

Since viral load monitoring is widely available in South Africa, decisions about switching regimens should be made for virologic failure, which usually precedes immunological and/or clinical deterioration. Ongoing antiretroviral therapy in the presence of failure leads to more resistance mutations. When a patient is failing virologically, always check the dosage and adherence. In infants and young children, the viral load nadir may only be reached by six months because of the higher values in children than in adults.

Viral resistance testing should be considered when VL>1000 on two consecutive occasions.

Usually patients failing first line NNRTI regimens will develop NNRTI, 3TC mutations and if the failing regimen is continued they may also accumulate other NRTI mutations, which may compromise even those NRTIs to which the patient has not been exposed.

As long as adherence issues have been addressed, a switch to a lopinavir/ritonavir based second-line regimen is warranted. Use at least two but preferably three new drugs.

Children failing first line lopinavir/ritonavir regimens may have no or few resistance mutations in which case perseverance with current regimen is warranted, with reinforced adherence counseling.

Children who received single protease inhibitors i.e. ritonavir according to prior recommendations for infants and/or TB co-infected children and subsequently failed treatment may have accumulated significant PI mutations warranting salvage therapy and consultation with an expert is warranted. (See Chapter 44: Adult antiretroviral therapy.)

Tuberculosis therapy and antiretroviral therapy

(See Chapter 16: Paediatric tuberculosis.)

Rifampicin reduces levels of most antiretrovirals through increased metabolism. This effect is blocked by adequate levels of ritonavir.

- Efavirenz is only minimally reduced by rifampicin but levels may be too low at currently recommended dosing.
- Efavirenz can be used with rifampicin: increase dosage by 50 mg (one capsule) to compensate for possible increased metabolism.
- Ritonavir-'boosted' lopinavir/ritonavir is recommended for children on rifampicin requiring lopinavir/ritonavir-based therapy. Add additional ritonavir until equal to lopinavir total dosage (*0.75 ml ritonavir for each ml of Kaletra®*).
- Although rifampicin reduces zidovudine and abacavir levels through enhanced glucoronidation, their dosages do not require modification.
- Avoid using nevirapine with rifampicin. Switching to efavirenz is warranted if virally suppressed and if over three years of age.

References and further reading

Coovadia, A., Abrams, E.J., Stehlau, R., et al. 2010. Reuse of nevirapine in exposed HIV-infected children after protease inhibitor-based viral suppression: a randomized controlled trial. *J Am Med Assoc*; 304(10):1082-90.

Eley, B.S. and Myers, T. 2011. Antiretroviral Therapy for Children in Resource-Limited Settings: Current Regimens and the Role of Newer Agents. *Pediatr Drugs*; 13 (5):303-316.

HIV/AIDS Treatment Information Service. Available: http://AIDSinfo. nih.gov

National Department of Health SA, South African National AIDS Council. 2010. *Guidelines for the management of HIV in children*, 2nd ed. www.doh.gov.za/

Paediatric European Network for the Treatment of AIDS. Available: www. ctu.mrc.ac.uk/PENTA

Palumbo, P., Lindsey, J.C., Hughes, M.D., et al. 2010. 'Antiretroviral treatment for children with peripartum nevirapine exposure'. *N Engl J Med*; 363(16): 1510-20.

Palumbo, P., Violari, A., Lindsey, L., et al. 2011. *NVP- vs LPV/r-based ART among HIV+ infants in resource-limited settings: the IMPAACT P1060 trial* [abstract no.129LB]. 18th Conference on Retroviruses and Opportunistic Infections; Boston (MA).

Southern African HIV Clinicians Society. Available: www. sahivclinicianssociety.org. E-mail: sahivsoc@iafrica.com

Violari, A., Cotton, M.F., Gibb, D. et al. 2007. 'Antiretroviral therapy initiated before 12 weeks of age reduces early mortality in young HIV-infected infants: evidence from the Children with HIV Early Antiretroviral Therapy (CHER) Study.' In: 4th IAS conference on pathogenesis, treatment and prevention Sydney, Australia: International AIDS Society; 2007.

Violari A, Cotton MF, Gibb DM, Babiker AG, Steyn J, Madhi SA, *et al.* 2008. 'Early antiretroviral therapy and mortality among HIV-infected infants'. *N Engl J Med*; 359:2233-2244.

WHO. Available: www.who.int

WHO. 2010. *Antiretroviral therapy for HIV infection in infants and children: towards universal access*. Recommendations for a public health approach: 2010 Revision. http://whqlibdoc.who.int/publications/ 2010/9789241599801_eng.pdf

Appendix 45.1 Antiretroviral therapy in adolescents

Introduction

Adolescents are a growing population of HIV-infected individuals due to the availability of life-prolonging antiretrovirals as well as the high incidence in adolescence. Therefore, HIV clinicians must be familiar with caring for HIV-infected adolescents. Many perinatally infected adolescents are already heavily experienced on ARVs and may already be on second or even third line therapy.

Regimens and dosing

Current first line regimens include tenofovir (TDF), zidovudine (AZT), and lamivudine as the NRTI backbone, with Lopinavir/ritonavir (LPV/r), efavirenz (EFV) or nevirapine (NVP) as the third drug. Avoid stavudine due to metabolic side effects (see below). Adherence may necessitate combinations such as Combivir®, Truvada®, or Atripla®, or once daily medication such as TDF or EFV. TDF can be used in adolescents older than 14 years with weight above 40 kgs and creatinine clearance above 80 with appropriate monitoring. Abacavir (ABC) is an option for younger adolescents. If choices are limited, TDF can be used as young as 12 years and 35 kgs, with caution. EFV should be avoided in adolescent females unless compliance with injectable contraceptives is demonstrated. Other ARVs that can be used once daily with caution are didanosine, LPV/r (if viral load low) and possibly NVP. Due to notoriously poor adherence during adolescence and probable exposure to multiple regimens for perinatally infected youth, resistance may necessitate the use of less-than optimal regimens.

Dosing

Use pediatric dosing for Tanner stages I, II and III, and adult dosing for Tanner IV and V. Generally it is advisable to not exceed the adult dose for larger children. Since this is a time of rapid growth, close monitoring for toxicity and virologic control is vital.

Side effects

Metabolic side effects of medications can become evident during child-hood and are common in adolescence. Since adolescence is a period of body image preoccupation and poor self-esteem, it may be necessary to change regimens to those with fewer metabolic side effects to promote adherence. Although stavudine is the most likely to cause metabolic side effects, all thymidine analog NRTIs, as well as PIs and EFV can do so to a lesser degree.

In summary, for adolescents already on antiretrovirals graduating from paediatric clinics, options are:

- maintain current regimen;
- if virally suppressed and on stavudine consider changing to a non-thymidine analogue NRTI. If on stavudine and lamivudine, consider changing to Combivir® or Truvada®;
- consider changing to a once daily or combination regimen e.g. Atripla®.

For adolescents who are horizontally infected therefore just starting antiretrovirals:

- choose a simple combination or once-daily regimen.

When to start

Start for WHO Stage III and IV regardless of CD4 count, or for CD4 =<350cell/mm³. Use co-trimoxazole as a training tool.

Comprehensive care

In order to ensure successful retention in care, adolescents require a confidential setting in which personnel are adolescent-friendly and non-judgmental. In addition, short waiting times and after-school clinic hours are necessary. It is preferable to have clinics for adolescents that are independent in space or time from those of adults and younger children. Transition to adult care may be facilitated by a step-wise transition, or through the use of shared staff.

Psychosocial needs

Clinics caring for adolescents with HIV should ensure the availability of social support, including referrals for sexual, physical, and substance abuse, and depression. Support for disclosure and adherence should be provided.

Additional adherence interventions may be needed in adolescents, such as cell phone reminders. Individual and group peer support is particularly effective in this age group.

Table 45.4 Pubertal staging

This involves an assessment of breast development in girls (B), genital development and testicular volume in boys (G), and pubic (P) and axillary (A) hair development in both sexes.

Breast staging

B1	Prepubertal
B2	Breast budding
B3	Development of actual breast mound
B4	Areola projects at an angle to breast mound
B5	Adult configuration

Genital staging

G1	Prepubertal penis (unstretched length 2.5–6 cm), scrotum and testes (volume <3 ml)
G2	Testes >4 ml and/ or scrotal laxity, but no penile enlargement
G3	Penile lengthening with further development of testes and scrotum

G4   Penile lengthening and broadening, testes usually 10–12 ml
G5   Adult genitalia, testes usually 15–25 ml

NB testicular volume should be measured using the Prader orchidometer.

Pubic hair staging

P1   No pubic hair
P2   Fine hair over mons and/ or scrotum/labias.
P3   Adult type hair (coarse, curly) but distribution confined to pubis
P4   Extension to near adult distribution
P5   Adult

Axillary hair staging

A1   No axillary hair
A2   Hair present but not adult amount
A3   Adult

Puberty begins after 9 years and usually not later than 14 years in males (corresponding ages in girls are 8 years and 13 years).
Sexual precocity: early sexual development.
Source: J. Tanner, 1962.

References and further reading

Tanner, J. 1962. *Growth and adolescence*. Oxford: Blackwell.

APPENDIX 45.2 — Antiretroviral Drug Dosing

Compiled by James Nuttall and the Child and Adolescent Committee of

	Abacavir (ABC)		Lamivudine (3TC)		Efavirenz (EFV)	Lopinavir/ritonavir (LP/rtv)
Target dose	8 mg/kg TWICE daily OR ≥10 kg: 16 mg/kg ONCE daily		40 mg/kg TWICE daily OR ≥10 kg: 8 mg/kg ONCE daily		By weight band ONCE daily	300/75 mg/m²/dmg dose LPV/rtv TWICE daily
Available formulations	Sol. 20 mg/ml Tabs 300 mg (not scored)		Sol. 100 mg/ml Tabs 150 mg (scored) 300 mg		Caps 50, 200 mg Tabs 50, 200, 600 mg (not scored)	Sol. 80/20 mg/ml Adult Tabs 200/500 mg Paeds Tabs 100/25 mg
Wt. (kg)	Currently available tablet formulations of abacavir, efavirenz, LPV/rtv and					
<3	Consult with a clinician experienced in paediatric ARV prescribing					
3–3.9	2 ml bd		2 ml bd		Avoid using when <10 kg or <3 years: dosing not established	*1 ml bd
4–4.9						
5–5.9	3 ml bd		3 ml bd			*1.5 ml bd
6–6.9						
7–7.9	4 ml bd		4 ml bd			
8–8.9						
9–9.9						
10–10.9	Choose only one option:		Choose only one option:		200 mg nocte (1x200 mg cap/tab)	2 ml bd
11–13.9	6 ml bd	12 ml od	6 ml bd	12 ml od		
14–16.9	8 ml bd	1 tab od OR 15 ml od	1/2 x 150 mg tab bd OR 8 ml bd	1 x 150 mg tab od OR 15 ml od	300 mg nocte: (200 mg cap/tab + 2x50 mg cap/tab)	Choose one option: –2.5 ml bd –100/25 mg paeds tabs: 2 bd –200/50 mg adult tabs: 1 bd
17–19.9						
20–24.9	10 ml bd	20 ml od	1x150 mg tab bd OR 15 ml od	2x150 mg tab od OR 1x300 mg tab od OR 30 ml od		Choose one option: –3 ml bd –100/25 mg paeds tabs: 2 bd –200/50 mg adult tabs: 1 bd
25–29.9	1x300 mg tab bd	2x300 mg tabs od	1x150 mg tab bd	2x150 mg tabs od OR 1x300 mg tab od	400 mg nocte: (2x200 mg caps/tabs)	Choose one option: –3.5 ml bd –100/25 mg paeds tabs: 3 bd –#200/50 mg adult tabs: 1 bd +100/25 mg paeds tabs: 1 bd
30–34.9						Choose one option: –4 ml bd –100/25 mg paeds tabs: 3 bd –#200/50 mg adult tabs: 1 bd +100/25 mg paeds tabs: 1 bd
35–39.9						Choose one option: –5 ml bd –200/50 mg adult tabs: 2 bd
>40					600 mg tab nocte	

od = once a day
bd = twice a day

*Avoid PLV/rtv solution in any full term infant <14 days of age and any premature infant <14 days after their due date of delivery (40 weeks post conception) or obtain expert advice.
#Children 25–34.9 kg may also be dosed with LPV/rtv 200/50 mg adult tabs: 2 tabs am; 1 tab pm

Chart for Children (2012)

SA HIV Clinicians Society in collaboration with the Department of Health

Ritonavir boosting (RTV)	Stavudine (d4T)	Didanosine (ddI)	Nevirapine (NVP)	Zidovudine (AZT)	
ONLY as booster for LPV/rtv when on Rifampicin TWICE daily (0.75xLPV dose bd)	1 mg/kg/dose TWICE daily	180–240 mg/m²/dose ONCE daily	160–200 mg/m²/dose TWICE daily (after once daily lead-in x 2 wks)	180–240 mg/m²/dose TWICE daily	**Target Dose**
Sol. 80 mg/ml	Sol. 1 mg/ml Caps 15, 20, 30 mg	Tabs 25, 50, 100 mg (dispersible in 30 ml water) Caps 250 mg EC	Sol. 10 mg/ml Tabs 200 mg (scored)	Sol. 10 mg/ml Caps 100 mg Tabs 300 mg (not scored)	**Available Formulations**
AZT are film-coated and must be swallowed whole and NOT chewed, divided or crushed					**Wt. (kg)**
for neonates (<28 days of age) and infants weighing <3 kg					<3 kg
1 ml bd	6 ml	Avoid	5 ml bd	6 ml bd	3–3.9
					4–4.9
1.5 ml bd	7.5 mg bd: open 15 mg capsule into 5 ml water: give 2.5 ml	100 mg od: (2x50 mg tabs)			5–5.9
				9 ml bd	6–6.9
	10 mg bd: open 20 mg capsule into 5 ml water: give 2.5 ml	125 mg od: (1x100 mg + 1x25 mg tabs)	8 ml bd		7–7.9
				1 cap bd OR 12 ml bd	8–8.9
					9–9.9
1.5 ml bd	15 mg bd: open 15 mg capsule into 5 ml water	150 mg od: (1x100 mg + 1x50 mg tabs)	10 ml bd		10–10.9
					11–13.9
2 ml bd	20 mg bd: open 20 mg capsule into 5 ml water (if the child is unable to swallow a capsule)	175 mg od: (1x100 mg + 1x50 mg + 1x25 mg)	1 tab am 1/2 tab pm OR 15 ml bd	2 caps am 1 cap pm OR 15 ml bd	14–16.9
				2 caps bd OR 20 ml bd	17–19.9
		200 mg od: (2x100 mg tabs)			20–24.9
3 ml bd	30 mg bd	250 mg od: (2x100 mg + 1x50 mg tab) OR 1x250 mg EC cap od	1 tab bd	1 tab bd	25–29.9
					30–34.9
4 ml bd					35–39.9
					>40

Weight (kg)	3–4.9	5–9.9	10–13.9	14–29.9	≥30
Cotrimoxazole Dose	2.5 ml od	5 ml od	5 ml od	10 ml or 1 tab od	2 tabs od
Multivitamin Dose	2.5 ml od	2.5 ml od	5 ml od	5 ml od	10 ml or 1 tab od

46 Prevention of mother-to-child transmission of HIV

Mother-to-child transmission of HIV (MTCT) is the leading cause of HIV infection in children. There are more than two million pregnancies in HIV-positive women each year, with an estimated 370 000 vertically infected children in 2009 which is a substantial reduction from earlier estimates of 500 000 annually. The overwhelming majority of these infections occur in the developing world, especially in sub-Saharan Africa. In several African countries, more than 30% of women attending antenatal clinics are HIV-positive. In South Africa, upwards of 300 000 HIV-positive women will become pregnant each year and, in the absence of effective prevention interventions, more than 70 000 children would be infected.

HIV contributes to child mortality in high HIV-prevalence countries and in 2009, 260 000 paediatric HIV deaths occurred. More than 16 million children have lost their mothers, or both parents, to AIDS, and this figure is likely to increase. HIV/AIDS has become a prime cause of maternal mortality in high-prevalence areas, and in South Africa is the leading cause of maternal mortality and accounts for 35% of deaths among children under five years.

The WHO has promoted a four-pronged approach to the prevention of mother-to-child transmission (PMTCT), entailing:

- The prevention of new infections in parents-to-be;
- The prevention of unwanted pregnancies in HIV-infected women;
- The prevention of transmission from an HIV-infected mother to her infant;
- Access to appropriate treatment and care.

Among these prongs, the prevention of new infections in parents-to-be and the prevention of unwanted pregnancies in HIV-infected women are frequently overlooked. Fertility desires of HIV affected couples need to be regularly explored. Where pregnancy is desired, strategies to reduce horizontal and vertical transmission should be optimized prior to pregnancy; where pregnancy is not desired, contraception should be provided (see Chapter 27: Contraception).

The use of antiretroviral regimens for PMTCT should be integrated with:

- Modifications to routine obstetric practice;

- Expanding access to care and support for HIV-positive mothers and their families;
- Treating opportunistic infections (OIs);
- Accelerating access to antiretroviral treatment of HIV for those in need.

Preventing MTCT has made significant advances, particularly in the past decade including increases in access to PMTCT prophylaxis. Despite this, in sub-Saharan Africa only 54% of pregnant HIV-infected women accessed PMTCT strategies and consequently improving access to services remains a key focus for reducing MTCT.

Mother-to-child transmission of HIV

In 1990, the HIV prevalence among pregnant women attending antenatal clinics in South Africa was <1%, but 10 years later, in 2000, the prevalence had risen to 24.5%, and by 2006 had reached 29% where it has remained static for the past five years (29.4% in 2011). Without any preventative interventions, up to 40% of children born to HIV-infected women will be infected. In well-resourced countries with access to appropriate treatment, transmission rates lower than 2% have been achieved.

Infection can take place *in utero*, during labour and delivery, or postpartum via breastmilk. The relative contribution of each of these routes will depend on whether, and for how long, the infant is breastfed and effectiveness and timing of PMTCT interventions.

Management of an HIV-infected woman during pregnancy

Many HIV-infected women will be identified for the first time during pregnancy, following provider initiated HIV counselling and testing (PICT) in antenatal care settings.

First visit

In addition to a comprehensive history and physical examination including examining for sexually transmitted infections, particular attention should be paid to sexual risk behaviour, current HIV-related symptoms, and medication. Financial circumstances, family history, and emotional and social support structures need to be assessed, and appropriate referrals organised. A CD4 cell count should be obtained to guide treatment decisions, and treatment options discussed with the woman.

Maternal follow-up visits

If there are no obstetric or medical complications, antenatal care visits do not need to be more frequent than normal. Once a month until 28 weeks, twice a month until 34–36 weeks and then weekly until delivery, is sufficient. Additional visits for follow-up counselling may be required.

Where available, a baseline maternal ultrasound at 16–18 weeks for accurate dating and to screen for anomalies should be performed. An earlier scan is required if the patient requests termination of pregnancy. Mothers with CD4 counts of <200 cells/µl or clinically advanced disease, i.e. WHO stage 3 or 4, or who show evidence of substance abuse, should be monitored closely, as adverse outcomes such as preterm delivery and low birth weight are common.

Laboratory tests

The level of laboratory investigation will depend upon the available resources. The following represents an optimal list of tests at the initial visit:

- Full blood count with a CD4 cell count;
- Routine antenatal blood screening (Rhesus screening, RPR);
- HIV-RNA (viral load) repeated six-monthly;
- Hepatitis B;
- Pap smear;
- All women who tested HIV-negative in pregnancy should have a repeat HIV test in their third trimester of pregnancy.

Invasive procedures

Invasive procedures such as amniocentesis, chorionic villus sampling, cordocentesis, and external cephalic version should be avoided, as they may be associated with an increased risk of transmission. If these procedures are unavoidable, full suppression of the HIV viral load with antiretroviral therapy prior to the procedure being performed is preferable.

Risk reduction counselling

The importance of safe sexual practices must be emphasised, including those who tested HIV negative. All women should be encouraged to disclose their HIV status to their partner/s. Partners should be tested for HIV and if they are HIV infected, they should be encouraged to access HIV care. Discuss infant feeding options during the antenatal period. The benefits of exclusive breastfeeding should be highlighted with advice on how to reduce transmission if breastfeeding is chosen (see Chapter 12: Infant feeding).

Intrapartum care

Elective caesarean section (CS), undertaken before rupture of membranes, has been shown to reduce the risk of perinatal transmission. However, it is not certain whether a CS offers additional benefits where the viral load is low in women on antiretroviral therapy. In most public health facilities in high prevalence settings, elective CS for all HIV-positive women will not be possible. In this situation, a CS should be considered for standard obstetrical indications. In all cases, the risks and potential benefits should be discussed with the mother during the course of the antenatal care. Prophylactic intravenous first generation cephalosporin given preoperatively is recommended for all CS. Alternatively, clindamycin with an aminoglycoside can be used in women with cephalosporin hypersensitivity.

During normal deliveries, the midwife or obstetrician should take universal precautions. Artificial rupture of membranes should be avoided, as there is an increased risk of transmission, especially if the duration of membrane rupture is more than four hours. Invasive foetal scalp electrode monitoring and blood sampling should be avoided, and episiotomy performed only where there is a strong obstetric indication. There is no current recommendation on the use of prophylactic antibiotics in vaginal deliveries.

Postpartum care

Ensuring the mother-infant pair continues to receive appropriate management and care is essential. Women on ART should be referred for ongoing treatment and those not on ART should be re-evaluated to determine the need for treatment. Women who tested HIV negative during the antenatal period should have their HIV status confirmed during the post-natal period. If a woman is newly identified as HIV infected she should be referred for appropriate care, and her infant tested for HIV infection. HIV-exposed infants should receive an HIV PCR six weeks after delivery, six weeks after breastfeeding cessation and at any age if they are suspected of being HIV infected due to ill health or poor development. All HIV-exposed infants not confirmed to be HIV infected should receive an HIV ELISA test at 18 months of age. An infant who is diagnosed as HIV infected should be initiated onto ART as soon as possible to reduce morbidity and mortality (see Chapter 10: Clinical assessment (paediatric)). Women who have chosen to breastfeed their infants should access ongoing interventions to reduce vertical transmission either through infant nevirapine adjusted according to age, or maternal ART. Contraception should be offered and provided to women. Cervical cancer screening should be conducted, and infants should receive standard immunization.

Prophylaxis for opportunistic infections (OIs)

Most recommendations for OI prophylaxis are based on studies in non-pregnant individuals. However, the progression of HIV disease and OI does not seem to be affected by pregnancy and, therefore, standard criteria for OI prophylaxis should be applied in pregnancy. Drugs should be selected taking into consideration the available information concerning safety during pregnancy and following local recommendations. Initiation of treatment may be delayed until after the first trimester, balancing maternal and foetal benefits and risks.

Antiretroviral treatment to reduce mother-to-child HIV transmission

Antiretroviral agents during pregnancy reduce MTCT and benefits are enhanced the earlier in pregnancy interventions are initiated. Strategies to benefit maternal health and survival should be prioritised. Women who require ART for their own health, determined clinically or immunologically (WHO stage 3 or 4 disease, CD4 count <350 cells/µl), should receive lifelong ART. Women who do not qualify for life long ART should receive either zidovudine (AZT) 300 mg twice daily from 14 weeks gestation (WHO option A) or alternatively ART to reduce MTCT (WHO option B). Advances in ART, including an understanding of reduced horizontal transmission and reduced morbidity with earlier treatment, the potential benefits of prescribing fixed drug combinations and programmatic challenges of access to appropriate PMTCT interventions, have shifted recommendations to include ART for all pregnant women, regardless of CD4 cell count (WHO option B). Women remaining on ART life long after completion of breastfeeding has become an option (WHO option B plus) (see Table 46.1). A number of countries in Africa have adopted this approach of prescribing ART for all HIV-infected pregnant women, regardless of stage of disease.

Table 46.1 WHOs three options for PMTCT programmes

	Women receives		Infant receives
	Treatment (for CD4 count ≤350cells/mm³)	Prophylaxis (for CD4 count >350cells/mm³)	
Option A[a]	Triple ARVs starting as soon as diagnosed and continued for life	*Antepartum:* AZT starting as early as 14 weeks gestation *Intrapartum:* at onset of labour, sdNVP and first dose of AZT/3TC *Postpartum:* daily AZT/3TC through 7 days postpartum	Daily NVP from birth through 1 week beyond complete cessation of breastfeeding; or, if not breastfeeding or if mother is on treatment, through ages 4–6 weeks
Option B[a]	Same initial ARVs for both[b]		Daily NVP or AZT from birth through 4–6 weeks regardless of infant feeding method
	Triple ARVs starting as soon as diagnosed and continued for life	Triple ARVs starting as early as 14 weeks gestation and continued intrapartum and through childbirth if not breastfeeding or until 1 week after cessation of all breastfeeding	
Option B+	Same for treatment and prophylaxis[b]		Daily NVP or AZT from birth through 4–6 weeks regardless of infant feeding method
	Regardless of CD4 count, triple ARVs starting as soon as diagnosed,[c] continued for life		

Note: Triple ARVs refers to the use of one of the recommended 3-drug fully suppressive treatment options.

[a] Recommended in WHO 2010 PMTCT guidelines

[b] True only for EFV-based first line ART; NVP-based ART not recommended for prophylaxis (CD4 count >350)

[c] Formal recommendations for Option B+ have not been made, but presumably ART would start with diagnosis

Source: World Health Organization. 2012. Programmatic update. Use of antiretroviral drugs for treating pregnant women and preventing HIV infection in infants.

Antiretroviral regimens may need to be adapted to pregnancy. All options have potential disadvantages and the choice should be discussed with women and a joint decision made. Regardless of ART regimen, the benefits of ART during pregnancy outweigh the potential harm. Efavirenz has been linked to neural tube abnormalities in animal studies and is classified as FDA class D. As such it has been avoided in pregnancy. However, there has now been sufficient first trimester exposure to exclude a doubling of congenital abnormalities linked to efavirenz use in pregnancy; consequently some international guidelines have advocated efavirenz use throughout pregnancy. Nevirapine has been associated with a higher risk of hepatotoxicity and with increased fatalities in women with CD4 counts above 250 cells/μl. Nevirapine-based antiretroviral regimens are best avoided in this subset of women with close monitoring. Protease inhibitors have been associated with low birth weight and premature delivery in some, but not all studies.

Reducing the risk of mother-to-child transmission of HIV

Several factors are associated with the risk of mother-to-child transmission of HIV – see Table 46.2.

Table 46.2 Factors associated with increased risk of mother-to-child transmission of HIV

	Strong evidence	Intermediate evidence	Limited evidence
Maternal factors	High viral load Immune deficiency Advanced disease HIV infection acquired during pregnancy or breastfeeding period No antiretroviral use	Chorioamnionitis Vitamin A deficiency Anaemia STIs Smoking	Frequent unprotected sexual intercourse Multiple sexual partners Intravenous drug use
Obstetric Factors	Vaginal delivery (compared with elective CS) Prolonged rupture of membranes	Invasive diagnostic procedures	Episiotomy
Infant factors	Mixed feeding Breastfeeding without prophylaxis	Prematurity	Lesions of skin and/or mucous membranes Oral thrush

Proven strategies to reduce or prevent MTCT include:

- Antiretroviral treatment or prophylaxis (see below);
- Elective CS;
- Replacement feeding for the infant;
- Exclusive breastfeeding rather than mixed feeding.

Antiretroviral prophylaxis

Women who do not yet need ongoing antiretroviral therapy should receive the most effective prophylactic antiretroviral regimen to reduce the risk of transmission to the baby.

Triple antiretroviral regimen should be used in pregnancy (as for ongoing treatment). In some settings, full antiretroviral therapy may not be available for PMTCT. In these settings, the most effective short course antiretroviral regimen should be used. A number of single drug and combination regimens have been shown to be effective. The WHO recommends AZT started from 14 weeks gestation. A single dose of nevirapine, together with either a single dose of truvada or the first dose of AZT/3TC should be given during labour. If AZT/3TC is chosen it should be continue for 7 days postpartum. Infants should receive daily nevirapine after birth which should be continued for 4–6 weeks regardless of feeding option. Infant nevirapine should continue for one week after breastfeeding cessation if the mother is not taking ART. Infant AZT for 4–6 weeks for women who received ART during pregnancy continued until breastfeeding cessation is an alternative option (see Table 46.1).

HIV infected women presenting for the first time in labour should receive a single dose of nevirapine together with either AZT/3TC for a week or a single dose of truvada. The infant should receive daily nevirapine until one week after breastfeeding cessation. Alternatively if not being breastfed the infant should receive daily nevirapine for 4–6 weeks or a single dose of nevirapine plus twice daily AZT for a week (See Table 46.1). Single dose nevirapine can select for NNRTI resistance mutations. If treatment is commenced within six months after single dose nevirapine there is an increased risk of virological failure.

Infant feeding

This is covered in Chapters 12 and 13.

Family planning and contraception

Appropriate family planning should be discussed antenatally and again before discharge. Lactational amenorrhoea may be a common method of contraception where breastfeeding is the norm, but is not a reliable method. Some women may undertake a period of abstinence after the birth of the child and may not wish to start contraception. They should be given information about how and where to obtain contraception for when they require it.

Postpartum care of the HIV-exposed neonate

Note the following points for the postpartum care of HIV-exposed neonates:

- The cord should be cut under a lightly-wrapped gauze swab to prevent blood spurting.
- All babies, irrespective of HIV status, should be kept warm post-delivery and should be handled with gloves until maternal blood and secretions are washed off.
- The new-born should not be suctioned with a nasogastric tube unless the liquor is meconium stained. Where suctioning is required, it is better to use a mechanical suction unit (at a pressure below 100 mmHg) or bulb suction, if possible, rather than mouth-operated suction.
- The baby should only be attached to the mother's breast if the mother has made a decision beforehand to breastfeed.
- If the mother has decided not to breastfeed, the baby should be placed on the mother's body for skin-to-skin contact. The mother should be educated on the correct use of formula feeding.
- Antiretroviral should be administered to the baby according to the antiretroviral prophylaxis regimen initiated.
- BCG should be administered according to the immunization guidelines of the World Health Organization.

References and further reading

BHIVA. 2012. BHIVA guidelines for the treatment of HIV-1 positive adults with antiretroviral therapy.

Chasela, C.S. et al. 2010. Maternal or infant antiretroviral drugs to reduce HIV-1 transmission. *New England Journal of Medicine*; 362(24):2271–81.

Cohen, M.S. et al. 2011. Prevention of HIV-1 infection with early antiretroviral therapy. *New England Journal of Medicine*; 365(6):493–505.

Ford, N. et al. 2011. Safety of efavirenz in the first trimester of pregnancy: an updated systematic review and meta-analysis. *AIDS*; 25(18):2301–4.

Jamieson, D.J. et al. 2012. Maternal and infant antiretroviral regimens to prevent postnatal HIV-1 transmission: 48-week follow-up of the BAN randomised controlled trial. *The Lancet*; 379(9835):2449–58.

Madder, L.S. et al. 2005. Risk factors for in utero and intrapartum transmission of HIV. *Journal of Acquired Immune Deficiency Syndromes*; 38(1):87–95.

Shapiro, R.L. et al. 2010. Antiretroviral regimens in pregnancy and breast-feeding in Botswana. *New England Journal of Medicine*; 362(24):2282–94.

UNAIDS. Know your epidemic. Available: http://www.unaids.org/en/dataanalysis/knowyourepidemic/ (accessed 26 Aug 2012.)

World Health Organization. 2012. *Programmatic update. Use of antiretroviral drugs for treating pregnant women and preventing HIV infection in infants* Geneva: World Health Organization.

Antiretroviral drug resistance

The mechanisms of antiretroviral drug resistance

HIV has a high viral turnover (10^8 to 10^{10} viruses per day) coupled with a high mutation rate (>1 for each new virus). Mutations resulting in changes in the amino acid sequence of the protein encoded for by an HIV gene may be neutral, conferring no impact on viral fitness; deleterious, causing the virus to replicate less well than the wild-type; or advantageous, conferring a replication advantage over the wild-type virus.

Antiretrovirals inhibit the function of essential viral proteins such as reverse transcriptase, integrase and protease. Mutations resulting in changes in the amino acid sequence at key sites in the antiretroviral target protein reduce the activity of the antiretroviral drug. This is known as resistance. Failure to achieve virological suppression on an antiretroviral regimen selects for drug resistant mutants, which rapidly become the predominant population if the antiretrovirals are continued. Antiretroviral drug resistance is not an 'all or nothing' phenomenon and in many instances the antiretroviral retains partial activity despite the presence of resistance mutations.

Most mutations conferring antiretroviral resistance are the result of amino acid substitutions. For example, substituting the amino acid valine for methionine at the 184th amino acid in the reverse transcriptase enzyme (conventionally abbreviated as M184V) confers high level resistance to the nucleoside reverse transcriptase inhibitors (NRTIs) lamivudine and emtricitabine.

Induced resistance

Most antiretroviral resistance is induced or secondary resistance, which means that the patient was infected with the 'wild type' HIV and resistance mutations were selected for following the use of antiretroviral agents by the patient. Resistance in this setting is the consequence of continuing an antiretroviral regimen with a viral load that is not suppressed, which selects for resistant mutations. More mutations accumulate that eventually convey resistance to all of the antiretroviral drugs the patient is taking. These mutations may also impair response to antiretroviral drugs that the patient has not yet taken (see notes on resistance to different antiretroviral drug classes below). The commonest cause of failure to suppress viral load is poor adherence (see Chapter 48: Adherence to antiretroviral therapy). But it is important to note that very poor adherence may not provide enough selection pressure for resistant mutations – this is especially seen with protease inhibitors.

Once resistance mutations have been selected for, they confer a survival advantage for the virus, and the mutant strain becomes dominant in the HIV population if the patient continues the antiretroviral regimen. However, if the antiretrovirals that have selected for the resistance mutations are removed the 'wild type' HIV population becomes the dominant population because it has greater fitness. The antiretroviral resistant mutant population will disappear from the circulation in weeks to months, and will no longer be detectable by resistance assays (see below). Unfortunately the resistance mutations are archived in long-lived populations of CD4+ T-cells and, if the antiretrovirals are reintroduced, the resistant mutant HIV rapidly becomes dominant again.

Primary resistance

Primary resistance occurs when the patient is infected with HIV that is resistant to one or more antiretroviral drugs in the absence of antiretroviral exposure.

Surveys in industrialized countries show that 5% to 20% of patients have primary resistance to one or more antiretroviral classes. The prevalence of primary resistance in southern Africa is currently low, but likely to increase with the burgeoning use of antiretroviral therapy.

Antiretroviral resistant mutations in primary resistance persist for much longer (a year or more) in the absence of antiretroviral drug selection pressure than in patients who have developed resistance after exposure to antiretroviral therapy. But eventually so-called back mutations occur that recreate the 'wild type'.

Resistance to specific antiretroviral drug classes

Mutations may be specific to individual agents, or may confer resistance to all or some drugs of the different antiretroviral classes.

Nucleoside reverse transcriptase inhibitors (NRTIs)

Multi-NRTI resistance mutations, also known as nucleoside analogue mutations (NAMs), accumulate slowly and resistance increases in a stepwise fashion. They eventually confer resistance to all NRTIs. Thymidine analogue mutations (TAMs) are a specific subset of NAMs that are selected by stavudine and zidovudine, the two currently available thymidine analogues. TAMs accumulate at a rate of approximately one mutation every six to twelve months in the presence of a failing thymidine analogue-containing regimen. The number and pattern of TAMs determines the degree of resistance, and several mutations need to be present before the NRTI's effect is significantly compromised.

The M184V mutation alluded to above confers high level resistance to lamivudine and emtricitabine, and also reduces the efficacy of didanosine and abacavir in the presence of other NAMs. However, the M184V mutation has some potential benefits (and lamivudine or emtricitabine are thus often continued despite documented resistance):

- Viral fitness is reduced by approximately 30%.
- The selection of TAMs is slowed.
- Susceptibility to tenofovir, zidovudine and stavudine is increased when NAMs are present.

Non-nucleoside reverse transcriptase inhibitors (NNRTIs)

NNRTI mutations are common soon after virologic failure on NNRTI-based regimens. Any one of several single mutations convey high level resistance, which affects both efavirenz and nevirapine. Thus, if resistance develops to nevirapine then efavirenz is also compromised. The second generation NNRTI etravirine retains activity against some of the resistant mutations selected for by efvire and neviarapine. NNRTI mutations do not significantly impair viral fitness. Ongoing use of NNRTIs after the selection of a resistant mutation will result in the accumulation of additional mutations, which may compromise the second generation NNRTIs that are currently in development.

Protease inhibitors (PIs)

PI-resistant mutations increase resistance in a stepwise fashion and up to 11 mutations need to be present to confer high level resistance to some of the newer PIs. There is a considerable degree of cross resistance with many PI mutations. Viral fitness is impaired by PI resistance.

Integrase inhibitors

Raltegravir has a relatively low genetic barrier to resistance. Two mutations are typically required to convey high level resistance.

Assays to detect antiretroviral resistance

Antiretroviral resistance can be measured either by sequencing the HIV genes of interest, (e.g. protease) to look for mutations that are known to confer resistance (genotyping), or by measuring the ability of the virus to grow in the presence of different antiretroviral drug concentrations (phenotyping). Virtual phenotyping is predicting the HIV phenotype from the genotype. Phenotype assays are technically demanding, extremely expensive, not available in our region and will not be discussed further.

There are several limitations to genotyping assays. Because resistant mutations fade after discontinuing antiretroviral drugs, it is essential that patients are taking their failing regimen at the time of assay. The assays can only detect a resistant population of viruses if these make up a significant proportion (exceeding about 20%) of circulating HIV. Important resistant mutations from prior antiretroviral regimens that are archived and will recur on re-exposure are not detected; it is therefore essential that a full antiretroviral drug history is available before interpreting genotyping results. The viral load must also be significantly elevated (>1 000 copies/mL) in order to detect resistance. A negative genotyping test in a patient with an elevated viral load is a very expensive way to demonstrate poor adherence, therefore the test should only be conducted after carefully assessing adherence. There is very little point in performing resistance assays in patients with <60% adherence. Finally, not all mutations or combinations of mutations conferring resistance are known.

Current guidelines from industrialized countries recommend antiretroviral resistance testing before starting antiretroviral therapy (to detect primary resistance) and at each episode of confirmed virologic failure. Genotyping is an expensive test. In southern Africa genotyping is currently unaffordable for public health programmes, but may have a role in selected patients if salvage therapy is introduced.

References and recommended reading

Bangsberg, D.R., et al. 2006. 'Adherence–resistance relationships for protease and non-nucleoside reverse transcriptase inhibitors explained by virological fitness.' *AIDS*; 20:223–231.

Clavel, F. and A.J. Hance. 2004. 'HIV Drug Resistance.' *New England Journal of Medicine*; 350:1023–1035.

Hamers, R.L., et al. 2011. 'HIV-1 drug resistance in antiretroviral-naive individuals in sub-Saharan Africa after rollout of antiretroviral therapy: a multicentre observational study.' *Lancet Infectious Diseases*; 11:750–9.

48 Adherence to antiretroviral therapy

Adherence

HIV is a chronic disease that eventually results in AIDS and death unless managed appropriately with antiretroviral therapy. Successful antiretroviral therapy results in suppression of HIV replication and halts clinical progression of the disease. There is a clear positive relationship between antiretroviral adherence and achieving and maintaining virological suppression. Non-adherence to antiretroviral therapy is associated with incomplete viral suppression and the selection of drug resistant virus that will eventually limit therapeutic options.

In the public health approach to antiretroviral therapy advocated by the World Health Organization, adopted by most resource-limited countries including South Africa, only two sequential antiretroviral regimens are available. With the limited antiretroviral options available, it is particularly important for antiretroviral programmes in southern Africa to achieve high levels of adherence.

What is sufficient adherence?

Adherence close to 100% is ideal and will minimise the risk of developing resistant virus for all treatment regimens. The percentage adherence required for virological suppression varies from individual to individual, with different antiretroviral classes, and over time (higher adherence is needed to achieve virological suppression than to maintain suppression). Adherence levels required in HIV are higher than in other chronic diseases, which are difficult to achieve.

The relationship between resistance and adherence

The relationship between adherence and the development of resistance is not linear. Patients with low adherence do not exert sufficient selection pressure to confer a replication advantage for drug-resistant mutants. Patients with high adherence suppress replication and mutations do not occur. Resistance is selected for by patients with moderate adherence.

While all antiretroviral drugs are susceptible to resistance, the degree of susceptibility varies. A single viral mutation results in complete resistance to the non-nucleoside reverse transcriptase inhibitors (NNRTIs), efavirenz and nevirapine. Similarly 3TC is rendered ineffective by a single mutation. In contrast, other nucleoside reverse transcriptase inhibitors (NRTIs) and the protease inhibitors (PIs) are more robust, requiring multiple viral mutations before resistance develops.

Because resistant virus is only generated if there is adequate drug pressure to drive the selection of these mutations, different antiretroviral classes are vulnerable at different adherence rates. Resistance to a PI is noted most frequently when adherence is between 80 and 95%, as high levels of drug are needed to create enough selective pressure to confer survival benefit on a virus with multiple mutations. Lower levels of drug do not create enough selection pressure and wild-type virus will remain the dominant virus.

Conversely, resistance to non-nucleoside reverse transcriptase inhibitors (NNRTIs) is more likely at <80% than at 80%–95% adherence. The single mutation that confers resistance to an NNRTI does not have an impact on the virus's ability to replicate.

Despite these complexities, the message to an individual on antiretroviral therapy remains the same. Long-term viral suppression will only reliably be achieved with near perfect adherence (>95%).

Measuring adherence

A number of methods are used to measure adherence. Such measures are usually classified as objective (data recorded independently of the patient) or subjective (in the opinion of the patient).

Objective assessments

Objective adherence assessments include:
- Pill counts: Counting returned medication in order to estimate the number of doses taken is a method frequently used to calculate adherence. To calculate adherence you need four variables:
  o the number of tablets returned (for each medicine), e.g. 9 3TC tablets left in the bottle;
  o the number of tablets dispensed (for each medicine), e.g. 60 3TC tablets;
  o the number of days between the visits, e.g. 28 days;
  o the number of doses of the medicine per day, e.g. twice a day for 3TC.

The adherence for this example would be = $\dfrac{\text{(no. tabs dispensed)} - \text{(no. tabs returned)}}{\text{(no. days between visits)} \times \text{(doses per day)}}$

$$= \dfrac{(60) - (9)}{(28) \times (2)}$$

$$= \dfrac{51}{56} = 91\%$$

Although valuable, this can be time consuming in a busy clinic. There is also a risk of people discarding their tablets to 'improve' their adherence, although this is not common. Surprise or unannounced pill counts at home may decrease the risk of pill-dumping, but would require a dedicated team of counsellors to visit clients at home, and is not practical when monitoring adherence on a large scale.

- Pharmacy refill data: Adherence as assessed by pharmacy refill data has been shown to predict virological failure and survival in Zambian and South African cohorts. This is the simplest method of objectively recording adherence and is best suited to monitoring adherence in large antiretroviral programmes. The number of times a patient receives medication over a fixed period, e.g. a calendar year, is expressed as a percentage of the number of times they should have collected medication, e.g. patient collected medication 11 times out of an expected 12 in the previous year = 92%.

- Electronic monitoring: The use of electronic devices that record each time a bottle is opened is rare outside of the research environment. These devices are expensive and require computers and software for downloading the information on return of the bottle. This method is, however, accepted as the best means of objectively assessing adherence.

- Therapeutic drug monitoring: Low plasma concentrations of anti-retrovirals may be due to poor adherence, malabsorption or drug interactions. Patients tend to adhere best around their clinic visit, so-called 'white coat adherence', so measuring drug concentrations over-estimates adherence.

Subjective assessments

Subjective adherence methods are notoriously insensitive, but better results are obtained by adopting non-judgmental attitudes and gaining the patient's trust. Subjective assessments include:

- Recall questionnaires: These are the most widely used tools to collect adherence data, usually asking the patient to recall doses missed over the past three days. Adherence percentage would be calculated based on the answer, e.g. missing one dose out of the six doses that should have been taken in the last three days means that five of six doses were taken, i.e. 83%.

Many people will not admit to missing a dose when asked by their healthcare team, and so a recall questionnaire often results in an over-inflated estimate of individual adherence. This method may be more useful as a research tool as more open, accurate responses might be expected when results are not reported to the clinical team.

- A 30-day visual analogue scale (VAS) of doses taken may be a faster and more efficient means of obtaining similar information to the recall questionnaire. (Figure 48.1)

Figure 48.1 Example of a visual analogue scale

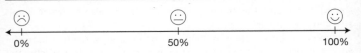

0%   50%   100%

Mark on the line how well you took your medication in the last month. Remember, 0% means you didn't take any medicines at all and 100% means you were perfect.

All measures of adherence remain approximations; however they can be used to target individuals who require more intensive adherence interventions.

Risk factors for poor adherence

Factors that may have either a positive or a negative impact on an individual's pill taking behaviour may be divided into three categories: patient-related, regimen-related and disease-related. These are tabulated below. With the simple regimens available as first line therapy, the major impact on adherence lies with the individuals on therapy and their interactions with their families, communities and their health carers. The more favourable these relationships, the more likely an individual is to remain adherent over time. The value of an individual accepting their HIV status and being properly prepared for therapy should not be underestimated.

Many people simply forget to take their medication. The use of devices such as pill boxes and diaries to remind them to take their antiretroviral therapy can be useful here. A number of studies have shown no change in adherence by level of education or gender. Adolescents and younger adults are less adherent than older adults. Disclosure of HIV status and support by a treatment partner or peer counsellor have been shown to have a great impact on adherence.

Interventions to improve adherence

Pre-treatment interventions

Individuals who start treatment should be well prepared. A standard module of information should be presented to all patients to ensure they have a basic understanding of HIV and antiretroviral therapy prior to starting antiretroviral therapy. This education should also be offered to the carers of children and of adults with mental illness. A 'treatment buddy' should be identified by the patient if possible and also educated about HIV and antiretroviral therapy.

People can be educated individually or in groups. Groups have the advantage of being more efficient in the context of large-scale antiretroviral therapy, as well as of allowing individuals to meet others with HIV, so perhaps encouraging acceptance of their status and disclosure.

Pre-treatment education should cover:

- a simple explanation of HIV, including what would be expected in each stage of the illness from stage 1 to 4;
- details of symptoms that would be of concern, (e.g. loss of weight, cough for >2 weeks);
- advice on living healthily with HIV (including nutritional advice) and how to prevent spread to other adults, (e.g. safe sex and condom use) and from mother-to-child;
- a short explanation of viral load and CD4 count;
- an explanation of antiretroviral therapy, including expected decrease in viral load and increase in CD4 count;
- a discussion on the importance of adherence to therapy, explaining that treatment is life-long;
- details of the actual antiretroviral therapy to be taken including names of the medications, colour and number of tablets per day, dosing, (e.g.12-hourly not twice a day) and what to do if a dose is missed;
- explanation of common or severe adverse effects and what to do or who to call if these occur.

Table 48.1 Factors influencing adherence

	Promoting adherence	**Reducing adherence**
Patient factors	• Comfortable with HIV-positive status • Motivated patient with a good sense of self-worth • Good understanding of HIV disease and therapy pre-treatment • Good understanding of importance of adherence • Education given in a patient's home language prior to and during therapy • Use of diaries, pill boxes etc. as reminders to take antiretrovirals	• Fear of disclosure of HIV status (to close family/friends) • Substance abuse, including alcoholism • Depression (or other affective disorder) • Anxieties or suspicions about the disease or therapy • Disorganized or disrupted daily routine, e.g. shift workers, truck drivers
Disease factors	• Late or symptomatic HIV disease	• Still healthy, i.e. early, asymptomatic disease
Therapy factors	• Simple regimen with a small number of tablets per day • Easy access to free therapy • Noting positive health benefits of therapy with few adverse events	• Large numbers of tablets or complicated therapy • Having to purchase therapy (financial constraints) • Severe or ongoing minor adverse events/reduced quality of life on treatment

This information can be given by a peer educator or counsellor over multiple group sessions, during the week or two weeks prior to starting therapy. Oral sessions should be accompanied by written information that is to be taken home and read at other times.

Before antiretroviral therapy is started, the individual's understanding should be checked with a few simple questions, e.g. how many different tablets must you take/what is a CD4 cell/how long must you take this treatment for? If knowledge is poor, provided the patient is not too ill, he/she should be encouraged to repeat the sessions before treatment starts. Although not ideal, if antiretroviral therapy is needed urgently, e.g. for PMTCT or very late stage disease, education can be repeated during the first month on therapy.

Interventions during treatment

The majority of 'treatment-ready' people (80–90%) who start therapy are adherent and might be expected to have a suppressed viral load by six months. However, some people never manage to take their pills correctly, and others tire over time and begin to miss doses due to pill-fatigue. These less adherent people need to be identified and targeted to receive more intensive adherence input.

Identifying those at risk means that the adherence must be monitored using at least one of the measures described above throughout an individual's time on antiretroviral therapy. Anyone who has an adherence approaching 80% or less, or who has a viral load that is not suppressed at any time after baseline, should receive attention from the health care staff. Step-up adherence interventions have been shown to result in more than 50% of those with a significant first viral load elevation (>1 000 copies/mL) again achieving suppression.

A stepped-up adherence intervention might include:
- time with a counsellor to discuss and resolve issues that may be leading to non-adherence or failure, e.g. non-disclosure, substance abuse, chaotic lifestyle;
- time with a clinician to discuss and resolve issues that may be leading to non-adherence or failure, e.g. wrong dosing or timing of doses, adverse events;
- repetition of the initial treatment information, with an emphasis on the importance of adherence;
- use of a pill-box (see photo 54) or dosing diary;
- a home visit by an adherence counsellor to assess home circumstances, where possible;
- dispensing medication and monitoring adherence monthly until adherence back above 80% or again virologically suppressed.

Expanding access to antiretroviral therapy across the resource-poor areas of the world remains a daunting prospect and there remains an anxiety that the clinical and political pressure to enroll large numbers of people onto antiretroviral programmes may adversely influence the quality of the service rendered. Both new and existing antiretroviral programmes need to maintain a focus on adherence and create systems and structures that withstand the process of expansion.

References

Bangsberg, D.R., Acosta, E.P., Gupta, R. et al. 2006. 'Adherence-resistance relationships for protease and non-nucleoside reverse transcriptase inhibitors explained by virological fitness.' *AIDS*; 20(2):223–231.

Mills, E.J., Nachega, J.B., Bangsberg, D.R. et al. 2006. 'Adherence to HAART: a systematic review of developed and developing nation patient-reported barriers and facilitators.' *PLoS Medicine*; 3(11):e438.

Mills, E.J., Nachega, J.B., Buchan, I. et al. 2006. ' Adherence to antiretroviral therapy in sub-Saharan Africa and North America: a meta-analysis.' *Journal of the American Medical Association*; 296(6):679–690.

Rosenbaum, M. et al. 2009. 'The risk of virologic failure decreases with duration of HIV suppression, at greater than 50% adherence to antiretroviral therapy.' *PLoS ONE* 4(9):e7196.

Drug-drug interactions

Combination antiretroviral therapy for HIV infection typically consists of three or more antiretroviral agents; two nucleoside reverse transcriptase inhibitors (NRTIs) and either a protease inhibitor (PI) or a non-nucleoside reverse transcriptase inhibitor (NNRTI). HIV-infected patients often also take other medication in addition to antiretroviral therapy; for treatment and prophylaxis of opportunistic infections, for co-morbid illnesses not directly related to HIV, and complementary or traditional remedies (often taken without the knowledge of the medical practitioner).

There is always a risk of drug-drug interactions with polypharmacy. However, this risk is especially high with antiretroviral therapy because the NNRTIs and the PIs inhibit and/or induce several key isoenzymes of the cytochrome P450 system, as well as being substrates of this system. In addition the PIs inhibit the key drug efflux pump P-glycoprotein. Inhibition of drug metabolism or transport increases concentrations, which may cause toxicity, while induction of drug metabolism may result in sub-therapeutic concentrations. When the drug-drug interaction causes sub-therapeutic antiretroviral concentrations this may result in treatment failure due to the development of viral resistance, which has serious consequences for the long-term management of HIV infection.

This chapter will outline the common mechanisms of drug interactions involving antiretroviral therapy. Clinical scenarios where interactions frequently occur will be discussed, together with practical management recommendations. Lastly, the exploitation of the inhibiting properties of the PI ritonavir, so called PI boosting, will be discussed. Useful information sources on individual drug-drug interactions are listed under references.

Mechanism of drug interactions

Drug interactions can be pharmacokinetic or pharmacodynamic. Pharmacokinetic interactions that are relevant to antiretrovirals predominantly involve changes in drug absorption, metabolism and excretion. Pharmacodynamic interactions may result from competition at receptor sites or activity of two drugs on the same physiological system. The effect on efficacy may be additive, synergistic or antagonistic (e.g. zidovudine and stavudine are antagonistic). Shared toxicity is another example of a pharmacodynamic interaction, (e.g. the additive risk of bone marrow suppression if ganciclovir and zidovudine are co-administered).

Drug absorption

The buffered formulation of the NRTI didanosine contains an antacid. The calcium and magnesium ions in the buffer may chelate concomitantly administered drugs. Plasma concentrations of drugs that require low gastric pH for absorption, (e.g. itraconazole, indinavir) are also reduced by concomitant administration with the buffered formulation. These interactions can be avoided by using the enteric-coated didanosine formulation or by dosing the drugs at different times.

Metabolic interactions

This is the major mechanism of antiretroviral drug interactions. A large number of drugs are metabolised by the cytochrome P450 system, which is located predominantly in the liver and in the enterocytes of the small intestine. Three families of cytochrome P450 enzymes (CYP1, CYP2 and CYP3) are important in human drug metabolism. Families are further subdivided into individual isoenzymes, for example CYP2B6 which metabolises efavirenz. The CYP3A isoenzymes are responsible for the metabolism of about half of the drugs metabolized by the cytochrome P450 system. A drug metabolized by the cytochrome P450 system will be a substrate of one or more isoenzymes. A drug may also act as an inhibitor or inducer of these isoenzymes.

Inhibition of metabolising enzymes is due to direct competition and typically involves one or a few CYP isoenzymes. Onset of enzyme inhibition is rapid and disappears when the inhibiting drug is metabolized. In contrast, enzyme induction is due to upregulation of many CYP genes (along with some drug transporters and conjugating enzymes), resulting in increased expression. The process of induction develops slowly and wanes slowly after the inducing drug is no longer present: induction is maximal after about 14 days and disappears slowly in about 14 days.

PIs are substrates of CYP3A4 and also inhibit this important isoenzyme. Ritonavir is the most potent inhibitor of the PIs; this is exploited in PI boosting (see below). Ritonavir also acts as an inducer of some P450 isoenzymes, which means that for most co-administered drugs ritonavir will increase concentrations (by inhibiting CYP3A4) but for some it will decrease concentrations, (e.g. by inducing CYP2C9). NNRTIs are also substrates of CYP3A4 and induce it. The NNRTI efavirenz may act as either an inducer or an inhibitor of CYP3A4. Thus, it is complex to predict what will happen when drugs are co-administered with PIs and NNRTIs and clinicians should always check before prescribing.

P-glycoprotein

P-glycoprotein is a trans-membrane efflux pump that actively transports many drugs. It is found at numerous sites: in the brush border surface of enterocytes (where its effect is to reduce absorption), where excretion occurs (the canalicular surface of hepatocytes and the apical surface of proximal tubular cells in kidneys), and in tissues known to have blood-tissue barriers (blood-brain-barrier, placenta, ovaries and testes). PIs and tenofovir are transported by P-glycoprotein. The PI ritonavir is an inhibitor of P-glycoprotein, which contributes to its PI boosting properties (see below). Some drugs that induce cytochrome P450 enzymes also induce P-glycoprotein (e.g. rifampicin).

Frequency of antiretroviral drug interactions

Potentially significant interactions with antiretroviral therapy occur frequently in clinical practice. A survey of South African private sector HIV-infected patients in a managed care scheme, who were on antiretroviral therapy as well as chronic medication for concomitant conditions, showed that 26% of patients receiving NNRTIs and 41% of patients receiving PIs were prescribed medication with potentially significant interactions. In many instances more than one interacting drug was prescribed.

Complementary and traditional medicines

Many patients on antiretroviral therapy also take complementary and traditional medicines, often without the knowledge of the treating doctor. Garlic and St John's Wort, a commonly used herbal remedy for depressive symptoms, are enzyme inducers, capable of significantly lowering PI concentrations. Recent *in vitro* studies of two South African herbal remedies that are promoted for HIV infection, *Sutherlandia* and *Hypoxis* (the so-called African potato), indicate that both preparations are inhibitors of P-glycoprotein and CYP3A4. There is a need for further research in this area.

Anticonvulsants

Anticonvulsants are often prescribed for HIV-infected patients because epilepsy is more common among these patients than in the general community. Anticonvulsants are also frequently used for neuropathic pain, which is common in HIV infection. The first-line anticonvulsants (phenobarbital, phenytoin and carbamazepine) are inducers of CYP3A4, and have the potential to decrease the concentrations of PIs and NNRTIs. Antiretrovirals also interact with some of the first-line anticonvulsants: carbamazepine concentrations are reduced by NNRTIs and increased by PIs (by inducing or inhibiting CYP3A4 respectively), and phenytoin concentrations are reduced by the PI ritonavir (by inducing CYP2C9).

Alternative anticonvulsants that do not induce cytochrome P450 should be prescribed for patients on antiretroviral therapy. Sodium valproate is the only first-line anticonvulsant that has minimal cytochrome P450 interactions. However, sodium valproate does increase zidovudine concentrations by interfering with glucuronidation. It is unclear whether the dose of zidovudine should be reduced. Close monitoring for zidovudine toxicity is recommended. The second-line anticonvulsants lamotrigine, gabapentin and levetiracetam are least likely to have significant interactions with antiretrovirals. If it is not possible to use anticonvulsants that are unlikely to have significant interactions with antiretrovirals then anticonvulsant and antiretroviral concentrations should be monitored (see therapeutic drug monitoring below).

Rifampicin

Rifampicin is a potent inducer of both cytochrome P450 enzymes and the drug efflux pump P-glycoprotein. This results in reduced concentrations of some NNRTIs and PIs. The reduction in concentrations of the NNRTI efavirenz is minimal and the trough concentrations remain therapeutic. There is a significant reduction in concentrations of the NNRTI nevirapine, and a large South African cohort study showed a greater risk of virological failure when nevirapine-based antiretroviral therapy was co-administered with rifampicin. However, PI concentrations are dramatically reduced to well below the therapeutic range, even when PI boosting (see below) is used. Additional ritonavir may overcome the inducing effect of rifampicin: either by using saquinavir 400 mg plus ritonavir 400 mg 12 hourly, by adding 300 mg ritonavir 12 hourly to the fixed dose lopinavir/ritonavir combination, or by doubling the dose of lopinavir/ritonavir. However, studies in healthy volunteers have shown high risks of hepatotoxicity when rifampicin is co-administered with adjusted doses of PIs. The minimal published data on the safety of adjusted dose PIs in patients with tuberculosis and local experience suggests that hepatotoxicity is uncommon. Nevertheless, liver function tests should be closely monitored in this setting.

Treating tuberculosis without rifampicin for patients on PIs is sometimes advocated, but this is not a realistic option in South Africa. Outcomes without rifampicin are not as good and antitubercular therapy must be prolonged. In developed countries the alternative rifamycin rifabutin (at reduced doses, as PIs lead to elevated rifabutin concentrations) is used instead of rifampicin. However, rifabutin is prohibitively expensive in South Africa and not available in the public sector. Thus the antiretroviral regimen should be tailored to be compatible with rifampicin wherever possible. If NNRTIs or PIs cannot be used due to resistance or intolerance, a triple NRTI regimen can be used for the duration of TB therapy.

Exploiting metabolic interactions: protease inhibitor boosting

PIs are substrates of CYP3A4 and P-glycoprotein, and ritonavir is a potent inhibitor of both CYP3A4 and P-glycoprotein. Ritonavir in therapeutic doses is poorly tolerated. However, small doses of co-administered ritonavir markedly increases the plasma concentrations and prolongs the half-lives of most PIs. The concentrations achieved may be high enough to overcome partial resistance. The prolonged half-life allows for less frequent dosing intervals, which improves adherence. This PI boosting effect has become the standard of care for PI use, and results in a better virological response. The PI lopinavir is only available co-formulated with ritonavir. However, PI boosting does increase toxicity.

Other interactions between antiretrovirals

There are some important interactions between NRTIs. Zidovudine and stavudine compete for the same intracellular phosphorylation pathway and antagonise each other – this combination is contraindicated. Tenofovir decreases the intracellular catabolism of didanosine, resulting in increased toxicity of didanosine – this combination should be avoided.

NNRTIs and PIs are occasionally co-administered, usually when severe hyperlactataemia has occurred from the NRTIs. NNRTIs induce the metabolism of PIs, and a dose increase of the PI may be necessary.

Therapeutic drug monitoring

In most instances where an interaction may occur with a co-administered drug and alternative agents are not available, clinicians need to dose cautiously and closely monitor response. Wherever possible drug concentrations of co-administered drugs (e.g. many anticonvulsants, digoxin), should be monitored. Therapeutic monitoring of antiretroviral drug concentrations should be considered when the co-administered drug alters the concentration of the antiretroviral drug.

References and further reading

Boulle, A., et al. 2008. 'Outcomes of nevirapine- and efavirenz-based antiretroviral therapy when co-administered with rifampicin-based antitubercular therapy.' *Journal of the American Medical Association*; 300:530–9.

Drug interaction information sources: http://www.hiv-druginteractions.org; http://hivinsite.ucsf.edu/InSite.jsp?page=ar-00-02

Medicines Information Centre, Division of Clinical Pharmacology, University of Cape Town (telephone 021-4066782) – ARV drug interactions for drugs used in the public sector available from their website: http://www.mic.uct.ac.za

Cooper, C.L., Van Heeswijk, R.P., Gallicano, K., Cameron, D.W. 2003. 'A review of low-dose ritonavir in protease inhibitor combination therapy.' *Clinical Infectious Diseases*; 36:1585–1592.

Liedtke, M.D., Lockhart, S.M., Rathbun, R.C. 2004. 'Anticonvulsant and antiretroviral interactions.' *Annals of Pharmacotherapy*; 38:482–489.

Maartens, G., Decloedt, E., Cohen, K. 2009. 'Effectiveness and safety of antiretrovirals with rifampicin: crucial issues for high burden countries.' *Antiviral Therapy*; 14:1039–43.

Mills, E., Foster, B.C., Van Heeswijk, R., Phillips, E., Wilson, K., Leonard, B., Kosuge, K., Kanfer, I. 2005. 'Impact of African herbal medicines on antiretroviral metabolism.' *AIDS*; 19:95–97.

Regensberg, L., Andrews, S., Pead, C., Maartens, G., Nortier, S. 2002. 'Unrecognised interactions between antiretrovirals and concomitant chronically administered medication in a managed health care program in Southern Africa (MoPeB3224).' 14th International AIDS Conference, Barcelona July 7–12.

Immune reconstitution inflammatory syndrome

The immune reconstitution inflammatory syndrome (IRIS) is a frequent early complication of antiretroviral therapy, particularly in patients who start antiretroviral therapy with low CD4 counts and established opportunistic infections. IRIS results from a pathological inflammatory response driven by the recovering immune system after antiretroviral therapy is initiated, causing clinical deterioration. The immunopathological response underlying IRIS is directed at pre-existing antigens from an infective agent or the host. A proposed case definition for IRIS is shown in Table 50.1.

Table 50.1 Proposed IRIS case definition

- HIV-positive
- Receiving combination antiretroviral therapy:
  - decrease in HIV-1 RNA level from baseline
  - increase in CD4+ cells from baseline (may lag behind HIV-1 RNA decrease)
- Clinical symptoms consistent with inflammatory process
- Clinical course not consistent with:
  - expected course of previously diagnosed opportunistic infection
  - expected course of newly diagnosed opportunistic infection
  - drug toxicity

Source: Shelburne, S.A., Montes, M., Hamill, R.J. 2006. 'Immune reconstitution inflammatory syndrome: more answers, more questions.' *Journal of Antimicrobial Chemotherapy*; 57:167–70.

Other terms used for IRIS are 'immune reconstitution/restoration disease (IRD)' and 'immune reconstitution syndrome (IRS).'

A classification of IRIS is shown in Table 50.2.

Infective forms of IRIS may manifest either as an 'unmasking' of a previously untreated infection, or as paradoxical clinical deterioration of an infective process for which the patient is on appropriate antimicrobial therapy. For example, patients who have active tuberculosis (TB) that is unrecognised prior to antiretroviral initiation may present with accelerated and inflammatory features of TB soon after antiretroviral initiation – 'unmasking' IRIS. Patients already on TB treatment when antiretroviral therapy is initiated may manifest with recurrence or worsening of their symptoms, signs and/or radiological manifestations after starting anti-

Table 50.2 Categories of IRIS

Category	Antigen target	Examples
Infective – unmasking	Antigen of an infection that is untreated (replicating organism)	Unmasking of cryptococcal meningitis
Infective – paradoxical	Antigen of an infection for which the patient is on appropriate treatment (dead or dying organism)	Paradoxical TB-IRIS
Auto-immune	Host	Grave's thyroid disease
Malignancies	Tumour	Worsening of Kaposi's sarcoma
Other inflammatory conditions	Range	Inflammation at site of tattoo; sarcoidosis

retroviral therapy – 'paradoxical' IRIS. Infective forms of IRIS may thus be due to an inflammatory reaction directed towards an untreated replicating organism (unmasking form) or towards dead/dying organism in patients who are on appropriate therapy for the infection (paradoxical form). Unmasking IRIS is characterized by atypical presentations such as localized inflammation (where disseminated disease is typical) or unusual degrees of inflammation.

Key factors that are likely to underlie the development of IRIS are:

- A pre-existing high infective antigen burden in patients with advanced HIV.
- Early rapid restoration of pathogen-specific immunity on antiretroviral therapy.
- A pro-inflammatory cytokine profile that characterises the recovering immune system.
- Deficient regulatory activity in the recovering immune system.

Most cases occur within three months of antiretroviral initiation during early rapid immune recovery. IRIS may also occur when a failing antiretroviral regimen is switched to a new regimen or when antiretroviral therapy is resumed after an interruption. Common forms of IRIS seen in southern Africa are listed in Table 50.3.

Table 50.3 Common forms of IRIS seen in southern Africa

Tuberculosis
Cryptococcosis
Acne
Molluscum contagiosum
Herpes simplex and zoster
Hepatitis B
Cytomegalovirus uveitis
Kaposi's sarcoma

Children

BCG IRIS is most frequent in children in the first year of life. It can present as local IRIS at site of injection and/or regional lymphadenitis (right axilla). Management is conservative. BCG and TB-IRIS often occur in the same patient.

Paradoxical TB-IRIS

Paradoxical TB-IRIS occurs in 8-43% of patients who are started on antiretroviral therapy while on TB treatment, typically one to four weeks after antiretroviral therapy is initiated. Common manifestations are return of TB symptoms, fever, lymph node enlargement with inflammatory features (see photo 55), worsening radiographic pulmonary infiltrates (see photo 56) and the accumulation of serous effusions. TB-IRIS is occasionally fatal, especially if there are neurological manifestations. Most cases of TB-IRIS are self-limiting within a few weeks. It is important to consider and exclude conditions that may mimic TB-IRIS, such as other opportunistic diseases or drug-resistant TB. Mild TB-IRIS can usually be managed supportively by educating the patient on what is causing the symptoms and symptomatic therapy. In patients with more severe TB-IRIS, corticosteroid therapy has been shown to reduce need for hospitalization. However, the additional immune suppression from corticosteroids may increase the risk of opportunistic diseases, notably fungal and herpes virus infections. Steroids should not be given to patients with Kaposi's sarcoma as this can result in fatal disease progression.

Paradoxical cryptococcal IRIS

Paradoxical cryptococcal IRIS occurs in patients who have had a diagnosis of cryptococcosis prior to starting antiretroviral therapy and are improving on antifungal therapy. Typically, after starting antiretroviral therapy they develop recurrent meningitis symptoms that may be associated with raised intracranial pressure. Other manifestations such as enlarging cryptococcomas, encephalitis and lymphadenitis are described. All cases with recurrent meningitis should have a lumbar puncture to measure and, if necessary, reduce raised intracranial pressure (serial lumbar punctures may be needed) and exclude alternative diagnoses.

Other manifestations of IRIS

A range of skin conditions can occur, recur or worsen with IRIS. These include HSV 1 and 2, shingles, warts, molluscum contagiosum, papular pruritic eruption and acne (see photo 57). It is important to differentiate these forms of IRIS from a cutaneous drug reaction.

Patients with chronic viral hepatitis B and C may present with a flare of their hepatitis due to IRIS. This can be difficult to differentiate from a drug-induced hepatitis.

Many patients with Kaposi's sarcoma (KS) experience partial or complete resolution of lesions with antiretroviral therapy alone. However, a minority of patients (7% in one cohort) develop KS-IRIS after starting antiretroviral therapy. This manifests with inflammation or enlargement of existing lesions, new lesions or the development of lymphoedema.

Diagnosis and management of IRIS

There is no confirmatory diagnostic test for IRIS. Instead the diagnosis rests on a suggestive history and clinical picture and the exclusion of possible alternative diagnoses to explain the patient's clinical deterioration – such as drug resistance (especially TB), drug reactions or new opportunistic infections.

In patients with 'unmasking' IRIS, antiretroviral therapy should be continued and effective treatment for the condition started. In paradoxical IRIS, antiretroviral therapy and effective OI therapy should be continued. In severe cases (especially those with CNS involvement) corticosteroids, (e.g. prednisone 1 mg/kg, duration dependent on response) should be considered in consultation with a specialist. In rare cases when the reaction is life-threatening and not responding to corticosteroids, it may be necessary to interrupt antiretroviral therapy.

References and further reading

French, M.A., Price, P., and Stone, S.F. 2004. 'Immune restoration disease after antiretroviral therapy.' *AIDS*; 18(12):1 615–627.

Murdoch, D. et al. 2007. 'Immune reconstitution inflammatory syndrome (IRIS): review of common infectious manifestations and treatment options.' *AIDS Research and Therapy*; 4:9.

Meintjies, G. et al. 2010. 'Randomized placebo-controlled trial of prednisone for paradoxical tuberculosis-associated immune reconstitution inflammatory syndrome'. *AIDS*; 24:2381–90.

Müller, M. et al. 2010. Immune reconstitution inflammatory syndrome in patients starting antiretroviral therapy for HIV infection: a systematic review and meta-analysis. *Lancet Infectious Diseases*; 10:251–261.

Shelburne, S.A., Montes, M., and Hamill, R.J. 2006. 'Immune reconstitution inflammatory syndrome: more answers, more questions.' *Journal of Antimicrobial Chemotherapy*; 57(2):167–170.

Principles of managing adverse drug reactions

ART is associated with considerable toxicity, some of which is life-threatening. However, less toxic drugs are now widely used and the burden of adverse drug reactions has decreased considerably. Clinicians need to be aware of common toxicities and their management. However, it is important to establish whether the adverse event is due to antiretroviral agents, other medication or co-morbid illness.

Many adverse drug reactions are mild and occur only in the first few weeks of therapy. If toxicity doesn't resolve or is severe then the offending drug should be substituted, as indicated below. It is essential to ensure that the viral load is suppressed before substituting a single drug, otherwise resistance might develop to the new drug, compromising future regimens. Single drug substitutions can safely be done in the first six months of ART without measuring the viral load.

It is rarely necessary to stop the whole ART regimen for toxicity. Switch only the culprit drug and continue the ART regimen. In certain life-threatening situations (e.g. hepatitis with liver failure, lactic acidosis) it may be necessary to stop all antiretrovirals. In patients with severe NNRTI-related toxicity a PI should be substituted or the NNRTI should be stopped and the two NRTIs continued for a week in order to reduce the risk of resistance to NNRTIs developing, which have a long half-life.

Haematological toxicity

Anaemia, thrombocytopenia and neutropenia all occur commonly in HIV infection without exposure to drugs. Patients on zidovudine, stavudine or cotrimoxazole may experience abnormalities in their full blood counts. Monitoring of full blood counts is only necessary with zidovudine – this should be monitored for the first six months of therapy and thereafter if clinically indicated (it is very unusual to see haematological toxicity occurring after six months). The main problem is anaemia and neutropenia – platelet counts generally rise with zidovudine. Macrocytosis is usual with both stavudine and especially zidovudine therapy; there is no need to measure B12 and folate concentrations and supplementation is ineffective. Significant bone marrow toxicity from cotrimoxazole generally only occurs with high doses used for treating opportunistic infections, but neutropenia is not uncommon with prophylactic doses.

Table 51.1 Guidelines for managing haematological toxicity associated with zidovudine

Hb	>8 g/dL Monitor	7–7.9 Repeat 4 weeks Reduce AZT* dose to 200 mg 12 hourly	6.5–6.9 Repeat 2 weeks Consider switching AZT	< 6.5 Switch AZT
Neutro-phils	1–1.5 × 10⁹/L Repeat 4 weeks	0.75–1 Repeat 2 weeks	0.5–0.75 Repeat 2 weeks Consider switching AZT	<0.5 Switch AZT

* Many experts would switch to alternative agents rather than reduce doses

3TC has rarely been associated with pure red cell aplasia, which presents with severe anaemia and low reticulocyte index. Parvovirus B19 infection should be excluded (request a plasma PCR, not a serological test). A bone marrow examination should be done to confirm red cell aplasia.

Hepatotoxicity

Drug-induced liver injury is potentially life-threatening, especially if it is symptomatic or accompanied by jaundice. Liver function tests (LFT) should be done at ART initiation and thereafter tailored to individual drug regimens. The full panel of LFT is expensive, therefore it is recommended that only the alanine transferase (ALT) is monitored as this is the most sensitive indicator of drug-induced liver injury. The full LFT profile should be requested in patients with symptoms suggestive of hepatitis. Transient mild elevations of ALT occur very commonly with many drugs. If the cannalicular enzymes are elevated more than ALT, or if conjugated bilirubin is elevated, a liver ultrasound should be conducted to exclude biliary obstruction. Many drugs, notably cotrimoxazole but not the anti-retrovirals, can cause cholestatic hepatitis.

Chronic viral hepatitis is a common co-infection in HIV-infected patients. In southern Africa hepatitis B co-infection is very common, ranging from 5% to 20%. Patients with underlying hepatitis B and C infection frequently experience a 'flare up' of hepatitis when ART is commenced, as part of the immune reconstitution inflammatory syndrome. Hepatitis B can also flare when antiretrovirals that have activity against hepatitis B (lamivudine, emtricitabine and tenofovir) are discontinued or if hepatitis B resistance develops. Therefore hepatitis B status should be determined before starting ART. If the hepatitis B status is unknown it should be determined in patients with suspected drug-induced liver injury. Hepatitis C is very uncommon in southern Africa, but should routinely be tested in intravenous drug users or haemophiliacs.

All antiretroviral agents available in our region may cause hepatotoxicity, but the most common is nevirapine (10 to 15% develop significant elevation of transaminases with laboratory monitoring, but only about 2% present with clinical hepatitis). Ideally patients starting nevirapine should have ALT checked at two, four, eight and 12 weeks after starting. If ALT monitoring is performed then there should be a system in place to obtain the result and an ability to contact the patient. In settings where the result will only be available when the patient is seen in two to four weeks or if the patient cannot be contacted then routine ALT monitoring makes little sense. In all patients starting nevirapine it is essential to educate the patient about the symptoms of hepatitis (nausea, vomiting, anorexia, malaise, jaundice, right upper quadrant pain) or drug rash (which is frequently associated with hepatitis). If such symptoms develop ALT should be done immediately and the result obtained urgently. Patients who develop a rash on nevirapine may develop hepatitis two weeks after the onset of the rash.

Hepatotoxic drugs should be discontinued at high levels of LFT abnormality (see table) or at low levels if any symptoms of hepatitis appear. Rechallenge may be considered in selected cases – consult a specialist. If hepatitis occurred together with a rash, or fever or other systemic involvement rechallenge should NOT be attempted.

NRTIs may cause fatty liver with prolonged usage, especially stavudine and didanosine. Typically ALT is elevated more than AST, and the cannalicular enzymes (GGT and alkaline phosphatase) elevated more than the transaminases. Non-tender hepatomegaly is present. Ultrasound or CT scan will show decreased hepatic density. The condition is not benign and fibrosis may occur in long-standing cases, which has been reported with long term didanosine use. Patients should be told to avoid alcohol. Patients on stavudine or didanosine who develop LFT abnormalities should be switched to safer NRTIs.

Isolated unconjugated hyperbilirubinaemaia (drug-induced Gilbert's syndrome) is associated with some PIs (indinavir and especially atazanavir). This is a benign condition, but is often cosmetically unacceptable to patients.

Many other drugs can cause hepatotoxicity, notably anti-tubercular therapy (including prophylactic isoniazid) and azoles. Cotrimoxazole is a rare cause of hepatitis, usually with a cholestatic picture.

Table 51.2 Guidelines for managing hepatotoxicity

Upper limit of normal (ULN)*	<2.5 x ULN	2.5 – 5 x ULN	>5 x ULN
ALT	Monitor	Repeat 1 week	Discontinue relevant drug(s)
Alk Phos	Monitor	Repeat 2 weeks	Ultrasound Consider biopsy
Bilirubin	Repeat 1 week	Discontinue relevant drug(s)	Discontinue relevant drug(s)

*Any elevations with symptoms of hepatitis (nausea, vomiting, right upper quadrant pain) should be regarded as an indication to stop relevant drugs

Hepatitis in patients on ART and TB therapy

Hepatitis is common in this setting and may be drug-induced or due to TB immune reconstitution inflammatory syndrome (TB-IRIS) with worsening granulomatous hepatitis. TB-IRIS typically presents a few weeks after starting ART in TB patients. The GGT and alkaline phosphatase are typically elevated more than the transaminases, bilirubin is predominantly conjugated and hepatomegaly may be present. However, this diagnosis is difficult to make with certainty as there is no diagnostic test. If the picture is predominantly cholestatic an ultrasound should be done to exclude post-hepatic cholestasis and a liver biopsy should be considered.

The priority in patients developing hepatitis on ART and TB drugs is to sort out the TB therapy first, followed by the ART. If hepatitis develops, as defined above, stop all antiretrovirals (if on a NNRTI-based regimen the NRTIs should be continued for a week), co-trimoxazole and all potentially hepatotoxic TB drugs (isoniazid, rifampicin & pyrazinamide). Three non-hepatotoxic TB drugs (streptomycin 15mg/kg daily, moxifloxacin 400mg daily/levofloxacin 750 mg daily and ethambutol 800–1200mg daily) should be started and continued throughout rechallenge to prevent the development of resistance and provide activity against TB. Once the ALT has settled to <100, rechallenge should be considered. It is important to review the diagnosis of TB before attempting rechallenge. If the diagnosis was not made on good grounds TB therapy should be stopped and the patient carefully monitored. If the hepatitis resulted in hepatic failure (encephalopathy or coagulopathy) then rechallenge should not be done – in this setting additional second line TB drugs may be necessary and treatment should be prolonged for 18 months – consult a TB specialist for advice. Other causes of hepatitis should also be excluded.

TB drug rechallenge has been found to be successful in 60 to 90% of patients and, provided ALT and symptoms are frequently monitored, it is usually safe. Several rechallenge regimens have been suggested and many local institutions have developed their own regimens. Many South African experts do not attempt rechallenge with pyrazinamide, but both the American and British Thoracic Society guidelines recommend this in certain circumstances. In severe forms of TB (e.g. meningitis), pyrazinamide rechallenge should be considered unless the intensive phase is almost complete. The first randomized controlled trial of different rechallenge regimens was recently published, but only HIV seronegative patients were studied. Three rechallenge regimens were tested, and all performed equally well. The three rechallenge regimens are listed below – choice of regimen (and whether to rechallenge with pyrazinamide) is up to the clinician:

- Rifampicin, isoniazid, & pyrazinamide (normal doses) from day 1.
- Day 1: Rifampicin (normal doses). Day 8: Isoniazid (normal doses). Day 15: Pyrazinamide (normal doses).
- Day 1: Isoniazid (100 mg daily). Day 4: Isoniazid (normal doses). Day 8: Rifampicin (150 mg daily). Day 11: Rifampicin (normal doses). Day 15: Pyrazinamide (500 mg daily). Day 18: Pyrazinamide (normal doses).

During rechallenge ALT should be monitored twice weekly, then every two weeks for a month, then monthly until three months.

The duration of TB therapy after rechallenge depends on how much TB therapy has been completed and which drugs were successfully rechallenged. The following durations are rough guidelines – contact a TB specialist for advice if necessary:

- pyrazinamide not rechallenged/not tolerated: stop moxifloxacin/levofloxacin and streptomycin, continue isoniazid, rifampicin and ethambutol for total duration nine months;
- rifampicin not tolerated: continue streptomycin (for two months) and moxifloxacin/levofloxacin, isoniazid, and ethambutol for total duration of 18 months;
- isoniazid not tolerated: stop moxifloxacin/levofloxacin and add ethionamide for total duration 12 months.

ART can be recommenced two weeks following rechallenge with TB therapy:

- If nevirapine was used this should be replaced with efavirenz.
- If efavirenz was used this should be recommenced.
- If double dose lopinavir/ritonavir was used this should be recommenced with slow dose escalation over two weeks.

Hyperlactataemia

NRTIs impair mitochondrial function by inhibiting the mitochondrial enzyme γ-DNA polymerase, which can result in the accumulation of lactate. Individual NRTIs differ in their degree of mitochondrial toxicity: stavudine/didanosine > zidovudine > tenofovir/emtricitabine/lamivudine/abacavir. The combination of didanosine and stavudine is associated with a high risk of symptomatic hyperlactactaemia or lactic acidosis (particularly in pregnancy) and this combination should be avoided. Symptomatic hyperlactataemia is typically seen in patients who have been on NRTIs for more than six months.

Risk factors for hyperlactataemia include:

- female sex;
- obesity;
- >6 months use of NRTIs;
- development of NRTI-induced peripheral neuropathy or fatty liver.

Asymptomatic elevated lactate is common in patients treated with NRTIs, but this does not predict the development of lactic acidosis and therefore it is unnecessary to monitor levels in asymptomatic patients.

Symptomatic hyperlactataemia has become less common and less severe with fewer patients starting ART with stavudine and with the use of lower doses of stavudine. However clinicians should remain vigilant in patients on stavudine and be aware that this side effect can occur with all the other NRTIs, although it is very uncommon with abacavir, tenofovir, 3TC and emtricitabine. Symptoms of symptomatic hyperlactataemia are non-specific and include: nausea and vomiting, abdominal pain, dyspnoea, fatigue and weight loss.

Lactic acidosis is a rare but potentially fatal side effect of NRTIs. A raised lactate of >5 mmol/L, together with metabolic acidosis confirms the diagnosis of lactic acidosis. Low serum bicarbonate (<20mmol/L) is the most sensitive marker of acidosis. Associated abnormalities include elevated AST and ALT, lactate dehydrogenase and creatinine kinase.

The treatment is supportive. High dose riboflavin and L-carnitine may be used, but there is no evidence for either intervention. Management of symptomatic hyperlactataemia depends on the lactate and bicarbonate concentrations:

- Lactate <5mmol/l and bicarbonate >20. NRTIs should be changed to agents less associated with hyperlactataemia: tenofovir or abacavir (if these are unavailable then zidovudine could be used) plus emtricitabine or lamivudine. Symptoms and serial lactate should be done for several months (note that lactate levels decrease slowly over weeks).

- Lactate >5mmol/L and bicarbonate >15. Discontinue NRTIs and the patient should be admitted. If the patient is on an NNRTI regimen, add a boosted protease inhibitor. If the patient has already failed an NNRTI and is on a boosted PI, add raltegravir and/or etravirine if available, or continue with boosted PI only. When lactate normalised switch to safer NRTIs as above.
- Lactate >5mmol/L and bicarbonate <15. Discontinue NRTIs and the patient should be admitted, preferably to an intensive care unit. If the patient is on an NNRTI regimen, add a boosted protease inhibitor. If the patient has already failed an NNRTI and is on a boosted PI, add raltegravir and/or etravirine if available, or continue with boosted PI only. Bicarbonate replacement is controversial, but most experts would partially correct severe acidosis with bicarbonate. Cover with broad spectrum antibiotic as sepsis can mimic NRTI-induced lactic acidosis (this can be discontinued if the procalcitonin is normal). On recovery, all NRTIs should be avoided in future regimens (some experts would be prepared to use safer NRTIs as above).

Dyslipidaemia

PIs, with the exception of unboosted atazanavir, can cause fasting hypertriglyceridaemia, low HDL cholesterol and elevated LDL cholesterol. Boosted atazanavir is associated only with mild dyslipidaemia. Stavudine and efavirenz can cause mild hypertriglyceridaemia. PIs are associated with the most marked elevation of triglycerides. Efavirenz can cause elevated LDL cholesterol. Fasting lipids should be checked after three months on a PI regimen. If normal at this stage it should be performed annually only in those with other cardiovascular risk factors (e.g. diabetes).

Diet and lifestyle modification should always be advised if dyslipidaemia occurs. Diet is much more effective for hypertriglyceridaemia than hypercholesterolaemia. It is essential that other cardiovascular risk factors should be addressed in patients on ART with dyslipidaemia.

Patients with severe hypertriglyceridaemia (>10 mmol/L) may develop pancreatitis. Urgent therapy is required. The fibrates are the drugs of choice. However, in HIV-uninfected patients with mild hypertriglyceridaemia fibrates have not been known to reduce the risk of cardiovascular disease. Thus it is unclear if triglycerides <10 mmol/L should be given.

Drug treatment for high cholesterol, especially high LDL cholesterol, should be considered on the basis of cardiovascular risk factor stratification as for HIV-uninfected patients. The standard tables based on age, smoking, sex, and blood pressure should be used. All type 2 diabetics and patients with established vascular disease need lipid-lowering therapy. If dyslipidaemia warrants therapy in patients on PIs they should be switched to boosted atazanavir, if possible, rather than adding therapy for the dyslipidaemia.

Many statins have interactions with PIs which can lead to potentially toxic concentrations of statins, with the exception of pravastatin and fluvastatin. Atorvastatin concentrations are significantly raised by PIs, but lower doses (e.g. 10 mg daily) can be used. Lovastatin and simvastatin should not be co-administered with PIs as their concentrations are dramatically increased.

Lipodystrophy

Long-term use of ART may cause chronic lipodystrophic changes with a change in body fat distribution. This can present either with fat accumulation (visceral obesity, breast enlargement, "buffalo hump", lipomata) or with fat loss (lipo-atrophy, presenting as facial, limb and buttock wasting) or with both fat loss and accumulation. Redistribution of body fat may be cosmetically unacceptable to the patient, resulting in discontinuing ART.

The thymidine analogue NRTIs (zidovudine and especially stavudine) are associated with fat loss. Lipoatrophy improves when stavudine/zidovudine is substituted with an NRTI less associated with such adverse effects e.g. tenofovir or abacavir, but resolution is very slow and incomplete. Therefore it is important to recognise lipoatrophy early or, better still, use NRTIs that are not associated with lipoatrophy.

Previously PIs were thought to be the cause of lipohypertrophy. However, more recent studies have shown that all classes of antiretrovirals are associated with fat gain to a similar extent. Furthermore, longitudinal studies comparing HIV-uninfected people with HIV-infected people on long term ART show that the extent and distribution of fat gain are similar. These data suggest that fat gain is a consequence of treating HIV. The appearance of the fat gain is particularly unsightly when accompanied by subcutaneous fat loss.

There is no good evidence to support switching antiretrovirals in patients with fat accumulation. Exercise helps to reduce abdominal fat. Surgery should be considered in selected cases with focal fat gain (e.g. those with prominent 'buffalo humps'), but recurrences are not uncommon. Metformin modestly reduces weight and improves insulin resistance in patients with the metabolic syndrome or isolated dysglycaemia. Visceral fat accumulation is associated with insulin resistance and dyslipidaemia in the same way that it does in HIV-uninfected patients. Other cardiovascular risk factors should be addressed in such patients (e.g. smoking, hypertension).

Hypersensitivity

Cutaneous hypersensitivity to drugs other than antiretrovirals, notably co-trimoxazole, is more common in HIV-infected patients. Some drug-induced skin rashes, notably Stevens-Johnson syndrome and toxic epidermal necrolysis, are life-threatening. Mucosal involvement is the hallmark of the Stevens-Johnson syndrome. Desquamation involving more than 30% of body surface area is termed toxic epidermal necrolysis. Rashes accompanied by systemic features are also potentially life-threatening. Patients with either Stevens-Johnson syndrome or toxic epidermal necrolysis should be admitted for treatment, preferably to a burns unit under the care of a dermatologist.

Rashes due to NNRTIs occur commonly in the first six weeks of therapy. Rashes are more severe and frequent with nevirapine. If a rash on NNRTIs is accompanied by systemic features (e.g. fever, elevated ALT, hepatitis), mucosal involvement or blistering, discontinue the NNRTI immediately and do not rechallenge. If the rash occurs without these features, the NNRTI can be continued and the rash treated symptomatically with antihistamines and possibly also topical steroids. Systemic steroids should not be used. Patients who develop rashes during the low dose nevirapine 'lead in' phase (200mg daily) must not have the dosage increased to 200mg 12 hourly until the reaction has completely resolved. This 'treat through' approach is only acceptable if the patient can be carefully observed, otherwise substitute for a drug from a different class.

There is a possible cross-reaction between nevirapine and efavirenz, although most studies report no evidence of this. It is acceptable to substitute efavirenz for nevirapine in the event of hypersensitivity, unless the reaction was life-threatening. There is hardly any data on substituting nevirapine for efavirenz in the event of hypersensitivity, so this substitution is not recommended.

Abacavir hypersensitivity is primarily a systemic reaction occurring within the first eight weeks of therapy. Fatalities may occur, especially on rechallenge. Abacavir must be discontinued and never rechallenged. The manifestations of hypersensitivity include: fever, rash, fatigue and abdominal or respiratory symptoms. If there is any doubt about the diagnosis (e.g. if the patient has a cough with fever) then the patient should be admitted for observation. Symptoms progress if hypersensitivity is present. The hypersensitivity reaction has been shown to be on a genetic basis, being virtually confined to the HLA-B*5701 allele, which is very uncommon in Africans. If affordable, this allele should be excluded prior to using abacavir.

Raltegravir and darunavir can both cause rashes. Stevens-Johnson syndrome has been reported with raltegravir. Darunavir has a sulphonamide moiety and is best avoided in patients with hypersensitivity to sulphon-amides.

Nephrotoxicity

A serum creatinine and urinalysis for proteinuria must be done at baseline in all patients to detect sub-clinical renal disease as there is an increased risk of renal failure in HIV infection due to a variety of causes. The dose of NRTIs, except abacavir, needs to be adjusted in renal failure.

In a minority of patients, tenofovir may cause a tubular wasting syndrome of phosphate, glucose and potassium. If patients on tenofovir develop muscle weakness or other muscle symptoms then check serum potassium and phosphate. Tenofovir can also cause acute renal failure, but this is uncommon. Finally, tenofovir is associated with a more rapid age-associated decline in renal function.

It is essential to estimate the creatinine clearance before commencing tenofovir, which should not be used if the clearance is <50 mL/min. The creatinine should be monitored at three months, six months, then six monthly in patients on tenofovir. In high risk patients (particularly those with co-morbidities) creatinine should also be checked at one and two months. Long term use of tenofovir with other nephrotoxic agents (e.g. aminoglycosides, NSAIDs) should be avoided. In patients where tenofovir is avoided because creatinine clearance is < 50 ml/min at baseline it may be possible to switch to tenofovir at a later point if renal function improves. This is often the case if patients have chronic diarrhoea or other opportunistic infections at the time of starting ART.

Neuropsychiatric toxicity

Efavirenz frequently causes neuropsychiatric effects in the first few weeks of therapy. This typically presents with insomnia, vivid dreams and dizziness. Both dysphoria and euphoria may occur. Fortunately these features subside in the majority of patients in the first six weeks. Psychosis may occasionally occur. If neuropsychiatric symptoms on efavirenz are not tolerated then switch to nevirapine. Zidovudine and raltegravir frequently cause headache when started, but this usually resolves.

Peripheral neuropathy is common in patients who have been on stavudine or, to a lesser extent, didanosine for more than six months.

Dysglycaemia

The older protease inhibitors, notably indinavir, cause diabetes. However, the newer PIs (atazanavir, darunavir and lopinavir) do not.

Efavirenz, stavudine and zidovudine have all been associated with mild dysglycaemia. Visceral fat gain, which occurs to a similar extent with all antiretroviral classes, is associated with insulin resistance and blood glucose should be serially checked in these patients as part of cardiovascular risk assessment.

Gynaecomastia

Gynaecomastia is the development of breast tissue, not adipose tissue, in men. It may be bilateral or unilateral. Serum testosterone should be measured and replacement therapy given if this is low. Gynaecomastia is most consistently associated with efavirenz and didanosine. Some cases resolve without a change in ART, but consider switching efavirenz to nevirapine or didanosine for another NRTI if gynaecomastia develops without testosterone deficiency.

Pancreatitis

Pancreatitis that is not due to alcohol or gall stones occurs more frequently in HIV-infected patients. Didanosine and stavudine can cause pancreatitis. PIs, notably lopinavir, can cause marked hypertriglyceridaemia, which can cause pancreatitis. 3TC has been suggested as a possible cause of pancreatitis, but this is not confirmed.

References and further reading

Boulle, A., Orrell, C., Kaplan, R., et al. 2007. Substitutions due to antiretroviral toxicity or contraindication in the first three years of ART in a large South African cohort. *Antiviral Therapy*, 12:753–760.

Dave, J.A., Lambert, E.V., Badri, M., et al. 2011. Effect of non-nucleoside reverse transcriptase inhibitor-based antiretroviral therapy on dysglycaemia and insulin sensitivity in South African HIV-infected patients. *J AIDS*, 57:284–289.

Dube, M.P., Shen, C., Greenwald, M., Mather, K.J. 2008. No Impairment of Endothelial Function or Insulin Sensitivity with 4 Weeks of the HIV Protease Inhibitors Atazanavir or Lopinavir-Ritonavir in Healthy Subjects without HIV Infection: A Placebo-Controlled Trial. *Clin Infect Dis*, 47:567–574.

Guaraldi, G., Squillace, N., Stentarelli, C., et al. 2008. Nonalcoholic fatty liver disease in HIV-infected patients referred to a metabolic clinic: prevalence, characteristics and predictors. *Clin Infect Dis,* 47:250–257.

Grunfeld, C., Saag, M., Cofrancesco, J., et al. 2010. Regional adipose tissue measured by MRI over 5 years in HIV-infected and control participants indicates persistence of HIV-associated lipoatrophy. *AIDS,* 24:1717–1726

Leung, V.L., Glesby, M.J. 2011. Pathogenesis and treatment of HIV lipohypertrophy. *Current Opinion in Infectious Diseases*, 24:43–49.

Mehta, U., Maartens, G. 2007. Is it safe to switch between efavirenz and nevirapine in the event of toxicity? A review of the evidence. *Lancet Infect Dis*, 7:733–738.

Mira, J.A., Lozano, F., Santos, J., et al. 2004. Gynaecomastia in HIV-infected men on highly active antiretroviral therapy: association with efavirenz and didanosine treatment. *Antiviral Therapy*, 9: 511–517.

Moyle, G.J., Sabin, C.A., Cartledge, J., et al. 2006. A randomized comparative trial of tenofovir DF or abacavir as replacement for a thymidine analogue in persons with lipoatrophy. *AIDS*, 20: 2043–2050.

Sanne, I., Mommeja-Marin, H., Hinkle, J., et al. 2005. Severe hepatotoxicity associated with nevirapine use in HIV-infected patients. *J Infect Dis*, 191:825–829.

Occupational post-exposure prophylaxis

Health care workers (HCWs) are at risk for occupational infections with blood-borne viruses, including hepatitis B virus (HBV), hepatitis C virus (HCV), and HIV. Occupational exposures result directly from accidental injuries, failing to comply with universal standard precautions (all patients should be treated as potentially infectious), and a breach of protective barriers. Table 52.1 lists infectious and non-infectious body fluids.

Most occupational exposures are preventable, and incidents should be reviewed by infection control teams and managerial staff regularly, to assess whether prevention programmes can be improved. Many occupational injuries occur after-hours or during emergencies or in the cleaning-up phase after procedures. Sharps containers should be easily accessible at the site of blood taking and procedures. Reducing the risk of exposure by changing the manner in which a task is performed promotes safer work practice. For example, recapping needles should not be performed but placed immediately into a sharps container. Although current concern for infection is focused on the risk of HIV infection, the magnitude of risk associated with parenteral occupational exposure to HIV is lower than that associated with either HBV or HCV. Tables 52.2 and 52.3 respectively summarize the factors predicting transmission of HIV to a HCW after percutaneous exposure, and the risk of transmission of occupational infections.

HCWs must be familiar with the procedures following an occupational exposure. In any health care setting, each exposure must be followed systematically, with immediate evaluation and counselling of the exposed HCW and source patient, investigation into the circumstances of the exposure, and periodic follow-up of the HCW. All hospitals and health care facilities should have a HIV exposure injury protocol in place and it should incorporate the following post-exposure management principles.

Management immediately after exposure

Treat all types of exposures as though they were equally serious and manage them in the same way.

Table 52.1 Infectious and non-infectious body fluids

Infectious body fluids	Non-infectious body fluids
All body fluids containing blood	Tears
Vaginal secretions	Faeces
Semen	Urine
Pericardial fluid	Saliva
Pleural fluid	Nasal secretions
Cerebrospinal fluid	Sputum
Amniotic fluid	Vomit
Peritoneal fluid	Sweat
Synovial fluid	

Source: Centers for Disease Control and Prevention, 1998.

Table 52.2 Factors predicting transmission of HIV to a health care worker after percutaneous exposure

	Adjusted odds ratio (95% CI)
Deep injury	16.1 (6.1–44.6)
Visible blood on needle/instrument	5.2 (1.8–17.7)
Needle used to enter blood vessel	5.1 (1.9–14.8)
Source patient has terminal AIDS	6.4 (2.2–18.9)
AZT prophylaxis used	0.2 (0.1–0.6)

Source: Centers for Disease Control and Prevention, 1998.

Table 52.3 Risk of transmission after percutaneous exposure

Virus	Risk
HIV	0.1–0.3%
Hepatitis B – eAg negative	2%
Hepatitis B – eAg positive	20–40%
Hepatitis C	1–10%

Source: Centers for Disease Control and Prevention, 1998.

Clean the exposed area immediately

Routine recommendations are that:
- *puncture wounds* should be washed with soap and large volumes of water;
- *mucosal exposures* involving the mouth and nose should be flushed vigorously with water; and
- *eyes* should be irrigated with clean water or eye irrigants.

Immediately inform the person in charge

The person in charge will institute management procedures and must urgently arrange to take blood from the source patient and injured HCW to test for HIV, HBV, and HCV. Syphilis and malaria are not routinely tested for, but may be indicated depending on the source patient's illness and the geographic setting or travel history in the case of malaria.

Counselling

HCWs occupationally exposed to HIV should be counselled and tested for HIV antibodies as soon as possible after the exposure. The need for counselling should not be underestimated, and one is likely to encounter fear, anger, sadness, depression, anxiety, and denial. Equally important is counselling and support around predictable side effects if antiretrovirals are used for prophylaxis. Counselling is perhaps the single most critical component of post-exposure management and it should involve informing the HCW's partner and discussing condom use. (See also Chapter 7: Counselling.)

Exposure report

All occupational exposures must be documented and reported in detail. Exposure to all body fluids and tissues, regardless of HIV risk, should be reported and evaluated to assess the risk of transmission and to determine the need for post-exposure prophylaxis (PEP). The exposed worker should provide accurate information about:
- the date and time of exposure;
- the type of exposure experienced (puncture, laceration, mucous membrane splash);
- the mechanism of exposure, and details of the procedure being performed (i.e. where, how, type of device);

- the source of the exposure (i.e. material, patient history, stage of disease);
- the type and amount of body fluid to which the worker was exposed (i.e. blood, bloody saliva, other body fluids); and
- whether gloves, eye protection, and masks were used at the time of exposure.

Rationale for post-exposure prophylaxis (PEP)

Macaque SIV infection studies have shown that tenofovir PEP started within 24 hours of exposure and continued for 28 days protected 100% of those infected from seroconverting. A single retrospective case-control study in the United States documented that zidovudine PEP reduced seroconversion by 81% following a percutaneous exposure involving HIV containing blood. After an occupational exposure, the source patient and the exposed HCW should be evaluated to determine the need for PEP. PEP is recommended only if the HCW has been exposed to blood or other HIV-containing body fluids through percutaneous injury, or exposure to broken skin and mucous membranes. Note the following:

- If the HCW is HIV-positive, no prophylactic medication for HIV is required. Many healthcare workers in southern Africa learn of their HIV status after an occupational exposure, and adequate counselling and rapid staging and referral for care should be anticipated.
- If the source patient is negative, then no prophylaxis is required.
- If the source patient is HIV-positive and the staff member is negative then it is recommended that PEP be taken.
- If the source patient's status is unknown and the staff member is negative, then it is recommended that PEP be taken.

Recommended prophylaxis

Recommendations for PEP should be explained to the HCW, together with the risks and benefits of receiving it. The PEP medication should be commenced as soon as possible after the exposure. PEP should not be given if more than 72 hours have elapsed following the exposure.

Low-risk exposures require the basic regimen of two nucleoside reverse transcriptase inhibitors (NRTIs). The nucleoside/nucleotide analogues recommended for PEP include either tenofovir (TDF), or zidovudine (AZT), together with emtricitabine or lamivudine (3TC). AZT is often recommended over the others as the only PEP study in humans used AZT. However, the efficacy of AZT in reducing transmission is considered to be due to its ability to inhibit HIV replication. Thus, any nucleoside/ nucleotide should be equally efficacious. AZT is also poorly tolerated in the PEP setting. A ritonavir-boosted protease inhibitor (atazanavir, lopinavir or darunavir) should be added if the risk of transmission is higher. Efavirenz may also be considered if a third drug is needed, but has a high frequency of rash and neuropsychiatric side effects. Nevirapine is not recommended, due to several case reports of severe toxicity following PEP. It must be stressed that there is no hard evidence that a second drug adds to the value of PEP, nor indeed that a third drug adds to the value of PEP. There is clear evidence that side-effects increase significantly with a third drug. Nevertheless all international PEP guidelines recommend two or three drug regimens as it is likely that these will be more effective than monotherapy. Data from animal studies show that PEP should be administered for four weeks. Frequent follow-up is recommended, so that if a HCW is experiencing side effects from the PEP medication, other medications can be substituted.

With the increasing use of antiretroviral therapy and the development of viral resistance, there is a risk of infection with viruses resistant to the standard PEP regimens. A drug history should be taken from every source patient, as the prophylactic regimen may need to be modified. Expert advice should be sought if resistance is suspected (national HIV & TB HCW hotline 0800-212506).

Table 52.5 summarizes practical guidelines for PEP against HBV within 48 hours of exposure.

Sustaining a needle-stick injury causes considerable psychological distress, often compounded by drug toxicity, and every effort should be made to attend to the HCW as quickly as possible and to provide appropriate follow-up and counselling.

Monitoring

Baseline creatinine and full blood count should be done if TDF or AZT respectively are used. Toxicity due to any drug used that cannot be managed symptomatically (e.g. nausea, headaches) should trigger a drug switch to an alternative. HIV antibody testing should be done at six weeks, 12 weeks, and six months. Note that PCR testing following occupational exposure is not recommended as it is not validated in this setting – most positive PCR results after occupational exposure will be false positives, which causes considerable distress. PCR should only be done, in consultation with an expert, if there are clinical features of seroconversion illness.

Table 52.4 Recommendations for PEP after exposure to infectious material (includes blood, CSF, semen, vaginal secretions and synovial, pleural, pericardial, peritoneal and amniotic fluid) from HIV-seropositive patients

Exposure	HIV Status of Source Patient		
	Positive	Unknown	Negative
Intact skin	No PEP	No PEP	No PEP
Mucocutaneous splash / Non-intact skin	2 drugs	2 drugs	No PEP
Percutaneous injury	3 drugs	3 drugs	No PEP

Table 52.5 Hepatitis B virus post-exposure prophylaxis

Status of HCW	Hepatitis B carrier status of source patient		
	Unknown	Negative	HBsAg (HBeAg) +ve
Unvaccinated or unknown	HBIG + vaccinate (3 doses)	Vaccinate (3 doses)	HBIG + vaccinate (3 doses)
Vaccinated. Titre of antibodies to HBsAg <50 units/L	Booster dose	Booster dose	HBIG + vaccine booster dose
Vaccinated. Titre of antibodies to HBsAg >50 units/L	No action	No action	No action
Non responder to vaccine HBsAg <10 units/L (3 doses of vaccine)	HBIG if available + 2 further vaccine doses	2 further vaccine doses	HBIG + 2 further vaccine doses
Non response to vaccine HBsAg <10 units/L (5 doses of vaccine)	HBIG if available	No action	HBIG

Source: Centers for Disease Control and Prevention, 1998.

Follow-up

HCWs with occupational exposure to HIV should receive follow-up counselling, post-exposure testing, and medical evaluation, regardless of whether or not they receive PEP. Counselling should cover the possibility of HIV seroconversion, the importance of starting prophylaxis, and behavioural changes that will have to be made for at least six months to prevent transmission of HIV to others. HIV-exposed HCWs should be advised to practice sexual abstinence or use condoms, avoid pregnancy, and refrain from donating blood, plasma, organs, tissue, or semen. Expert advice should be sought for HCWs who are pregnant or breastfeeding (national HIV & TB HCW hotline 0800-212506).

Summary

Post-exposure management of a HCW should include:

- immediate wound management;
- a report to the person in charge and a detailed record of the incident;
- a risk assessment;
- a blood sample from both the HCW and the source patient along with the necessary pre-test counselling and informed consent;
- a decision on whether to initiate PEP;
- active side-effect management;
- counselling, including advice on PEP, an explanation of monitoring, and safe sex;
- monitoring;
- follow-up at two weeks, four weeks, six weeks, 12 weeks, and six months; and
- post-test counselling.

References and further reading

Centers for Disease Control and Prevention. 2001. Updated U.S. Public Health Service Guidelines for the Management of Occupational Exposures to HBV, HCV, and HIV and Recommendations for Postexposure Prophylaxis. *MMWR*, 50 (No. RR-11):1–53.

Centers for Disease Control and Prevention. 2005. Updated U.S. Public Health Service guidelines for the management of occupational exposures to HIV and recommendations for Postexposure Prophylaxis. *MMWR*, 54 (No. RR-9):1–19.

Guidelines on occupational and non-occupational exposure from the Southern African HIV Clinicians Society, published in 2008, are available from their website http://www.sahivsoc.org/

PART 6

Holistic patient care

53 Primary care approach 553
54 Integrating HIV and TB services 569
55 Palliative care 576
56 Women's health 596
57 Gay sex and sexuality 602
58 Ethical issues 608
59 Health care worker burnout 624
60 Micronutrient and complementary
   therapies 629

Primary care approach

Healthcare workers (HCWs) in primary care facilities in sub-Saharan Africa grapple with the challenges of managing large numbers of HIV-infected patients, and must deal with the far-reaching impact of the HIV/AIDS epidemic in the communities in which they work. Expanded access to antiretroviral therapy has transformed the focus of HIV care at primary care level from palliation to long term chronic care.

As with the management of other chronic diseases, management at primary care level requires a multidisciplinary team, including counsellor, pharmacist, social worker, dietician, nurse and doctor. In many parts of sub-Saharan Africa, doctors are a scarce resource, and the bulk of the load of HIV care in the public sector falls on nurse practitioners. Support of nurse practitioners in the form of training and efficient referral systems is critical. The extent of the HIV epidemic means that all medical practitioners should have a working knowledge of HIV medicine and the skills to provide primary care to HIV-infected patients.

This chapter looks at the specific tasks, obstacles, and opportunities facing HCWs at primary care level, in both public and private sector practice.

Primary care goals

The goals of primary care include:

- implementing effective strategies to prevent HIV transmission;
- implementing efficient systems for diagnosis and clinical staging of HIV-infected patients;
- providing ongoing clinical care of HIV-infected patients (including pre-antiretroviral care, antiretroviral initiation, follow up on antiretroviral therapy, adherence support, and management of adherence problems);
- providing ongoing care to families of HIV-infected patients;
- making cost-effective and optimal use of limited resources;
- engaging in patient advocacy;
- conducting relevant audits and research appropriate to the needs of the local community.

Strategies to prevent HIV transmission include:
- providing information about HIV to the community;
- encouraging voluntary counselling and testing;
- providing information to patients on safer sexual practices;
- ensuring that both male and female condoms are readily available and that patients know how to use them;
- providing support and encouragement for patients to disclose their HIV status to their sexual partners;
- facilitating access to safe male circumcision;
- providing accessible and effective treatment for sexually transmitted infections;
- implementing strategies to prevent mother-to-child transmission (MTCT); and
- effective use of antiretroviral therapy.

Important aspects of care for HIV-infected patients and their families are:
- diagnosis and treatment of acute and ongoing problems;
- providing 'safety net' care, including careful instructions on how to deal with common side-effects, and walk-in emergency treatment;
- prompt identification of patients requiring antiretroviral initiation - this requires good pre-antiretroviral follow up and support;
- provision of antiretroviral therapy, and prophylaxis and treatment for opportunistic infections (reliable drug supply to primary care clinics is critical);
- counselling and support;
- nutritional and lifestyle advice;
- assistance with social problems, including applications for disability, child support, and care dependency grants when appropriate;
- preventative medical care such as screening (e.g. Pap smears) and contraception, and management of other common primary care conditions (such as diabetes, hypertension and epilepsy);
- provision of accessible clinical care – this may include evening or weekend clinics for people who are employed;
- patient education, including education about the significance of laboratory investigations and the possibility of drug side-effects;
- appropriate referral for investigation or admission; and
- appropriate initiation and provision of palliative care.

Challenges facing primary care practitioners include:
- Developing efficient systems to cope with large numbers of HIV-infected patients.
- Continuing medical education in a new field, with many varied problems and complex treatment regimens.
- Overcoming personal fears of HIV infection, and prejudice towards patients with a serious sexually transmitted infection.
- Treating large numbers of young patients presenting for the first time with advanced disease.
- Dealing with community apathy and stigmatization and with the rejection of HIV-infected individuals.
- Coping with lack of political support at local, regional and national levels.

The primary care HIV clinic

See Table 53.1 and Appendix 53.1 for a summary of the important considerations when setting up an HIV clinic.

Primary care management requires a multidisciplinary approach. The primary care practitioner needs to identify and make use of existing resources within the community, and to be proactive about encouraging the development of resources for education, care, and support. Creating a clinic community advisory board (comprised of clinic staff and community representatives including HIV-infected people and/or their families) may be useful in order to involve the community in decisions around clinic management, identify problems, gauge the attitudes to HIV and treatment in the community, and address community apathy and stigmatization.

In order to make optimal use of valuable and limited resources, HIV clinics in both the public and private sectors need to be financially well managed. HIV management is labour intensive, and requires more time, on average, than management of other primary care patients. Careful time management is, therefore, essential. Using structured clerking notes helps with efficient identification and ongoing management of problems, and with the development of an appropriate standard of practice guidelines. Patient-carried records may be valuable. Scheduling regular clinical team meetings, where charts and management decisions of clinical problems and deaths are reviewed, are valuable in identifying quality of care problems, and identifying areas of need for continuing medical education (CME) or training.

A pleasant and well-equipped working environment improves patient care, and reduces the stress levels of all staff members. Adequate working space is important (see text box) and basic medical equipment is essential (see Appendix 53.1).

> Space needs in the HIV clinic are:
> * a comfortable and non threatening waiting area;
> * a private space for counselling;
> * a secure pharmacy;
> * a private and secure consulting room;
> * a space for support groups to meet;
> * a staff room.

Table 53.1 Considerations when establishing an HIV practice

The primary care team	Time constraints in the medical consultation	Financial planning needed
Medical doctor	History taking*	Infrastructure (see Appendix 54.1)
Professional nurse	(often multiple problems)	Salaries for qualified staff
Pharmacist	Assessment of counselling needs	Billing for longer consultation times
Trained lay counsellor	Time for the patient to undress	Administration time
Social worker	Examination of more than one body region	Additional telephone and faxing costs
Dietician	Completing forms for investigations and managed care schemes	Staff time for continuing medical education
Interpreter (if necessary)	Accessing laboratory results	Staff time for debriefing
	Telephone consultations	Computers, appropriate software, and Internet access
	Referring patients	
	Patient education	
	Adherence evaluation	
	Dealing with social problems	

*Social and background history taking can be spread over several consultations if necessary.

Patient booking

Adherence to clinic appointments should be reinforced and 'walk-in' visits should be restricted to patients who are acutely ill, or who are running short of antiretroviral therapy due to unavoidable social issues. Clinic policy for patients who habitually disregard appointments should have buy-in from all staff members and should be uniformly applied. Doctor's leave should be scheduled well in advance to avoid overloading colleagues while away.

Antiretroviral waiting list

Most under-resourced antiretroviral clinics will have a waiting list of patients who want to start treatment. A uniform policy will need to be developed in consultation with staff members, referring clinics and district management to ensure that access to treatment is as equitable as possible. The needs of patients who test early and book before developing AIDS-defining conditions should be weighed against the needs of patients who may not have good access to health care and present for the first time with very advanced disease.

Patient referral

It is important to establish a good referral network. Referring patients is often very frustrating, particularly in the public sector. There is often resistance when referring patients for admission as hospitals in high-prevalence areas are overwhelmed with ill HIV-infected patients, with late disease. Waiting lists for out-patient clinic appointments are long. Close liaison with colleagues working in hospital practice enhances patient care enormously.

Infection control

Nosocomial transmission of tuberculosis in crowded clinic waiting rooms is likely. The waiting room should have open windows, plenty of sunshine and fans directing airflow outside. Cough hygiene should be encouraged, and coughing patients should be offered surgical masks to cover the mouth and nose. Crowding should be reduced by giving patients a time- and date-specific appointment (this can be for morning or afternoon sessions if patient transport is an issue).

Indications for referral

Refer patients for specialist assessment or for investigation by a hospital-based medical team, for:
- suspected symptomatic hyperlactataemia or lactic acidosis on anti-retroviral therapy (see Chapter 20: Common emergencies);

- investigation of persistent fever or unexplained weight loss if two (induced) sputum specimens are smear negative for acid-fast bacilli and the chest radiograph is normal (see Chapter 21: Evaluation of fever);
- lymph node biopsy in a patient with asymmetrically enlarged lymph nodes, if a wide-needle aspiration biopsy has not been helpful (see Chapter 21: Evaluation of fever);
- dermatological conditions that are refractory to primary care treatment (see Chapter 40: Dermatology); and
- cervical dysplasia, for colposcopy (see Chapter 26: Gynaecology).

Dealing with diagnostic and management uncertainty is a fundamental component of primary care practice. 'Safety-net' instructions to patients, telephonic consultations, and policies for common problems help to improve patient care and reduce caregiver anxiety. Policies should be developed that take into account local resources, expertise and preferences. Try to get input from a representative number of interested health care workers to ensure widespread acceptance and implementation.

For in-patient management refer:
- any patient with an acute, potentially reversible illness (e.g. Stevens-Johnson syndrome, lactic acidosis, hepatitis, pancreatitis, severe sepsis, PCP, meningitis, pyelonephritis, dehydration, altered mental status, status epilepticus, or new focal neurological signs).

Note:
- HIV-positive status is not in itself a criterion for referral to a specialist centre.
- The decision to refer a patient for admission or investigation should take into account the patient's baseline level of function. For patients with advanced disease that does not improve clinically on antiretroviral therapy it may be most appropriate to initiate palliative care and refer the patient to a home-based care organization (see Chapter 56: Palliative care).

Communication

When writing a referral letter to a hospital team, the following are important points:
- Include the patient's name and date of birth.
- Clearly state the problem and document significant clinical findings.

- Summarize the HIV background, including the World Health Organization (WHO) clinical stage (with staging conditions).
- Give details of the prophylactic medications.
- Supply details of current and previous antiretroviral therapy, with CD4 count and viral load results.
- Give relevant past medical and surgical history, allergies, contraception, and current medications (including vitamins, antacids, sleeping pills, over-the-counter and traditional remedies).
- Request a detailed reply.

The reply from the referral hospital should give details of:
- the problem with which the patient was referred;
- new diagnoses made during the patient's admission and/or out-patient visits;
- results of relevant investigations (e.g. CD4 count, haemoglobin and differential, white cell counts, renal function, virology, histology, and microbiology reports);
- new medications and duration of treatment;
- psychosocial interventions (e.g. ongoing post-test counselling, disability grant applications, hospice referral);
- arrangements made for further specialized follow-up; and
- prognosis.

Advantages and disadvantages of dedicated HIV clinics at primary care facilities

Advantages

- Reliable uninterrupted drug supply is often easier to ensure in dedicated clinics. This is critical for antiretroviral provision.
- Patients network at the clinic while waiting to be seen, providing an informal support group and facilitating the exchange of valuable information.
- Most primary care facilities are overstretched and overcrowded. Dedicated clinics may make care more accessible, particularly to ill patients with advanced disease.
- Patients develop an ongoing therapeutic relationship with their primary-care providers and HIV care team.
- A clearly visible and well-run service encourages others to come forward to be tested, in order to access care.

- Dedicated HIV clinics facilitate a thorough and systematic approach to HIV-infected patients, set standards of care, and provide ongoing assessment of whether these standards are realistic and have been maintained.
- Dedicated clinics provide sites to train HCWs in the principles of HIV management.

Disadvantages

- It is very difficult to maintain confidentiality and patients may feel exposed. All patients attending a facility rapidly learn where and when the HIV clinic is operating.
- Dedicated clinics may perpetuate the myth that HIV patients are different from other patients and need different treatment.
- The burden of HIV care is placed on selected HCWs, while others abdicate responsibility. This leads to frustration, burnout, and resentment. Management of acute problems may be delayed until the dedicated clinic day.

In practice, a compromise is often the most practical solution - often both options may exist within a facility. Patients with symptomatic disease (WHO Stage 3 and 4) and numerous HIV-related medical problems often prefer to be seen in a dedicated clinic. Patients with early disease will often not want to attend a dedicated clinic because of issues of confidentiality. Patients should be given the choice, where possible.

Issues of confidentiality

In a primary care facility, many members of staff live in the community that the facility serves. Often, patients know members of staff socially. Many people have access to a patient's medical record.

Confidentiality in this setting refers to confidentiality within the facility (i.e. all staff within the facility must understand and practise the ethos that no information gained within the facility will be discussed outside the facility), rather than simply confidentiality between doctor and patient.

It is difficult, if not impossible, to guarantee patients complete confidentiality. This needs to be explained to patients as part of pre-test counselling. Some patients will find this unacceptable and may want to attend another facility away from where they live, in order to be more anonymous. The patient's choice should be respected.

Arrange that all staff members in the facility, including non-professional staff, receive education about HIV generally, and about issues of confidentiality. It may be useful to get all members of your multidisciplinary team to agree to and sign a clinic confidentiality agreement. (See also Chapter 58: Ethical issues.)

Disclosure

Often, the primary care practitioner is the health care provider for the family of an HIV-infected patient. Issues of non-disclosure of HIV status to sexual partners can be very problematic, especially when the sexual partner is also your patient! In this context, pre-test counselling should always include an explicit discussion of feelings about disclosure. The doctor should explain his or her obligation to disclose a patient's status to contacts at risk. It is helpful to get explicit consent from the patient for disclosure to his or her partner, and to document this clearly in your notes. (See Chapter 58: Ethical issues.)

Working with interpreters

Interpreters are often members of the community and are an invaluable source of information about local culture and belief systems. Interpreters are often members of the community that your facility covers, and may know patients socially. It is very important to discuss a policy of confidentiality with the interpreter.

HIV-related consultations may take longer than other consultations in your facility, and your interpreter is often requested to ask quite detailed and probing personal questions on your behalf, including questions about the patient's sexual behaviour. It is important to spend time with the interpreter explaining why you ask the questions that you do, and what their importance is in the management of your patients.

Remember that your interpreter is vulnerable to burnout – he or she needs debriefing and support.

Burnout

The burnout rate in HIV clinicians is high, and preventing burnout in essential staff is a cost-effective use of resources (see Chapter 59: Health-care worker burnout).

Decanting antiretroviral patients to nurse-based primary care

The South African antiretroviral rollout is doctor-based. This limits access to antiretroviral therapy as there are not enough doctors to meet the needs of all patients who want treatment. One solution is for stable patients on antiretroviral therapy to be decanted to nurse-based primary health care clinics for continued care.

Leadership and logistic organization is required to effectively establish ongoing patient management in nurse-led clinics. Important role players include:

- district management;
- the antiretroviral clinic manager;
- the hospital and district pharmacy service;
- the district medical manager;
- the HIV coordinator;
- the laboratory service;
- non-governmental organizations that may be in a position to employ contract staff and provide infrastructure such as computers and clinic equipment;
- activists working on community mobilization (non-discrimination and non-stigmatization, and promotion of openness and disclosure).

Nurses working in clinics that refer large numbers of patients for antiretroviral initiation should preferentially receive antiretroviral training.

Patients who meet the following criteria should be considered for referral back to their local clinic:

- on antiretroviral therapy for more than six months;
- improved clinically;
- an undetectable viral load and a rising CD4 count;
- fully adherent to treatment;
- social issues (specifically social grants through social services) and nutritional issues are resolved.

The primary health care nurse should dispense patients' pre-packaged antiretroviral therapy monthly, and screen for antiretroviral side-effects. Visiting clinicians can review symptomatic patients when necessary. Important side-effects include hyperlactaemia (requires a handheld lactate meter), peripheral neuropathy associated with stavudine, and anaemia caused by zidovudine (requires a handheld haemoglobinometer). The CD4 count and viral load should be repeated every six months (or when clinically indicated), and the results checked by the clinician. The repeat prescription for antiretroviral therapy should be written by the clinician at the same visit. The pharmacy service (especially pharmacy assistants) plays a central role by pre-packing antiretroviral therapy and transporting treatment to the clinics two to four weeks in advance. The transport system should promptly return the renewed prescription card to the pharmacy, and deliver pre-packaged medication and laboratory results back to the clinic, using infrastructure established for other chronic medications.

Children should be reviewed by the clinician frequently as medication doses need to be adjusted as the child gains weight.

Patients should be referred back to the antiretroviral clinic for:
- clinical deterioration including antiretroviral adverse drug reactions;
- virological failure or falling CD4 count;
- loss of developmental milestones in children.

The HIV coordinator plays an essential role:
- identifying challenges and finding practical solutions;
- ensuring the smooth delivery of medications and results to clinics;
- continuing in-service training.

Clinics should be visited regularly to ensure that the system is functioning as smoothly as possible. In-service training and forward planning is essential. Poverty alleviation and nutritional support should be an integral part of the service, and requires ongoing input from the social worker and dietician.

Systematic improvements

Once the decanting system is established consideration can be given to:
- local clinics maintaining a buffer stock of antiretroviral therapy;
- visiting clinicians being able to modify antiretroviral therapy according to clinical guidelines;
- clinicians starting patients on antiretroviral therapy at the primary care clinics;
- primary care nurses starting antiretroviral therapy for selected patients.

Working with community services and donor organizations

Primary care services need to be integrated into the community. Governmental structures and non-governmental organizations offer a variety of services and clinicians need to be aware of available resources. Community responses are an integral part of holistic care for HIV- infected and -affected individuals and families, offering support and access to care that many patients would not be able to access via traditional health service structures. Inter-sectoral links and collaborations are the single most important component of any community programme. The over-riding principle is the provision of comprehensive services (including health and social services) by formal and informal caregivers in the home, in order to promote, restore, and maintain a person's maximal level of comfort, function, and health. It includes a concern for death with dignity.

Members of the community take responsibility for their own health and are empowered to plan, implement, monitor, and evaluate projects, ensuring that children and families have access to health and social welfare services. Programmes aim to be person-centred and culture-sensitive, respecting patient privacy and dignity. Sustainable and cost-effective practices are essential. Importantly, community leadership structures differ widely between urban and rural areas. It is essential to involve traditional healer representatives.

Caregivers and communities should understand the needs of the communities they serve, as well as the needs of the service providers. Health care workers can play an initial leadership role in rationalizing and standardizing clinic services, and may form a bridge between NGOs and local government. In the longer term, responsibility should be handed over to elected officials in the community.

Social workers are an integral part of the extended healthcare team, and have detailed insight into community dynamics. The best medical care will be ineffective if the patient has no food, no home, and no form of income. Medical professionals should complete a disability grant form for patients with symptomatic HIV infection (WHO Stage 3 or 4 or a CD4 count of <200 cells/μl). The social worker, besides providing counselling skills, is invaluable in:

- assisting with applications for identity books, disability grants, child support grants, and care dependency grants;
- drawing up wills;

- liaising with church groups supplying food parcels for patients;
- organizing funeral insurance to relieve a patient's fear about funeral costs; and
- initiating plans for orphan placement, i.e. planning for the future care of potential orphans and arranging guardianship.

Community projects are usually NGO or church led, caring for anything from 10 to 100 patients. Care could include the medical, nursing, social, educational, and spiritual aspects. Examples include: ongoing counselling; help with cooking and/or cleaning; food parcels; material support; wound care; basic hygiene; supervision of drug taking; pain management; identification of OIs; and treatment of tuberculosis (TB) using directly-observed therapy (DOTS).

Various infrastructures that are able to provide different models of care include:
- drop-in centres or support groups;
- outreach and home visiting programmes; and
- comprehensive home-based care (HBC).

A simplistic example of an integrated home or community model would be a care centre situated in the community, attached to a church or school, which houses various facilities (including voluntary counselling and testing [VCT] and continuing education) and provides infrastructure and administrative support (e.g. telephones, fax machines, or computers with Internet access). A Department of Health and Welfare liaison official would play a pivotal role in providing support and guidance, as well as a direct link to the local health care facilities.

Focus is essential when planning an effective service, and a programme may concentrate on only one of the following areas:
- education and prevention;
- people with AIDS;
- support groups;
- HBC-training and manual distribution;
- orphans; or
- mother-to-child transmission (MTCT) and antiretroviral therapy.

The following aspects should be considered when establishing a new programme:
- Identify needy communities.
- Conduct a situational analysis.
- Mobilize communities.

- Establish local funding and implementing structures.
- Identify beneficiaries.
- Involve the community and local and district government in planning, implementing, and evaluating.
- Build capacity at all levels (provide technical assistance).
- Mobilize resources and plan for sustainability.
- Monitor and evaluate.
- Funding and income generation.

It is essential to:
- submit sustainable funding proposals to local government and overseas organizations;
- to monitor delivery and feedback from sponsors; and
- to support group income generation.

Some income-generating ideas include:
- beadwork;
- food gardens and poultry;
- soup kitchens; and
- alliances between richer and poorer communities, e.g. sponsoring a carer.

To strengthen an existing initiative:
- Identify existing interventions.
- Perform a needs assessment of these programmes.
- Strengthen programmes by identifying long-term sources of funding and investing in human resources.
- Plan for sustainability.
- Develop minimum standards and best practices.
- Monitor and evaluate.

Examples of important role players are:
- HCWs in the public and private sectors;
- the Red Cross;
- churches, which provide buildings, infrastructure, and leadership;
- home-based care organizations;
- activists;
- the education sector, including schools and school nurses;
- the welfare section, especially Child Welfare; and
- local government (i.e. elected councillors) and local business.

Ideally, programmes should provide a sustainable salary to key carers and activists.

Activist groups such as the Treatment Action Campaign help to focus attention on neglected areas, mobilize the community and obtain buy-in for new initiates.

An up-to-date index of resources in the community, with current contact details, is essential and should be widely available to all health care workers.

Clinicians may also have a role in raising funding and obtaining support from donor organizations. Potential donors can have complex agendas determined in part by political considerations and funders' requirements. Donations and offers of support may not be entirely philanthropic and could have a 'Trojan horse' element intended to advance business interests. It is very important to obtain detailed written confirmation of the support offered, with timelines, associated costs, and duration for which support can be expected. Consulting with established services in other parts of the country is very helpful.

References and further reading

Evian, C. 1997. *Primary AIDS Care*. Cape Town: Jacana.

http://www.knowledgetranslation.uct.ac.za/work.htm (For annually updated algorithms to guide clinical nurse practitioners in primary care HIV management).

Appendix 53.1 Essential equipment for an HIV Clinic

Clinic equipment

Examination couch, linen and screens
Desk, chairs
Sharps container
Running water and soap
Paper towels
Waste bin for medical materials
Gloves, both sterile and non-sterile
Dressing packs
2% lignocaine
10% povidone-iodine solution, 0.5% chlorhexidine solution in 70% alcohol
Gynaecology lamp
Vaginal speculums
Lockable drug cupboard
Refrigerator
Syringe driver
Patient information posters and leaflets
Intravenous cannulae and fluid administration sets, Ringers-lactate, normal saline 5% dextrose
Nasogastric tubes
Condom catheters
Foley catheters
Urinary bags
Plastic linen savers

Diagnostic equipment

Weight scale
Height ruler
Stadiometer
Tape measure
Glucometer
Haemoglobinometer
Lactate meter
Urine dipsticks
Urine pregnancy tests
Stethoscope
Baumanometer
Pulse oximeter
Diagnostic set
Tongue depressor
Patella hammer
Syringes, needles, laboratory tubes
Alcohol swabs, cotton wool, plaster
Specimen jars
Pus swabs
Spatulas for Pap smears
Glass slides
Cytofixative
Punch biopsy
Mosquito forceps
Scalpel blade
Alcohol and formalin
Lumbar puncture needles
CSF manometers
Ultrasonic nebuliser
5% saline, sterile water
Disposable masks and tubing

Administrative equipment

Notepaper, envelopes, forms (sorted into labeled pigeon-holes)
Telephone
Fax machine with an adequate paper supply
Photocopier with adequate paper supply and back-up toner cartridges
Reliable filing system for patient notes and laboratory results

Related infrastructure

Regular access to pathology laboratory services with consistent results retrieval system
Accessible radiology facilities
Reliably stocked pharmacy

Integrating HIV and TB services

Sustainable integration of TB/HIV services is the single greatest challenge facing primary health care services in southern Africa. Fundamental to the successful implementation of an integrated service is a stable group of well supervised healthcare professionals supported by coherent national policies, realistic strategic planning and appropriate budgeting, and responsive district management.

Core services should include:
- clinical staff trained in TB/HIV care;
- intensified tuberculosis case finding;
- adequately staffed sputum microscopy laboratory;
- voluntary counselling and testing for HIV infection;
- access to chest radiography and experienced medical practitioners;
- adherence training programmes for both antituberculous therapy and antiretroviral therapy;
- reliable supply of first-line antituberculous drugs, co-trimoxazole, isoniazid preventative therapy, and antiretroviral therapy;
- effective patient registration, monitoring, reporting and defaulter tracing;
- infection control procedures;
- other essential primary care services including syndromic treatment of sexually transmitted infections and contraception;
- staff support including debriefing and feedback.

Appendix 54.1 gives details of the WHO's DOTS strategy, and Appendix 54.2 gives the details for monitoring antituberculous therapy. Refer to Chapter 22: Primary prophylaxis, Chapter 24: Adult tuberculosis (the section on antiretroviral therapy), Chapter 50: Immune reconstitution inflammatory syndrome and Chapter 53: Primary care approach.

Diagnosing and treating HIV in tuberculosis patients

Between 60%–80% of tuberculosis patients are co-infected with HIV, and most are unaware of their HIV sero-status. The diagnosis of tuberculosis is a unique opportunity for healthcare workers to offer voluntary counselling and testing for HIV infection. Potential benefits for the patient include:

- an opportunity to learn about safer sexual practices;
- co-trimoxazole preventative therapy;
- measurement of CD4 count;
- screening for other HIV-associated conditions (e.g. oral thrush, pre-cancerous lesions of the cervix);
- antiretroviral therapy;
- ongoing isoniazid preventative therapy after completion of anti-tuberculous therapy.

All tuberculosis patients should be offered HIV testing repeatedly during treatment, preferably on-site by the same healthcare team. A well-functioning programme could consider introducing 'opt-out' testing. Patients who test HIV-positive should be offered empathetic post-test counselling, and be encouraged to consider disclosing the result to trusted family members and friends.

Diagnosing, treating and preventing tuberculosis in HIV-infected patients

Tuberculosis is the commonest cause of death in patients living with HIV, and it is appropriate to focus healthcare resources on prompt diagnosis and treatment. Intensified case finding refers to the WHO strategy of screening every HIV-infected patient for tuberculosis symptoms at the time of diagnosis and at every subsequent contact with a health care worker.

The set of questions used to screen for tuberculosis has not been standardised but should include:

- cough (usually for more than two weeks);
- drenching night sweats;
- weight loss and loss of appetite;
- unusual fatigue;
- swollen lymph nodes;
- shortness of breath;
- chest pain, and abdominal pain or swelling.

Routine chest radiograph should be reserved for symptomatic patients with negative sputum smears or non-productive cough. Symptomatic patients should be referred for further assessment.

A minimum of six months of isoniazid preventative therapy can be considered for patients who have no tuberculosis symptoms, have stable weight and reliable clinic attendance. Importantly, this should be given by the HIV Wellness Clinic and not by the tuberculosis programme, due to the substantial risk of well HIV patients becoming infected by patients with active pulmonary tuberculosis.

Immune reconstitution following the initiation of antiretroviral therapy can unmask previously occult tuberculosis. New pulmonary infiltrates, lymphadenopathy and effusions are common, and should initially be investigated with sputum staining for acid-fast bacilli, and aspiration of prominent nodes and effusions. Corticosteroids are indicated for tuberculous meningitis, pericarditis, lymphadenopathy obstructing important anatomical structures, and for miliary disease.

Infection control procedures

The most important drawback to an integrated TB/HIV service is the substantial risk of transmission of tuberculosis in the clinic. Effective policies and procedures are the best way to reduce transmission. Policies should focus on:
- ensuring healthcare worker vigilance for active tuberculosis;
- encouraging patients to request screening for tuberculosis at every visit;
- triaging coughing patients out of the general clinic queue and obtaining sputum specimens for acid-fast bacilli;
- obtaining specimens in a well-ventilated area;
- ensuring a rapid turn-around time for sputum specimens;
- ensuring waiting rooms and consulting rooms have open windows and receive plenty of sunlight;
- monitoring and evaluating the infection control programme.

Caring for TB/HIV healthcare workers

Primary healthcare workers usually live in the local community and will have similar HIV sero-prevalence. Staff will be continually exposed to tuberculosis and are at high risk of developing active disease. Management should ensure that staff have ready access to a confidential staff health service that includes regular screening for tuberculosis symptoms, voluntary counselling and testing for HIV infection, and access to antiretroviral therapy, antituberculous therapy and isoniazid prophylactic therapy. It is appropriate to offer ongoing isoniazid prophylactic therapy to asymptomatic HIV-infected staff-members, to consider initiating antiretroviral therapy at a CD4 count of <350 cells/μl, and to send sputum cultures for drug susceptibility testing for all staff members with newly diagnosed tuberculosis.

Finally, the morale of healthcare workers should be supported by regular meetings with management, regular feedback on the performance of the TB/HIV programme, and ongoing in-service training.

References and recommended reading

Bock, N. et al. 2007. 'Tuberculosis infection control in resource-limited settings in the era of expanding HIV care and treatment.' *Journal of Infectious Diseases*; 196: S108–113.

Bonnet, M. et al. 2006. 'Tuberculosis after HAART initiation in HIV-positive patients from five countries with a high tuberculosis burden.' *AIDS*; 20:1275–1279

Dong, K. et al. 2007. 'Challenges to the success of HIV and tuberculosis care and treatment in the public health sector in South Africa.' *Journal of Infectious Diseases*; 196: S491–496.

Harries, A. et al. 2006. 'Providing HIV care for tuberculosis patients in sub-Saharan Africa.' *International Journal of Tuberculosis and Lung Disease*; 10: 1306–1311.

Interim policy on collaborative TB/HIV activities. 2004. Stop TB Department and Department of HIV/AIDS. WHO. Available: http://whqlibdoc.who.int/hq/2004/who_htm_tb_2004.330.pdf

The five elements of DOTS. 2007. WHO. Available: http://www.who.int/tb/dots/whatisdots/en/print.html

Uebel, K. et al. 2007. 'Caring for the caregivers: models of HIV/AIDS care and treatment provision for health care workers in southern Africa.' *Journal of Infectious Diseases*;196:S500–S504.

Appendix 54.1: The WHO's DOTS strategy

- Government commitment to ensuring sustained, comprehensive TB control activities.
- Case detection by sputum smear microscopy among symptomatic patients self-reporting to health services.
- Standardized short-course chemotherapy using regimens of six to eight months for at least all confirmed smear-positive cases.
- Good case management includes directly observed therapy during the intensive phase for all new sputum-positive cases, the continuation phase of rifampicin-containing regimens and the whole re-treatment regimen.
- A regular, uninterrupted supply of all essential anti-TB drugs.
- A standardized recording and reporting system that allows assessment of case-finding and treatment results for each patient and of the TB control programme performance overall.

Source: World Health Organization, International Union against Tuberculosis and Lung Disease and Royal Netherlands Tuberculosis Association. Revised international definitions in tuberculosis control. *International Journal of Tuberculosis.*

Appendix 54.2 Monitoring patients on antituberculous therapy

Adapted from *'TB/HIV: A Clinical Manual'* Second Edition. Stop TB, Department of HIV/AIDS, WHO. 2004

Table 54.1 Monitoring of patients with sputum smear-positive PTB

When to monitor	8-month treatment regimen	6-month treatment regimen
At time of diagnosis	sputum smear	sputum smear
At end of initial phase	sputum smear	sputum smear
In continuation phase	sputum smear (month 5)	sputum smear (month 5)
During last month of treatment	sputum smear (month 8)	sputum smear (month 6)

Sputum smear at end of initial phase

The vast majority of patients have a negative sputum smear at the end of the initial phase. If the sputum smear is still positive at the end of the initial phase, continue initial phase treatment with the same four drugs for four more weeks. If you check the sputum smear again at this point, it is unlikely still to be positive. Go on to the continuation phase (even if the sputum smear after the extra four weeks of initial phase treatment is still positive).

Recording treatment results in sputum smear-positive PTB patients is vital to monitor patient cure and NTP effectiveness.

Sputum smear in continuation phase

In eight-month regimens, a positive sputum smear at five months (or any time after five months) means treatment failure. In six-month regimens, a positive sputum smear at five months (or any time after five months) means treatment failure. A common cause of treatment failure is the failure of the programme to ensure patient adherence to treatment. The patient's treatment category changes to Category 2 and the re-treatment regimen starts. Sputum culture should be sent for drug susceptibility testing.

Sputum smear on completion of treatment

Negative sputum smears in the last month of treatment and on at least one previous occasion mean bacteriological cure.

Recording treatment outcome

Sputum smear-positive PTB patients

At the end of the treatment course in each individual patient, the district TB officer (DTO) should record the treatment outcome as follows:

- cured patient who is sputum smear-negative in the last month of treatment and on at least one previous occasion;
- treatment completed patient who has completed treatment but does not meet the criteria to be classified as a cure or a failure;
- treatment failure patient who is sputum smear-positive at five months or later during treatment;
- died: patient who dies for any reason during the course of treatment;
- defaulted: patient whose treatment was interrupted for two consecutive months or more;

- transferred out: patient who has been transferred to another recording and reporting unit and for whom the treatment outcome is not known.

Treatment success is the sum of patients cured and those who have completed treatment. In countries where culture is the current practice, patients can be classified as cure or failure on the basis of culture results.

Sputum smear-negative PTB and extrapulmonary TB patients

All patients diagnosed with smear negative or extrapulmonary tuberculosis should have at least one specimen sent for culture. Failure to convert from culture-positive to culture-negative constitutes treatment failure. Patients who are culture-negative at the initiation of therapy should be followed clinically for deterioration, which should lead to referral for further investigation. Four of the above standard outcome indicators are applicable to adults and children with smear-negative PTB or extrapulmonary TB. These indicators are treatment completion, death, default and transfer out, which the DTO should record in the district TB register. Record as a treatment failure a patient who was initially smear-negative before starting treatment and became smear-positive after completing the initial phase of treatment.

Palliative care in children

Effective paediatric palliative care (PPC) requires a multidisciplinary approach that includes the family and makes use of available community resources: it can be successfully implemented in tertiary care facilities, in community health centres and even in the child's own home.

> The Association for Children with life-threatening or Terminal conditions (ACT) defines paediatric palliative care as 'an active and total approach to care, embracing physical, emotional, social and spiritual elements. It focuses on quality of life for the child and support for the family and includes the management of distressing symptoms, provision of respite and care through death and bereavement. It is provided where curative treatment is no longer the main focus of care and may extend over many years'.

PPC includes all stages of HIV from diagnosis through active treatment, death and bereavement. It also contributes to the care of HIV-affected orphans (whether infected or not) through addressing bereavement.

The main focus is to maximize the patient's quality of life by providing relief from distressing symptoms. PPC ensures good end of life care and a comfortable, dignified death. Predominant symptoms occurring in HIV-infected children include:

- pain;
- cough;
- dyspnoea;
- excessive secretions;
- painful swallowing;
- nausea and vomiting;
- chronic diarrhoea;
- anorexia, wasting and weakness;
- depression and anxiety;
- pruritis and other painful skin conditions.

Symptom control

General palliative care principles:
- Determine and treat underlying cause including non-physical causes.
- Relieve the symptom without creating new symptoms and unwanted side-effects.
- Consider different types of interventions: drug and non-drug.
- Consider whether the treatment is of benefit to the individual patient.

Pain

Pain is 'what the patient says hurts'. It may be difficult to determine in pre-verbal children. In 2001 Wong et al developed the 'QUESTT' acronym for assessing pain in childhood.

Q: Question the child if verbal and parent/caregiver in both the verbal and non-verbal child.
U: Use pain rating scales if appropriate.
E: Evaluate behaviour and physiological changes (tachycardia, raised blood pressure, palmar sweating, and so on, although often absent in chronic pain).
S: Secure parent/caregivers' involvement.
T: Take the cause of pain into account.
T: Take action and evaluate results.

Questions

Site of the pain, radiation (if relevant), severity (intensity), duration, precipitating and relieving factors. Descriptions of pain help to classify pain which also guides its treatment. Type of pain include:
- *Nociceptive pain* (sharp well localized pain originating in diseased areas and dull poorly localized pain originating in diseased visceral organs) responds best to opioid or non-opioid analgesics.
- *Neuropathic pain* (burning pain often described as 'pins and needles' originating from damaged nerves) responds best to adjuvants (e.g. tricyclic antidepressants and carbamazepine).

- *Sympathetic pain* (burning pain associated with hyperaesthesia and trophic changes from damaged sympathetic nerves) may require nerve blocks.
- *Psychogenic pain* (headaches, abdominal pain, muscle aches; usually with anxiety and depression) and requires psychotherapy and/or psychotropic drugs.

Pain scales:
- *quantitative* (a number out of ten); *or*
- *qualitative* (e.g. colour scale, drawing).

Qualitative scales give a better idea of suffering. Pain scales are useful in evaluating response to treatment, but should always be interpreted with caution. Children may lie about pain because they may fear that the acknowledgement of pain may lead to hospitalization and/or the performance of a painful procedure. Different scales have been designed for use in different age groups.

Many of the pain rating scales were developed for children with chronic pain caused by underlying malignancies. The Red Cross Comfort scale is a South African scale developed by Albertyn et. al. to quantify levels of discomfort specifically in HIV-infected children.

Pain should be treated:
- *By the clock*: regular dosing prevents having to first experience pain before it is treated. Regular dosing decreases the total daily analgesic requirements. Dosing intervals are determined by the duration of action of the drug.
- *By the WHO ladder** (see below).
- *By the appropriate route*: the oral route is preferred although if not possible may be given buccally, via a nasogastric tube or subcutaneously. IMI analgesia is not recommended as it is painful. The IV route may be used if IV access is available and the severity of pain warrants it.
- *By the child*: with the same pathologies children may have different experiences of pain.

The WHO pain ladder (Figure 55.1) was designed for the management of chronic cancer. Although some HIV-infected children do have chronic pain, they more often experience acute intermittent pain often caused by intercurrent infections.

Figure 55.1 Three step WHO analgesic ladder: Note: Step 1 and 2 drugs can be combined. When a strong opioid (e.g. morphine) is started (step 3) the weak opioid should be discontinued. Step 2 can be skipped for rapid control of severe pain.

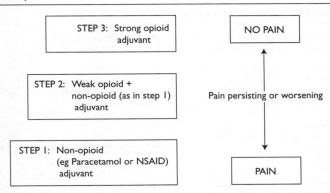

Procedural pain is an important cause of distress. Children do not get 'used to' repeated procedures and have considerable 'anticipatory anxiety'. It can be addressed by counselling cognitively competent children, using distraction techniques and/or local anaesthetics, (e.g. Emla cream®). Paracetamol can be given after the procedure. Vallergan forte is often used prior to procedures but has sedative properties without analgesia.

Cough

Most acute coughs will resolve once the underlying pathology (infections, allergies) has resolved. Chronic cough, (e.g. bronchiectasis) may cause considerable distress for the child and his/her family. It becomes pathological when it interferes with sleep, rest, eating and social functioning. The child may also be exhausted from coughing and also may have associated chest pain.

Antitussives are unnecessary with acute cough. Some cough mixtures (those with atropine, alcohol and high doses of antihistamines) may even be harmful. For pathological cough a cough suppressant is indicated. There is a 'cough ladder' starting with a simple linctus (which can be a home made remedy of hot water, honey and lemon – IMCI), codeine linctus, morphine linctus, codeine phosphate and eventually morphine sulphate. Non-drug measures include physiotherapy and saline nebulization.

Dyspnoea

The table below provides some assistance with determining whether infants and children are feeling short of breath.

Table 55.1 Assessment of dyspnoea

Infant and young child: What does dyspnoea look like?	Older child and adolescent: What does dyspnoea feel like?
Often associated with tachypnoea	Gasping or panting
Signs of respiratory distress	Feeling of drowning or suffocating
Difficulty feeding	Feeling of tightness in the chest
Restlessness (hypoxia)	Aware of every breath
Other associated signs of respiratory disease	Associated headache or light headedness
Wide eyed anxious look on face	Frightened

Figure 55.2 'Blow-by' oxygen administered on a mother's lap.

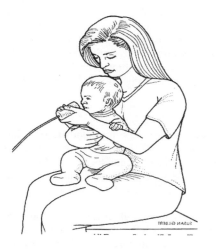

Dyspnoeic children are also anxious about their breathlessness. Adults and older children often describe a feeling of 'impending death'. Anxiety should also be addressed through counselling and occasionally anxiolytics. Some treatments for dyspnoea, (e.g. an oxygen mask) may be frightening and can aggravate dyspnoea. Oxygen needs to be administered in a non-threatening manner (Figure 55.2). Once children learn that their dyspnoea is relieved by the oxygen they often settle.

Non-pharmacological treatments for dyspnoea include exploring the psychological influences on breathlessness (especially anxiety and fear), using relaxation techniques in older children, correct positioning, suctioning and exploring complementary therapies such as aromatherapy and music therapy. A fan that blows cold air on the child's face may help to relieve breathlessness by stimulating the V2 branch of the fifth cranial nerve causing a central inhibitory effect on the sensation of breathlessness.

Morphine is the drug of choice for the management of dyspnoea. It decreases the sensitivity of the respiratory centre to carbon dioxide thereby deceasing the awareness of breathlessness. In heart failure it causes vasodilatation, decreasing the load on the heart and its sedative effect reduces anxiety. Many doctors are scared to use morphine because of respiratory depression. Respiratory depression is rare in patients with pain as they develop tolerance to this side effect and pain is the pathological antagonist to the CNS depressant effects of morphine.

For breathlessness alone oral morphine should be prescribed at a third to one half of (i.e: 0.1–0.25 mg/kg/dose) of the usual oral starting dose for pain. Nebulised morphine may be beneficial, with the advantage of being rapidly effective while producing fewer systemic side effects. The starting dose is 2.5–5 mg via a nebulizer. If bronchospasm develops, it should be discontinued.

Excessive secretions

Excessive secretions and drooling are often prominent in dying patients, who are unable to swallow due to a depressed level of consciousness. Manage with gentle suctioning and hyoscine butylbromide (Buscopan) given orally, intravenously or subcutaneously via a syringe driver. As oral absorption of Buscopan is poor, IV or subcutaneous administration is preferred.

Painful swallowing

Oral pain is most often the result of oral candidiasis, herpes stomatitis or dental caries. Treatment includes aggressive management of the underlying infection with systemic and occasionally intravenous or nasogastric medication when oral intake is not possible.

Avoid hot spicy or acidic foods such as tomatoes and oranges. Paracetamol should be given regularly (four to six hourly) before meals. Other topical treatments include ice, teething gels or local anaesthetic mouth washes. Vaseline or soft paraffin should be applied to painful cracked lips.

Nausea and vomiting

This may occur with infection or medication. Psychogenic nausea and occasionally vomiting may also be seen in children with anxiety and depression. Avoid spicy, sweet or fatty foods. Exclude hepatitis, lactic acidosis and raised intracranial pressure. Tolerance to antiretroviral therapy often develops within a few weeks. Many drugs (not buffered didanosine) can be given with food to decrease GIT intolerance. Where anti-TB treatment and antiretrovirals are given simultaneously, the anti-TB medication can be given later in the day. Ethionamide dosage may be split to avoid gastritis.

Antiemetics should be selected according to the most likely mechanism (i.e. central vs. peripheral). Corticosteroids have antiemetic properties and also assist with relieving nausea associated with raised intracranial pressure (TB meningitis, cryptococcal meningitis, brain tumours). Antiemetics under two years of age have a high side effect profile (extrapyramidal and anticholinergic).

Drug interactions exist between some anti-emetics (especially prochlorperazine, chlorpromazine and promethazine) and some antiretrovirals (especially Kaletra and nevirapine) and adjustments to the dosing schedules need to be made.

Chronic diarrhoea

See Chapter 15: Diarrhoea.

Perineal and buttock excoriation cause considerable discomfort and should be managed by the liberal use of barrier creams such as Fissan paste* or zinc and castor oil. Exposing the excoriated area to the air as well as applying corn flour can also provide relief. Treat *Candida albicans* with topical antifungal cream.

Anorexia, wasting and weakness

Apart from appropriate antiretroviral therapy use:

- antiemetics for nausea;
- appetite stimulants (more often used in adults);
- treatment for malabsorption and intestinal overgrowth (described in the section on chronic diarrrhoea);
- growth hormone;
- thalidomide (decreases cytokine levels).

Mothers should be adequately counselled and supported. Practical tips on how to feed an ill child (including nutritionally complete liquid meals) and giving an extra meal a day during the recovery phase of any illness should be provided. Clinics should also provide nutritional supplements (e.g. Pilane porridge) and multivitamins.

Depression and anxiety

Depression occurs in 20% of chronically ill children (compared to 2%-5% of normal children) and 40% of chronically ill adolescents. 28% of ill adolescents attempted suicide in one study. Depression is especially common in children where insight and intellect are maintained in the presence of deteriorating health.

Many of the 'vegetative features' are similar to those of the primary disease, (e.g. anorexia, insomnia and so on). Maintain a high index of suspicion. Young children commonly present with more somatic complaints (abdominal pain, headache), psychomotor agitation, restlessness and mood congruent hallucinations, whereas older children commonly have more 'negative features of depression' including apathy, hopelessness, psychomotor retardation, delusions and nihilism.

Occasionally bereavement may be complicated by clinical depression (usually diagnosed after two months).

Address psychosocial stressors where possible, counsel the child (where cognitively competent) and use antidepressants where indicated. Selective serotonin re-uptake inhibitors (SSRIs) are preferable to tricyclic antidepressants (with their higher side effect profile) in children.

Anxiety may exacerbate other symptoms, (e.g. dyspnoea and diarrhoea). It should be managed by adequate counselling where the child is given the opportunity to discuss his/her concerns and to regain a sense of control where possible. Anxiolytics may be used carefully.

Pruritis and painful skin conditions

Bed sores are less common than in adults mostly because young children weigh comparatively less. Pressure sores related to nasal cannulae, naso-gastric tubes and monitors, (e.g. saturation probes) should be prevented by careful skin care, (e.g. using granuflex under nasal cannulae if receiving long term oxygen therapy)

Drugs for pruritis include aqueous cream, and oral antihistamines. Calamine lotion may aggravate pruritis by drying the skin.

Palliative and end of life care

Decisions to withdraw aggressive treatment in end stage disease and to provide exclusively palliative treatment are difficult. Health professionals generally err on the side of optimism. Although good, it should not detract from ensuring that children in whom death is inevitable can die comfortably and with dignity.

There are some basic guidelines that can be used to decide whether aggressive treatment is in the child's best interest or not:

- Irreversible end organ damage may make antiretroviral therapy futile. Examples include: extensive bronchiectasis, severe cardiomyopathy, advanced HIV encephalopathy, PCP diagnosed late and not responding to treatment.
- Avoid futile treatments especially if invasive when they cannot improve quality of life.
- Where antiretroviral therapy causes an intolerable pill burden or side effects, a decision to stop therapy should be entertained in advanced disease.

A decision to withdraw active treatment and to enter into an exclusively palliative phase should be made by more than one medical professional. If difficult, an expert consultation (even telephonic) should be sought with a professional in a tertiary HIV care centre. The child's family as well as the child him/herself (if cognitively competent) should also be involved in the decision making process. Hero stories have proven to be an effective intervention in the support of children affected and infected by HIV.

End of life care

The setting should be chosen by the family and if possible, by the child. Assist families wishing to take a dying child home. Supervised home-based care teams should provide the necessary drugs (including morphine) to ensure a comfortable death. Local hospices and their community-based outreach teams should also be utilized.

Routes for drugs at the end of life include buccal, sublingual, rectal, subcutaneous and nasogastric. Staff providing end-of-life care should be familiar with a syringe driver, even in the child's own home. All professional staff should be familiar with distressing end-of-life symptoms such as terminal seizures, restlessness, respiratory panic and death rattle. They should predict these and prepare parents and caregivers for these symptoms.

The family should also be supported after the death of the child and through bereavement.

Palliative care in adults

Palliative care is an essential part of comprehensive HIV care and it is important that the principles and practice of palliative care are integrated into the delivery of care to people living with HIV from the time of diagnosis of the infection and throughout the continuum of illness.

The World Health Organization (WHO) defines palliative care as an approach that improves the quality of life of patients and their families facing problems associated with life-threatening illness, through the prevention and relief of suffering, the early identification and impeccable assessment and treatment of pain and other problems, physical, psycho-social and spiritual. The WHO definition further states that 'palliative care is applicable early in the course of illness, in conjunction with other therapies that are implemented to prolong life'. In order that patients receive the benefit of comprehensive care, it is important that primary health care practitioners and specialists also develop the knowledge, attitude and skills to deliver appropriate palliative care alongside disease-specific treatment, in this case antiretroviral therapy. Palliative care is an integral part of every health care professional's role and effective palliative care is best delivered by involving an interdisciplinary team, including nurses, social workers, doctors, pastoral workers, physiotherapists, community care workers, and other professionals and volunteers. All members of the palliative care team should receive ongoing training and support in palliative care.

South African hospice programmes provide palliative care for patients with advanced HIV infection. Palliative care in HIV goes far beyond care of the dying patient. The focus of palliative care is quality of life and aggressive management of opportunistic infections and support of antiretroviral treatment are key components of hospice programmes.

Hospices are also points of entry into voluntary counselling and testing with family members and neighbours choosing to test for HIV as a result of the care the patient is receiving and the counselling that is a part of hospice services. Hospice careworkers take advantage of the most powerful teaching moment of caring for a seriously ill HIV-positive person to emphasise the importance of prevention of infection. Many HIV clinicians are using hospice in-patient units to admit patients with low CD4 counts to start their antiretroviral treatment under hospice care to manage possible immune reconstitution. Home-based carers provide strong treatment support to promote adherence to antiretroviral therapy.

Home-based care (HBC) is the cornerstone of palliative care, and aims to be compassionate and patient-centred, and to empower the family to care for the patient at home. Short-stay admission for control of symptoms or for family respite may be required, but the aim is to discharge the patient to the home care programme, when his or her condition is controlled. The complexity of the HIV epidemic has meant that effective patient care is best achieved by partnerships between various care agencies in the formal and informal health care sectors, including faith-based agencies.

Even with effective prevention (a goal we are far from achieving) and universal access to antiretroviral treatment, patients will still die from HIV-1-related causes. The estimate of 320 000 deaths in adults and children in South Africa in 2005 (UNAIDS 2006 Report on the Global AIDS Epidemic) does not describe the suffering preceding those deaths.

Physical care

The most important step in palliative care is a comprehensive assessment of the patient's condition: physical, psychosocial and spiritual. Once the cause and severity of symptoms are established the first management step is to treat the cause. Palliative care clinicians institute aggressive management of opportunistic infections alongside symptom control for the best possible outcome for the patient.

Symptom control

Pain

Pain is a highly prevalent symptom in HIV and AIDS with patients experiencing up to 7 different types of pain at one time.

Table 55.1 Sites of pain reported by South African adults with AIDS

Site	Percentage experiencing pain
Lower limbs	66.0
Mouth	50.5
Head	42.7
Throat	39.8
Chest	17.5
Muscles	14.6
Abdomen	12.6
Genitals	12.6
Backache	11.6
Generalized	11.6
Upper limbs	7.8
Rectum	3.9
Skin	2.9

Adapted from: Norval DA 2004. South African Medical Journal. 94:450–454.

Pain is an unpleasant sensory and emotional experience associated with actual or potential tissue damage. Pain is always a subjective experience: remember that 'pain is what the patient says hurts'. The perception of pain is modulated by the patient's mood, morale, and the meaning the pain has for the patient. Total pain is an interaction of physical, emotional, psychosocial, and spiritual pain (see Figure 55.3).

An accurate history is essential, including precipitating and relieving factors, quality of pain, radiation of pain, severity, and duration of pain. A simple pain scale from 1 to 10 allows pain to be quantified, and the response to therapy to be monitored. It is important to explain to the patient the cause of the pain, realistic goals for the control of pain and the use of medication to control pain, both analgesics and adjuvants. Non-drug measures of pain control can be used to supplement conventional therapy, (e.g. relaxation, psychotherapy, distraction or stimulation, reflexology, aromatherapy, TENS, or acupuncture).

The WHO recommends that analgesics be given:

- by mouth (it is preferable to give oral medication);
- by the clock (chronic pain requires regular medication - prescribing medication to be given 'as needed' is irrational and inhumane); and
- by the ladder (see Figure 55.1).

Use of morphine

Morphine is the most widely used strong opioid analgesic and should not be withheld from patients experiencing severe pain. Morphine may be administered orally (morphine oral solution, controlled release tablets), or by injection – most commonly by subcutaneous infusion using a syringe driver. Oral morphine solution must be given four hourly, starting

Figure 55.3 Causes of pain in advanced HIV infection (adapted from Saunders, 1967)

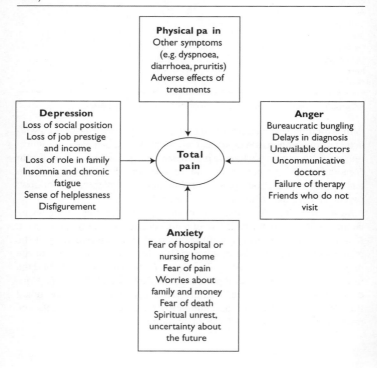

at 10 mg per dose, titrated upwards, depending on the patient's analgesic requirements. When the pain is controlled, the patient can switch to slow release tablets, with the total daily dose given in two divided doses. Physiological addiction is not seen, as inflammatory mediators block the receptor that mediates the euphoric effect of recreational drugs. Caution should be used, however, when prescribing for patients with pre-existing drug addiction.

Side effects of morphine include:
- drowsiness or confusion;
- nausea and/or vomiting; and
- constipation.

Note:
- Tolerance occurs to all the side-effects of morphine except constipation, so laxatives must also be prescribed.
- Oral morphine does not cause respiratory depression when given at recommended doses.
- Myoclonus may be a problem at the end of life, owing to renal failure and the accumulation of metabolites. This can be managed by reducing the dose.
- Pethidine should *not* be used in the treatment of chronic pain.

Adjuvant analgesics

- NSAIDS are useful for inflammation, bone pain, or serosal pain.
- Corticosteroids reduce inflammation and oedema.
- Tricyclic antidepressants treat neuropathic pain and tension headache.
- Anticonvulsant medication treats neuropathic pain.

Cough and dyspnoea

Respiratory secretions can be reduced with hyoscine butylbromide 10–40 mg eight hourly and expectorated with physiotherapy. Bronchodilators can be given for associated wheeze. Dyspnoea responds to low-dose morphine oral solution or dexamethasone. Significant pleural effusions should be drained.

Diarrhoea

Rehydration fluids should be given orally to prevent dehydration. Milk and high-roughage foods exacerbate diarrhoea, and should be avoided, and fruit juices should be diluted. High-energy soft foods, such as maize meal, bananas, rice, white bread, peeled potatoes, and grated apple are suitable. Antidiarrhoeals, such as loperamide and codeine phosphate, can be given on a regular basis.

Constipation

Add roughage to the diet if the patient is able to eat properly. Fresh fruit and vegetables, stewed fruit, prune juice, grated beetroot, high-fibre cereals, and oats porridge are good choices. Extra fibre may be added to cereals, porridge, or soup. If extra fibre is added, the patient must drink extra fluids. Laxatives include stimulants such as senna or bisacodyl. Liquid paraffin (one tablespoon in orange juice), sorbitol, lactulose, or glycerine suppositories can be used to soften stool. Many patients use home remedies such as marula jam and Black Forest Tea, and can continue to do so if the remedy is effective. Impaction can be treated by softening the stool with 100 ml warm olive oil instilled rectally for one hour, followed by a gentle warm water enema. Manual removal of faeces may be indicated to make the patient feel comfortable.

Anorexia, nausea, vomiting

Maintain good oral hygiene and adequate fluid intake. Keep the mouth fresh with a mouthwash of one teaspoon of salt, vinegar, or lemon juice in one litre of water. Meals should be small, unspiced, and frequent, and should be given with extra fluids. Avoid foods with strong odours. Try small amounts of alcohol before meals as an appetite stimulant. Low-dose steroids may be used to stimulate appetite. Antiemetics include metoclopramide for nausea of gastrointestinal origin, haloperidol for drug- or anxiety-induced nausea, and cyclizine with dexamethasone for raised intracranial pressure (see below). Dietary and vitamin supplements should be considered.

Pruritus and other skin conditions

Pruritus and other skin conditions should be treated as follows:
- Maintain good hygiene with soap and water.
- Keep the skin soft with aqueous cream.

- Protect reddened pressure areas with clear dressings (e.g. Tegaderm® or Opsite®).
- Treat seborrhoeic dermatitis and papular urticaria with topical corticosteroids.

Promethazine 10–25 mg at night can be used as an antipruritic. Additional infection should be treated with topical antiseptics or antibiotics.

Mouth care

Brush teeth with a small, soft toothbrush and fluoride toothpaste after each meal and at night (a baby's toothbrush is ideal). If brushing is not possible due to pain or bleeding, use foam sticks, soft sponges, cotton buds, a gloved finger wrapped with gauze or a soft wash cloth.

Use a mouthwash after each meal and at night. Mouthwashes are used in addition to brushing, not as a substitute. Avoid mouthwashes that contain alcohol as these dry out the mouth. Regular sips of water are important to keep up fluid intake. Keep lips clean, soft, lubricated and intact as far as possible. Apply petroleum jelly or moisturising lotion to lips regularly. Check the mouth, palate, gums, tongue and teeth often to catch and manage any problems early.

Suggestions for mouthwash:
- saline – 500 ml boiled, cooled water and 1 teaspoon salt;
- sodium bicarbonate mouthwash – 500 ml boiled, cooled water and 1 teaspoon bicarbonate of soda;
- 1 teaspoon of vinegar or lemon juice in 1 litre of water;
- 0.2% chlorhexidine gluconate mouthwash;
- 1% povidone-iodine mouthwash.

Rinse with 15 ml for 60 seconds.

The palliative management of xerostomia

- good oral and dental hygiene;
- treatment of infections such as candidiasis and herpes simplex;
- review drug regimen – reduce dosage or change the drug if possible;
- artificial saliva products are costly, 'home made' saliva (methylcellulose + lemon essence + water is a possibility, but methylcellulose is often unavailable).

- in patients with advanced disease, lubricating jelly (KY jelly) applied to the tongue and oral cavity has been shown anecdotally to be an affordable and effective means of keeping the oral cavity moist and lubricated;
- use lip moisturisers, e.g. petroleum jelly or flavoured lip gels;
- frequent sips of cold water, if patient is very ill, spray cold water into the mouth using a spray bottle or use a sponge stick;
- offer a mouthwash 2-hourly and avoid mouthwashes that contain alcohol as it dries out the mouth;
- eat soft, liquid foods that are easy to chew and swallow and during eating, lubricate the inside of the mouth with a little butter, margarine or salad oil;
- humidify the room in areas where the air is very dry;
- suck ice cubes, vitamin C tablets, sugar-free lemon-flavoured sweets or sour sweets;
- chew sugar-free gum;
- chew or suck fresh pineapple chunks (avoid if open sores in mouth).

Denture care

Patients who wear dentures may experience problems due to severe weight loss. Dentures may no longer fit properly and ill-fitting dentures make eating, chewing and talking difficult. Patients may also develop denture stomatitis, which needs to be treated with antifungal agents. After every meal, dentures must be thoroughly cleaned to remove all food particles and plaque. Dentures should be regularly disinfected using a denture cleaning solution. Patients must be advised to always remove their dentures before sleeping, and store them in water or a denture sterilising solution.

Pressure care

It is essential that professional health care workers and other carers are aware of the causes and risk of pressure sores and the imperative to prevent pressure sores where possible. The following measures will assist in the prevention of pressure sores:
- vigilance of nursing staff:
  o inspect the skin every time the patient is moved;
- care of the skin and pressure areas:
  o the skin should be washed and dried regularly, including bed bath for the bed bound patient;

o maintain suppleness of skin by regular massage with skin lotion;
o avoid trauma – no restraints, lift patients do not drag them to move them in the bed.
- regular positional change, if patient is not able to lift and shift their weight 3–4 times an hour, family or hospice/hospital carers should assist in changing the patient's position every 2–4 hrs depending on patient's risk factors;
- special mattress to distribute body weight more evenly;
- keep the bed linen dry and free from creases;
- keep the patient well nourished and well hydrated.

Delirium and dementia

It is important to explain the reason for the patient's symptoms to the patient and family. Take advantage of lucid intervals. Agitation and anxiety can be treated with haloperidol 0.5–1.5 mg 12 hourly, increasing to 5–10 mg 12 hourly if necessary. Cerebral oedema responds to dexamethasone. Start with a dose of 16 mg in the morning and at midday (dexamethasone at night may interfere with sleep). Reduce it to a maintenance dosage of 2 mg daily or 12 hourly when symptoms are controlled.

Incontinence

Incontinence can be treated as follows:
- Keep the patient clean and dry.
- Preserve the integrity of the skin with protective creams, such as Vaseline° or Fissan paste°.
- Use adult disposable nappies or large towelling nappies.
- Protect the bed with plastic sheeting.
- Incinerate disposable nappies.

Treat unpleasant odours by giving oral charcoal 50 g in 200 ml water, or by placing vanilla essence in the room.

Anxiety and insomnia

Psychosocial support and spiritual counselling (if wanted) are essential. Avoid alcohol and stimulants in the evening, and give warm milk or herbal tea at night. Aromatherapy, massage, reflexology, and relaxation techniques may be very helpful. Anxiolytics such as diazepam 5 mg eight hourly orally or midazolam 5–15 mg daily, given subcutaneously with a syringe-driver, are very useful. Oxazepam 10–15 mg can be given as a sedative at night.

Fatigue and weakness

Depression may cause fatigue, and requires counselling and appropriate antidepressant medication. Anaemia (haemoglobin <7 g/dl) may be treated with transfusion if the patient is ambulant and symptomatic; iron, folate, and vitamin B12 deficiencies should be treated. Adequate nutrition and nutritional supplements are important, and patients with poor nutritional status appear to do better with a multivitamin supplement. Caregivers should assist with daily activities of living such as bathing, dressing, and feeding, and encourage the use of wheelchairs, walkers, and bath aids. Ensure a safe environment and supervision when a patient is in danger of falling. Teach the patient to 'listen to his or her body' and to rest when tired.

Psychological and social support

Patients and their families or carers need ongoing emotional support and empathy. Always tell the truth, but in a gentle manner. Common emotions include fear, denial, guilt, anger, bargaining, sadness, depression, resignation, and acceptance. Memory boxes may be put together by a parent for his or her children, or by the children themselves. Support groups for people with AIDS, for caregivers, and for family members are fundamental. Social and financial issues need to be addressed. In any setting, it is appropriate that care is delivered in the patient's own language, in the patient's own home and community. Where possible, carers from the patient's own culture should be involved in the patient's care. HBC is the most appropriate model of care to provide for a patient's emotional and spiritual needs, while providing quality physical care. Carers should be sensitive to, and have respect for, other cultures, and have an awareness of cultural rituals regarding death, dying, and funeral arrangements. Ask about spiritual support, and determine whether the patient wishes to involve trained clergy, or spiritual leaders from the community, who can deliver spiritual counselling while respecting the patient's own faith and spiritual views. The challenge for the patient at the end of life is to make sense of, and come to terms with, illness and impending death, in relation to the patient's own world view or understanding of God.

Caring for the carers

Caring for a patient with AIDS can be emotionally exhausting, especially as the caregivers themselves are exposed to multiple losses because of the nature of their work. To prevent burnout, all those providing care need access to some form of support, either through regular support groups, or via individual counselling sessions. Caregivers who receive adequate initial and ongoing training, and who are professionally supervised, gain fulfilment from providing quality care to patients. The morale of the care team needs to be sustained and enhanced by sharing their experiences and expertise.

References and further reading

Doyle, D. et al. 1999. *The Oxford textbook of palliative medicine.* 2nd edition. Oxford: Oxford University Press.

Evian, C. 1997. *Primary AIDS care.* Cape Town: Jacana Education.

Gibbon, C. J. 2000. 'Prescribing in palliative care'. *South African medicines formulary.* Cape Town: South African Medical Association.

Gwyther, E., Merriman, A., Mpanga Sebuyira, L., Schietinger, H. A. 2006. *Clinical Guide to Supportive and Palliative care for HIV/AIDS in sub-Saharan Africa 2006 edition.* Available: http://www.fhssa. org/i4a/pages/Index.cfm?pageID=3359

Hospice Association of South Africa. *Clinical Guidelines 2006.*

International Association for Hospice and Palliative Care. 2002. Available: http://www.hospicecare.com [19 July 2002].

Saunders, C. 1967. *The management of terminal illness.* London: Edward Arnold.

World Health Organization (WHO). 1990. *Cancer pain relief and palliative care.* Technical Report Series 804. Geneva: WHO.

Selwyn, P. and M. Forstein. 2003. 'Overcoming the False Dichotomy of Curative vs Palliative Care for Late-Stage HIV/AIDS'. *Journal of the American Medical Association*; 290:806–814.

Women's health

In the early 1980s AIDS was largely a disease affecting gay men in the developed world. At the start of this millennium, new HIV infections in women have surpassed those in men. This is largely because of the burgeoning HIV epidemic in the developing world and in the inner cities of large, urban areas in developed countries, where most of the infected women are young, indigent, and face social challenges that often pose more of an immediate threat to their well-being and that of their families than HIV does. Countless women are not able to determine their sexual experiences or partners and they are often prevented from learning about, or using, safer sex techniques. For these reasons, approaches to the control of the AIDS epidemic should be gender sensitive.

At the end of 2006, the global estimate of the number of individuals infected with HIV was approximately 40 million people, with over 25 million resident in sub-Saharan Africa. Over 50% of those infected were women (http://www.unaids.org). This has profound implications for women and society as a whole, particularly with regard to vertical transmission to offspring, AIDS orphans, and the sick women's ability to care for her family, which is often compromised, as well as creating significant economic uncertainty and instability in society.

Epidemiology and transmission in women

Globally, most women have acquired the HIV infection via vaginal intercourse. The efficiency of HIV transmission during vaginal intercourse is greater from men to women than vice versa. This is reflected in the South African epidemic, where gender ratios of infection are 13 women: 10 men.

Blood transfusions administered for obstetric reasons represented a significant risk factor in the mid-1980s before widespread HIV screening of blood supplies, and remain a risk in some developing countries today.

Spread of HIV through sharing of infected needles and syringes in illegal drug use is becoming more important in developing countries.

Natural history of HIV infection in women

Although early studies reported significantly shorter survival time in women, more recent studies have shown that women have less access to routine HIV care and best current therapies than men. This is a major confounder in assessing biological differences in survival. The pattern of opportunistic infection (OI) differs minimally between men and women. Oesophageal candidiasis, cytomegalovirus disease, and herpes simplex virus infection appear to occur more commonly in women. Kaposi's sarcoma was thought to be rare in women, but there is anecdotal evidence that this may not be the case in Africa.

Laboratory testing and monitoring

Multiparous women have a higher frequency of false positive enzyme-linked immunosorbent assay (ELISA) tests and indeterminate Western blots because of the presence of human leukocyte antigen antibodies formed as a consequence of immunization through pregnancy. Where doubt exists, other definitive tests should be employed. (See Chapter 5: Laboratory investigations.) No evidence exists for gender differences in CD4 count or viral load.

Antiretroviral therapy in women

There has been concern that women may respond differently to antiretroviral therapy. Few pharmacokinetic trials have included enough women for subgroup analysis, but recent studies have shown no difference in drug efficacy. Protease inhibitors may alter blood levels of oral contraceptives and so, in this setting, an alternative form of pregnancy prevention should be advised (see Chapter 27: Contraception).

Indications for starting antiretroviral therapy are not influenced by the patient's gender.

Gynaecological disease in HIV-infected women

Cervical dysplasia and invasive cervical cancer are more prevalent in HIV-infected women and this correlates with the level of immune suppression. Pelvic inflammatory disease is frequent in HIV-infected women, but the causal role of HIV is difficult to tease out, because of the known association of PID with early multiple sexual partners and sexually transmitted infections, which are factors associated with HIV infection.

Many menstrual abnormalities have been reported among women with AIDS, but a recent, large, well-controlled study showed no difference in intermenstrual bleeding, irregular bleeding, or amenorrhoea in HIV-positive women. Vaginal candidiasis may occur earlier than oral thrush and may serve as an earlier marker for HIV infection. (See Chapter 26: Gynaecology.)

A detailed sexual and gynaecological history should be obtained from all women, and a pelvic examination and cervical smear performed. Contraceptive advice should be given and safer sex techniques explained. Women should not rely on condoms alone for pregnancy prevention.

HIV infection and pregnancy

The risk of pregnancy-related HIV disease progression is low, at least in women with largely asymptomatic HIV infection. However, the frequency of bacterial infections in HIV-infected women is higher during pregnancy and the peripartum period. Successful maternal outcomes depend on effective prophylaxis and therapy for HIV-related OIs and, where possible, antiretroviral therapy. The greatest maternal danger occurs when HIV infection is not detected, or when inadequate prenatal or routine HIV care is received.

Vertical transmission of HIV

See Chapter 46: Prevention of mother-to-child transmission (PMTCT) of HIV.

The impact of HIV on women's health care

HIV infection within a family is often diagnosed when a vertically infected child presents for medical care. The child's mother, whose partner may also be infected, usually becomes the primary care giver, and often her own needs are ignored.

Despite the family nature of the illness, care is fragmented. Women with HIV may have limited access to appropriate medical care, as they are often from socio-economic groups that rely on poorly resourced clinics. Much HIV-related education is given at the workplace, so the woman tending the home may not receive information regarding HIV and AIDS, and will be unaware of risk factors in her sexual partner.

Rural women are at risk as a result of migratory labour practices, where men are infected at their place of work and bring the infection home when they are on holiday. In poor areas, women are turning to commercial sex work as a way of providing food and basic necessities for needy family members.

Prevention of HIV infection in women

Prevention programmes largely focus on condom usage and voluntary changes in sexual behaviour, but for women these issues are often much more complex. A woman cannot force her partner to use a condom and may suffer domestic and sexual violence if she insists. The female condom is now licensed for contraception and safer sex, but still needs the partner's agreement, since it is not totally unobtrusive and needs further development to improve comfort. Other female-controlled contraceptive and safer sex devices are urgently required. The spermicide nonoxynol-9 destroys HIV *in vitro* but also increases HIV transmission, owing to vaginal wall irritation. Other less irritant microbiocidal agents are currently being tested, with and without spermicidal properties. The latter may be important in societies where childbearing is considered imperative. Importantly, topical vaginal microbiocides do not need the partner's cooperation.

In sub-Saharan Africa heterosexually transmitted HIV infection occurs from the age of 12 years in the female population. Education, therefore, needs to start at primary school level, to influence choices about sexuality before sexual debut. Peer pressure among young people is enormous, and educational programmes should include peer educators and peer opinion leaders. Another problem in Africa is the practice of older men having casual sex with young, and often barely pubertal, women. Young women are lured by the social and economic status that goes with relationships with older men, but are readily infected and, consequently, HIV is transmitted to the next generation.

HIV testing in women

All pregnant women should be offered counselling and testing for HIV since the option of PMTCT may reduce the risk of HIV transmission to an urban child. However, while vigorously promoting testing, health care providers should be mindful of its possible negative consequences. Women who reveal their positive serostatus to abusive partners may be harmed physically or emotionally. A positive test, especially if done rapidly, with little time for thinking about the consequences, nor the opportunity to discuss outcomes with other family members, may lead to social and emotional isolation and severe risk to the woman's well-being.

Domestic violence

Domestic violence is a very common event that is frequently undetected by medical professionals. Domestic violence is defined as physical, verbal, sexual, emotional, and/or economic abuse of a woman by her (usually male) partner.

Diagnosis

Women may complain directly of violence at home, but more frequently a woman presents to a casualty department with injuries she will claim originated in 'falling down the stairs,' or some other kind of accident. Domestic abuse should always be suspected when a woman presents with injuries. However, she may present with more indirect symptoms such as chronic pelvic pain, depression, minor menstrual abnormalities and so on.

Management

Women who are victims of domestic violence frequently suffer from low self-esteem, poor trust, chronic anxiety, and fear. Establishing trust and developing a relationship between the doctor and patient is an essential first step. Listening in a non-judgemental way to her story is the second step. Unsolicited and uninformed advice can be very dangerous. For example, a typical reaction from health professionals is to say things like, 'why don't you leave him?' This kind of statement implies that she chooses (and, therefore, enjoys) being in the relationship. It also exhibits a very poor understanding of the helpless and economically dependant situation in which many battered women find themselves.

For many women, the decision to leave an abusive partner takes months of planning and courage. It has been well documented that the most dangerous time for a battered woman is the time during which she decides to leave the abusive relationship. This move frequently provokes the batterer to lethal violence in a last attempt to maintain control. The role of the health professional is to recognize the problem and to provide maximum support, practical advice, and information to the woman, especially by referring her to an appropriate agency, shelter for battered women, or social work network. The health professional can neither solve the problem for the woman, nor can she or he force the woman to follow her or his advice. This can often be a frustrating experience for doctors, who frequently see themselves as 'problem solvers'. The problem of domestic violence is a complex one, which may take weeks or months for the woman to resolve. Patience is required, not value judgements like 'I cannot help you if you will not help yourself'. Such judgements only serve to further undermine these vulnerable and battered women. The development of a trusting and respectful relationship between patient and doctor may initiate the healing process and improve a woman's self esteem.

References and further reading

Hirsch, J.S. et al. 2002. 'The social constructions of sexuality: Marital infidelity and sexually transmitted disease - HIV risk in a Mexican migrant community'. *American Journal of Public Health*; 92 (8):1221–1237.

Maman, S., et al. 2002. 'HIV-positive women report more lifetime partners violence: Findings from a voluntary counselling and testing clinic in Dar es Salaam, Tanzania'. *American Journal of Public Health*; 92 (8):1331–1337.

Martinez, A. et al. 2002. 'Posttraumatic stress disorder in women attending human immunodeficiency virus outpatient clinics'. *AIDS patient care standards*; 16 (6):283–291.

Rosenfield, A. and K. Yanda. 2002. 'AIDS treatment and maternal mortality in resource-poor countries'. *Journal of American Medical Women's Association*; 57 (3):167–168.

Tschann, J. M. et al. 2002. 'Relative power between sexual partners and condom use among adolescents'. *Journal of Adolescent Health*; 31 (1):17–25.

Worth, D. 1998. 'Sexual decision-making and AIDS: Why condom promotion among vulnerable women is likely to fail'. *Studies in Family Planning*; 20 (6 Pt 1):297–307.

57 Gay sex and sexuality

Issues relating to HIV infection among gay men and women differ from those occurring in heterosexual populations. Cultural attitudes and prejudice mean that issues relating to gay sexuality and relationships are often poorly understood and not freely discussed. Patients may be uncomfortable exploring matters of gay sexuality especially with counsellors who have little training in issues specific to the gay community. These issues do, however, need to be discussed to impact positively on the lifestyle and health of the gay patient who presents for HIV testing or management.

Issues of gay sexuality

The 'gay' community in South Africa is extremely diverse. Many people who engage in same-sex sexual activities may not identify themselves as gay and may not fit the usual cultural stereotypes. Examples of this include some male sex workers and prisoners. While many gay people openly express their sexuality, there is still pressure for gay men and women to conform to heterosexual societal norms and this leads to guilt and shame, reflected in the high suicide rate among gay teenagers.

HIV and the gay community

HIV first struck the gay community over 25 years ago, and prompt responses from this community in the USA led to the promotion of safer sexual practices in the late 1980s, and a fall in transmission rates. Many teenagers engaging in gay sex today have had no contact with the history of HIV and feel distant from the HIV epidemic. This, combined with the feeling of invincibility common to most youth, may lead to dangerous risk-taking behaviour. Barebacking (unprotected anal sex) is rising in the gay community and has been associated with a rise in the HIV incidence. Ongoing counselling and education is needed to counteract high-risk behaviour.

Gay sex between men and the risk of HIV infection

Certain gay sexual practices increase the risk of contracting HIV infection. Gay men have a reputation for sexual promiscuity but this is not universal and many gay people enjoy long-term monogamous relationships. However, the 'code of ethics' that exists for heterosexual marriage is different in gay relationships. Also heterosexual children learn societal norms regarding relationships from their parents; this guidance is lacking for the gay teenager. Expectations and norms in gay relationships are different from those of the general society. There is less pressure for monogamy and this may promote sexual promiscuity and increase the risk of HIV.

Common sexual practices and the risk of HIV transmission

Very low risk:
- kissing;
- hugging and rubbing (with unbroken skin);
- masturbation.

Low risk:
- oral sex with exposure to pre-ejaculate fluids only.

Medium risk:
- oral sex with exposure to semen.

High risk:
- insertive anal intercourse.

Very high risk:
- receptive anal intercourse;
- rough sex play (cutting or piercing) where there may be trauma and bleeding from skin or mucosal surfaces.

The risk of HIV transmission may be enhanced by the use of recreational drugs during sex, which is common in the gay community.

Condom use should be promoted for anal sex and preferably for oral sex as well. Suitable water-based lubricants must be used to reduce the risk of condom breakage and abrasion.

Lesbian sex and safer sexual practices

Woman-to-woman transmission of HIV has been reported, but transmission risks have not yet been well studied. Research data is urgently needed. Risk factors are thought to include:

- sex during menstruation;
- contact with white blood cells in vaginal discharge caused by vaginitis (bacterial vaginosis is common);
- genital ulceration due to sexually transmitted infections (STIs);
- traumatic sexual practices, including shaving, cutting, and piercing.

Safer sexual practices include:

- wearing gloves for genital contact, especially if the fingers have cuts or sores;
- covering the vulva with plastic wrap and wearing a latex dental dam during oral sex;
- avoiding genital sex during menstruation; and
- covering sex toys with a condom and not sharing them.

Some women who have sex with women also have sex with men, increasing the risk of STI transmission, including HIV. Safer sex information given to lesbian women should emphasize the importance of regular Pap smears.

Counselling gay patients for HIV testing

Counselling should be gay affirmative and non-judgmental. Being gay is not a disease and no attempt should be made to 'cure' a person of being gay or from engaging in gay sex. HIV is a preventable infection, and this message should be promoted both by medical professionals and by the gay community. Most heterosexual health care workers (HCWs) and counsellors are poorly informed about the details of gay sexuality, and, while it is unnecessary for them to know the intimate details of gay sex, counsellors need to be able to identify and modify risky sexual practices among gay patients. Practitioners who are uncomfortable dealing with gay patients should refer them to a gay-affirmative professional for further counselling and testing.

Assessing risk

Always ask why the patient is presenting now for an HIV test, as there may have been a recent high-risk sexual incident. Important issues in the sexual history include the number of sexual partners, episodes of unprotected sex, and the types of sex acts that the patient engages in. Ask about unprotected oral and anal sex, whether the patient is the insertive or receptive partner, and if there has been any contact with paid sex workers. Co-factors for risk-taking behaviour should also be sought, e.g. clubbing, drug taking, alcohol use, visiting saunas, and multiple sex partners. These practices are often part of accepted gay culture. Ask about previous STIs and any symptoms of a current STI. Previous HIV tests are relevant.

Assessing support systems and ability to cope

HIV pre-test counselling should include an assessment of the patient's support system in case of a positive test result. Gay social structure is different to that of heterosexual society, and gay patients may lack support from conventional sources such as the nuclear family. Relationships with family and friends should be explored, and it is worth finding out whether patients are 'out' to their families and whether their families are supportive.

Ensure that the patient is aware of gay-friendly support groups in the area. Inquire about previous psychiatric illnesses such as depression, and attempt to identify high-risk patients for suitable ongoing counselling and management.

Discussing a positive HIV test result

Do not delay giving the result and be clear about the result. Lengthy discussions regarding HIV and AIDS may not be useful at the time of conveying a positive result – information is unlikely to be retained during this time of crisis. Emphasize the fact that treatment exists for HIV and AIDS. Demonstrate that you have good knowledge of HIV and AIDS and that you are able to make a plan to ensure that the patient's health needs are met.

Treatment options, and the financial implications, should be discussed. Educate patients about their legal rights in the face of an HIV-positive diagnosis. Our constitution protects individuals against discrimination on the basis of their HIV status and sexual orientation. Antiretroviral therapy is available free of charge to South African citizens in the state health care sector.

Repeated advice on safer sexual practices is essential. (See Chapter 7: Counselling.)

Education

This should preferably be given prior to HIV testing. HIV and its spread in the gay community should be discussed. The patient should be informed about high-risk behaviours for HIV transmission. Give the facts – euphemisms should be avoided. It is important to remain positive about gay sex practices, but risky behaviour must be discussed and modified if possible. The option of celibacy is likely to be met with little enthusiasm. Advice about reducing risk through ensuring safer sex practices should be offered. Types of sex acts should be discussed; not all intimacy needs to involve high-risk sexual acts. The ideal of the single monogamous relationship should be encouraged, and the risks associated with casual sex partners should be conveyed. Patients should be encouraged to ask about the HIV status of their sex partners. Patients should be educated about other STIs, including hepatitis B, and C and should be immunized if necessary where possible. Recreational drug and alcohol use compromise safer sex decision-making and should be discouraged. Sex toys should, ideally, not be shared and should always be used with condoms and water-based lubricant. Condoms make sex safer but do not eliminate the risk of HIV transmission completely.

Counselling and testing gay men and women for HIV infection requires time and commitment. The end result is an informed patient who is able and willing to practise safer sex.

Care of the man who has been raped

Male rape is not uncommon and is probably under-reported. The same management principles outlined in Chapter 28: Sexual assault, should be used for male rape survivors. Accurate documentation of perianal and perineal injuries, and prompt collection of forensic specimens, should be performed in all cases. The risk of HIV transmission is high, and patients should be counselled on the probable benefits of post-exposure prophylaxis, as well as the transmission of other STIs.

Further information

Triangle Project (Cape Town): www.triangle.org.za

Triange Project Clinic Bookings: clinic@triangle.org.za

Mother City Men's Health Project: www.desmondtutuhivcentre.org.
 za/men.htm

Gay Health: http://www.gayhealth.com

Gay South Africa: http://www.gaysouthafrica.org.za

Lesbian STIs: http://depts.washington.edu/wswstd

General HIV Information: www.thebody.com

HIV/AIDS raises many ethical issues relating to basic rights and fair treatment of people infected with HIV. Regrettably, the ongoing myths and misconceptions about HIV/AIDS have lead to fear, discrimination, and stigmatization of infected persons and their carers. HIV denial, both by individuals and society, and failure to confront the extent to which social and behavioural factors shape the pandemic, have been important contributory forces.

Health care workers (HCWs) are expected to be role models of acceptance and treatment of those infected with HIV and their loved ones. They should be knowledgeable regarding HIV management and provide appropriate education to those who require it. HCWs also need to be informed about policy related to professional conduct, and should work towards reducing denial and stigma. This applies to all medical conditions and is not specific to HIV. When policies are not yet in place, HCWs must consult guidelines relevant to the daily problems faced at the bedside and in the clinic. This chapter is based on the guidelines of the Health Professionals Council of South Africa and the South African Medical Association's Human Rights and Ethical Guidelines on HIV and AIDS, a manual for medical practitioners, developed in 2001 and revised in 2006.

Rights and responsibilities

The South African Constitution, which is based on the underlying notion of human dignity, grants every person:

- the right of access to health care services;
- the right to equality and freedom from unfair discrimination;
- the right to freedom and security of person (bodily integrity and autonomy);
- the right to privacy (confidentiality); and
- the right to an environment that is not harmful to their health and well-being.

Several ethical rules are applicable to health professionals registered with the Health Professionals Council of South Africa (HPCSA).

The ethical rules of the HPCSA make the following provisions:

- They protect professional confidentiality: Patient information may only be divulged with the patient's express, and preferably written, consent. For children <14 years, the consent of a parent or guardian is required. If the patient is deceased, then the written consent of the next-of-kin or executor must be obtained.
- There is a requirement for reporting (including self-reporting) of impairment in a student or health professional. This usually applies to intellectual impairment or addiction. However, HIV infection may be viewed as an impairment. Health care practitioners must ensure that the risk of HIV transmission is prevented during the course of their work.

The World Medical Association (WMA) International Code of Medical Ethics states:

- that a physician shall protect the rights of patients, of colleagues, and of other health professionals and shall safeguard patient confidences; and
- that practitioners have an ethical duty to act in the best interests of their patients at all times (WMA 1983).

HIV testing

Any medical test, including an HIV test, may interfere with a person's rights to freedom, the security of their person, and privacy. Therefore, a person may only be tested:

- at their own request;
- after they have given informed consent, or
- if the test is authorized by legislation or a court order.

However, early diagnosis of HIV may therefore be of both public health and individual survival benefit. On September 22nd 2006 the United States National Center for HIV/AIDS published revised recommendations for HIV testing of adults, adolescents and pregnant women to facilitate HIV testing as a normal part of medical practice similar to screening for other treatable conditions. HIV screening for all patients in US health-care settings is now recommended unless the patient declines (i.e. 'opt-out screening'). Separate written consent for HIV testing is no longer required and general consent for medical care will be considered sufficient to encompass consent for HIV testing. Prevention counselling will not be required with HIV diagnostic testing or as part of HIV screening programmes in health care settings. The objective of the revised policy is to increase HIV screening of patients and pregnant women in health-care settings to foster earlier detection of HIV infection, identify and counsel individuals with unrecognized HIV infection and link them to clinical and prevention services. The WHO and UNAIDS encourage expansion of HIV testing and counselling as an important strategy in addressing the HIV/AIDS epidemic and as a means to attain the fulfilment of the right to the highest possible level of health. The WHO and UNAIDS recognize four types of HIV testing, client initiated voluntary counselling and testing (VCT); diagnostic HIV testing of those with symptoms and signs of HIV-related disease; routine health care provider initiated testing and mandatory screening of blood destined for transfusion or manufacture of blood products.

Before testing

Before testing, ask the following:
- Are there laws that regulate HIV testing, e.g. prisons, schools, workplace, insurance policies etc.?
- Is there a clinical indication?
- Has the patient been fully informed and, thereafter, consented?
- Is confidentiality assured?

In the absence of a test, emergency treatment may not be withheld. In certain well-defined high-risk or exposure-prone procedures, the patient should be informed and asked to consent. If a patient declines, they should be managed as if positive. Testing an existing blood sample is allowed only with informed consent.

A general poster in the ward or clinic room that 'all patients will be tested for HIV' does not constitute informed consent. It is the tester's responsibility to check the patient's willingness and information prior to taking blood.

Testing is permitted as part of research only with the participants free and informed consent, and the principles and regulations in relation to medical research must be adhered to (see the Helsinki Declaration). Unlinked and anonymous testing is permitted by the South African Department of Health if it is done by a national or local health authority, and when applicable as part of research.

Post-test counselling

The responsibility for post-test counselling falls on the practitioner who commissioned the test. (See Chapter 7: Counselling.)

Case I

A 24-year-old man presents to the surgery six weeks after a hospital admission for an appendectomy. He developed post-surgical skin sepsis, and, according to him, an HIV test was done 'routinely' as part of the investigation for this condition and found to be positive. He is angry, but withdrawn, and counselling regarding his illness proves difficult. He does not return for a follow-up visit.

Telephonic contact with the surgeon concerned confirms the patient's story. It further transpires that the skin sepsis had been associated with an abscess, severe pyrexia, and short-term delirium. The surgeon argues:

- that the patient's delirium made it impossible to obtain informed consent in this case and that the HIV test was essential to the patient's management at that time;
- that the requirement for informed consent for HIV testing is inappropriate anyway, as 'we don't ask for informed consent when doing a VDRL';
- that requiring informed consent in such cases (as well as other surgical cases) compromises the better management of the patient, as he would have been more aggressive in his antibiotic prophylaxis originally if he had done a routine HIV test prior to embarking on the appendectomy; and
- that the potential infringement of the patient's rights in doing an HIV test without informed consent is outweighed by the rights of both the surgeon and the surgical team.

Response

Many would argue that this patient's rights have been violated and his adverse response to further HIV counselling reflects this. There is no evidence for additional antibiotic cover in patients with HIV. The same strict adherence to sterile technique applies, regardless of HIV status. Some may argue that HIV testing should be on a par with other 'routine' blood tests but the consequences of an HIV test are more profound, and the current guidelines state that it is preferable for a patient to give consent and be counselled before testing. The argument of contagion to the surgical team is unwarranted, since universal precautions should be practised with all patients, and appendectomy is not considered a particularly high-risk procedure. In the case of a temporary inability to provide consent, the case is less clear where treatment of HIV-infected patients is compromised while health care workers 'await' a mental state that is conducive to counselling and testing. The health care practitioner must ask him/herself whether knowing HIV status in a comatose/semi-comatose patient would assist with diagnosis and management. Not testing a patient in this scenario violates the patient's right to excellent health care in favour of his/her privacy rights.

HIV testing in children

Children of 14 years and older can independently provide informed consent for an HIV test. Confidentiality must be maintained, but the child should be advised of the importance of disclosing to a responsible adult, e.g. as soon as feasible to parents, caregivers or partners. Children under 14 years old can only be tested if their parents or legal guardians have provided informed consent. Schoolchildren may not be tested without the consent of a legal guardian, and a teacher or principal may not provide such consent.

Testing the unaccompanied child

Regardless of a child's presentation, the diagnosis of HIV is seldom an emergency. If it is, there might not be time to wait for a test result. In a true emergency, assume the diagnosis that is in the child's best interest:
- Assume that the child is negative in the case of life-saving interventions.
- Assume that the child is positive in the case of a likely HIV-specific complication, and begin appropriate treatment.

Confidentiality

Patient confidentiality is an integral part of medical practice. It is the cornerstone of the doctor-patient relationship and enables patients to share intimate medical and personal information that is essential for good medical care. The Supreme Court of Appeal recognized the right of the HIV-positive person to confidentiality in the well-known case of Jansen van Vuuren vs. Kruger, 1993. The ethical duty of all doctors to safeguard the confidences of their patients is further upheld by the South African constitution, the WMA, SAMA, and HPCSA.

It is recognized that in reality, health care teams may be large, with multidisciplinary involvement, and communication may be verbal or written. Confidentiality, therefore, becomes more complicated, and requires careful attention. The HPCSA recommends specific policy formation regarding this.

In the discussion that follows, we address specific areas where maintaining confidentiality may be a particular problem.

Sexual partners

All patients taking an HIV test should have pre- and post-test counselling that includes information on the need for partner notification. This should continue throughout the entire therapeutic relationship. Legal and other risks associated with abusive or other inappropriate sexual behaviour must be stressed. Duties regarding harm to others and patient confidentiality need to be balanced. On identification of a third party at risk, the patient should be encouraged to disclose, and an offer should be made to assist in the process of disclosure. Clinicians should recognize that, in some cases, source patients may believe that their lives would be endangered if they were to disclose their HIV status to their partners. Under these circumstances, since the practitioner's primary duty is to protect the life of the patient, the HIV status should not be disclosed. If, however, a patient is simply unwilling to disclose, despite repeated counselling, then the doctor should notify the partner, but only if:

- the partner is a known and identified person;
- that partner is at risk of infection, i.e. it is known that no precautions for safer sex are being taken;
- the index patient has been informed that these steps are being taken by the practitioner (some patients may then choose to be involved); and
- the partner is offered testing, and pre- and post-test counselling are given.

It is important to stress that these types of disclosure should be dealt with very carefully, and that all steps taken should be documented, since there is no case law and doctors run the risk of legal action by the patient. Having all the facts and good documentation may provide some protection.

Case 2

A 23-year-old man, well known to the family practice, is diagnosed with HIV, following an episode of shingles. He is married, and has no children. His wife is also a patient at the practice. He initially refuses to inform anyone of his diagnosis, and, despite repeated counselling over the next six weeks, refuses to disclose his HIV status to his wife.

Scenario 1

He informs the doctor that he and his wife consistently use condoms, a fact that is confirmed by his wife at her next clinic visit. Should the doctor inform the wife of his HIV status?

Response

While it is still advisable for this man to reach the point of disclosing his status to his wife, she is not in immediate danger, and continued encouragement and support of the husband to do so is all that is required.

Scenario 2

He informs the doctor that he and his wife consistently use condoms. His wife presents to the clinic 10 days later, having missed her last period, and requests a pregnancy test. She tells the doctor that she and her husband have been actively trying to have a baby for over six months. Should the doctor inform the wife of his HIV status?

Response

In this case there is an identified person at risk of infection, and the husband should be confronted, counselled again, and offered help with the disclosure. Failing this, after informing the husband, it is reasonable to inform the wife, and offer her testing and counselling support.

Notifying family members

A family does not have the right to know the patient's HIV status. However, the advantages of telling one's family should be pointed out during counselling, before the patient becomes ill. A major difficulty for doctors dealing with patients who are ill with, or dying of, HIV is what to tell family members. Patients should be informed that next of kin or another third party may obtain access to his or her medical records after death. The principal member of a medical aid has no right to obtain the medical records of his or her dependants. Doctors are often harassed by third parties to provide information on a patient's HIV status, or to state whether tests were done. These parties should be informed that patient-doctor confidentiality is safeguarded by legislation and ethical rules, and that unless the patient (or his or her next of kin in the case of death) provides consent, no medical information may be divulged.

Case 3

A 32-year-old man is brought to casualty unconscious, with a Glasgow Coma Scale rating of 5. He is brought into casualty by his sister (26 years) and mother (61 years). On examination, among other findings, the casualty doctor discovers oral hairy leukoplakia. HIV disease is strongly suspected. In the absence of first-person informed consent, the doctor struggles with the dilemma of whether the family members can provide a substituted judgement, and consent for testing, in a case that is potentially devastating to their own lives. He also debates whether the family has the right to know of his suspicions, and, once the patient is confirmed HIV-positive, of the diagnosis.

Response

This covers two aspects, i.e. consent to HIV testing, and disclosure to family members. Since the confirmed diagnosis of HIV infection may assist in determining the cause of the unconscious state, it is more advisable to get next-of-kin consent for testing, rather than simply to do the test on medical grounds. This, however, will also mean that the family will need to be informed of the outcome. Under these circumstances disclosure by the doctor would be justified. If the patient were fully conscious and able to give consent, he should first be asked whether he wished to have an HIV test and, if the test were positive, whether he wished his family to be informed.

Healthcare workers

In all cases, universal precautions should be taken in all medical procedures.

When referral to other members of the health team is required, the HIV status may not be disclosed without the prior consent of the patient. The patient should be informed that not disclosing his or her HIV status to other relevant practitioners may compromise his or her health care. Once informed, all other members of the health team are duty-bound to maintain confidentiality.

Case 4

Scenario 1

A 44-year-old man is admitted to the medical ward with community-acquired pneumonia (CAP). While on the ward, he confides in his doctor that he is HIV-positive, and has been for three years. He requests that no other member of the medical staff be informed of his diagnosis.

Response

This is only a reasonable request if staff don't need to know his HIV status to treat him optimally. This is relatively unlikely in the case of CAP. If divulging the information would serve that patient's best interests, discussions should enable him to understand the need for sharing information, with his consent.

Scenario 2

A 44-year-old man is admitted to the surgical ward for a routine haemorrhoidectomy. While on the ward (and prior to his surgery) he confides in his doctor that he is HIV-positive, and has been for three years. He is not on any form of antiretroviral therapy. He requests that no other member of the medical staff be informed of his diagnosis.

Response

This is only a reasonable request if the staff don't need to know his HIV status in order to treat him optimally, and if he poses no risk to them. This is unlikely in this case, where other members of the health team will be required to make decisions and carry out the procedure. If either of the latter applies, he should be appropriately informed, and discussions should be held to enable him to understand the need for sharing information with his consent.

Medical certificates

The ethical guidelines regarding what should be written on a medical certificate include 'a description of the illness, disorder, or malady in layperson's language'. A medical practitioner is not permitted to write false information on a certificate. However, the practitioner may state that the employee is, in his or her opinion, not capable of work, owing to injury or illness, for a period of time, without disclosing the sensitive nature of the illness. Information may only be made available to the employer if the employee-patient consents.

Insurance issues

An insurance contract is binding between the insurance company and the policyholder. The contract may (with patient consent) authorize a medical practitioner to test a patient who is a policyholder and/or to make medical information known. In the absence of such consent patient confidentiality prevails. Medical practitioners may require proof of such contracts. There is a duty on any policyholder (and not on the doctor) to disclose material facts that affect the risk to the company.

Case 5

A 31-year-old woman comes to the day hospital, and reveals that she is HIV-positive, diagnosed 18 months previously during an insurance investigation. She is married, with two children, one of whom was born eight months ago. She has not revealed her status to her husband, and does not understand why this is necessary. She remembers signing a form prior to having her blood drawn for the insurance test, but says that 'the doctor was very busy' and did not explain the test to her. She appears to have no understanding of her illness at all.

Response

Her rights and responsibilities should be explained to her. She needs to understand the implications of the HIV test that was done when she applied for insurance, and the implications of her HIV status for her baby. The 'busy' doctor described here, even if working on behalf of the insurance company, has the responsibility to ensure that the client is fully informed and receives pre- and post-test counselling when ordering HIV tests. The client may then refuse the test and, consequently, the insurance will be refused. Inadequate counselling often leaves patients ill-prepared, and subsequently they require much more counselling. Better counselling would enable her to understand the good reasons for sharing her HIV test results with her husband, so that she would be in a better position to understand the situation and take responsibility for her decisions.

Employment issues

The Employment Equity Act of 1998 prohibits unfair discrimination against any employee based on his or her HIV status. In the case of Hoffman vs. SAA, 2000, the South African Constitutional Court found that discrimination against a prospective HIV-positive employee is unfair. An employer may only conduct pre-employment testing with the informed consent of every employee. The HIV test and the results must remain confidential, even where the employer has paid for the test. It is unlawful for a practitioner to test an employee solely at the request of the employer, and to make the results available to the employer. If the employee agrees that the employer may be informed, the employer must keep those results confidential, unless the employee gives permission for disclosure.

Under the Occupational Health and Safety Act of 1993, all employers have to adopt measures to reduce the risk of HIV transmission at work. Employees should also have access to medical aid schemes that must provide a minimum benefit to people living with HIV/AIDS.

In terms of HIV-positive practitioners, the HPCSA guidelines state that no doctor is obliged to disclose his or her HIV status to an employer or co-employee. Infected doctors may continue to practise, but must seek counselling and advice on how to adjust their professional activities so as to protect their patients. Some aspects of medical training or practice may be inadvisable for medical students or doctors, and more appropriate professional choices should be made, with effective counselling.

Case 6

Scenario 1

A 27-year-old man is sent to his doctor by his employer for a full medical examination and HIV test (the patient has freely consented). The employer is paying for the procedures. The HIV test is positive, and the patient (who is a long-distance truck driver) is found to have

Grade I dementia, probably related to his HIV. The doctor struggles with the ethical dilemma of whether to inform the employer of the driver's HIV status and early dementia.

Response

While confidentiality is important, doctors also have a duty to the public at large. If the patient is considered unfit to drive, action needs to be taken to prevent him from doing so. Although the patient came for the examination consentingly, it is clear that the cerebral involvement may have reduced his decision-making capacity, and that it would not be in his best interests to reveal the test result directly to the employer. If the patient has reduced decision-making capacity, the doctor should discuss the problem with family members first, and seek permission to reveal the test result to the employer. Involving the family strengthens their ability to obtain a reasonable settlement from the employer if employment is terminated. Payment for the test by the employer does not afford the employer any special rights to the results, and the same rules for confidentiality apply.

Scenario 2

A 27-year-old man comes to see his primary care doctor for a full medical examination and HIV test (with his consent and at his request). The patient is paying for the examination. The HIV test is positive, and the patient (who is a long-distance truck driver) is found to have Grade I dementia, probably related to his HIV. The doctor struggles with the ethical dilemma of whether to inform the employer of the driver's HIV status and the early dementia.

Response

While confidentiality is important, doctors also have a duty to the public at large. If the patient is considered unfit to drive, action needs to be taken to prevent him from doing so. The doctor should discuss the problem with family members first and seek permission to reveal the test result to the employer. Involving the family strengthens their ability to obtain a reasonable settlement from the employer if employment is terminated.

Scenario 3

A 27-year-old man comes to see his primary care doctor for a full medical examination and HIV test (with his consent and at his request).

The patient requests, and is paying for, the examination. The HIV test is positive and the patient (who is a long-distance truck driver) is otherwise found to be well and to have a CD4 count of 550. The doctor struggles with the ethical dilemma of whether to inform the employer of the driver's HIV status.

Response

There is no ethical responsibility to break confidentiality if the patient's HIV status does not pose a risk to the public at large.

Death certificates

In South Africa new regulations on death certificates were passed in 1998. The new death certificate has two pages, which are detachable. The first page, which the family sees, allows for notification of death to the Department of Home Affairs. On this page it is necessary only to indicate the death as 'natural' or 'unnatural'. The second page is confidential and should be placed in a sealed envelope – this is to provide the Department of Home Affairs with data for statistical and public health purposes. On this page the medical cause of death must be stated, and the page should be sent directly to Home Affairs, and not given to another person – not even a family member. Because envelopes containing this information have been opened by funeral directors and family members, this can only be prevented by their being sent directly to Home Affairs by the institution notifying the death. Funeral directors should not need access to this information, as they too are advised to practise universal precautions in all cases.

Occupational injury

Universal precautions should be taken with all patients, regardless of their HIV status. All provinces have their own occupational exposure policies that should be available in all state facilities. An injured employee may claim for compensation from the Compensation Commissioner. Employees must not be denied, or hampered from obtaining, access to post-exposure prophylaxis (PEP). (See Chapter 52: Occupational post-exposure prophylaxis, for PEP guidelines.)

Testing the source patient in cases of occupational exposure is a complex issue. It should only be undertaken with the informed consent of the patient. If consent cannot be obtained, e.g. where the patient is unconscious or legally incapable of consenting, and testing is required as a matter of urgency, an existing blood sample may be used or legitimate proxy consent obtained (i.e. family members or legal guardian). If the patient is unwilling and refuses consent, forcefully drawing blood or drawing blood under false pretences should not be undertaken. If this occurs it may result in legal action against the health worker concerned. In these cases it is preferable to do rapid testing on the HCW who has been exposed, and to presume that the patient is positive.

Access to treatment

Every patient has the right to access treatment. The basic duty to realize this right rests on the state. Doctors may not hamper a patient's access to treatment, and should provide HIV-infected patients with the same standard of treatment as other patients. They may not refuse to treat a patient on the basis of HIV status alone. Where a patient refuses to follow the advice and treatment of the medical doctor, the doctor may advise that the patient see a different doctor, as long as other facilities exist. A doctor may not refuse any patient emergency care. Medical practitioners have the right to treat patients without undue pressure or victimization from employers or government institutions. Medical practitioners have an ethical duty to act in the best interests of their patients at all times.

Notification

HIV/AIDS is not a notifiable condition, and medical practitioners are under no obligation to inform the authorities if a patient is HIV-positive or has AIDS.

HIV/AIDS and research

All the same issues apply, i.e. patients should receive adequate counselling to enable them to give informed consent to participate in a trial. Researchers should consider the following:
- the Helsinki Declaration, amended 2000, updated 2002 and 2004; and
- the South African Department of Health's Research Ethics Guidelines (Ethics in Health research: Principles, structures and processes) 2004.

Due consideration should be given to how the patient will be treated after completion of the trial. In the case of antiretroviral agents, it is necessary to negotiate with the funding agencies, prior to the study, to ensure the best possible treatment plan for the patient on completion of the trial.

Other ethical considerations before conducting research

Before testing an individual, it is beneficial to all to ask the following questions (this is especially significant in prevention of mother-to-child transmission and voluntary counselling and testing programmes, where patients are counselled and rapid tests are performed on the same day, without much opportunity for deliberation):

- Is the patient really fully informed?
- Is consent being given without coercion and incentives?
- Has an opportunity been provided for the patient to deliberate with his or her family?
- Is appropriate health care available should the result be positive?
- Will positive HIV status lead to victimization of this patient's health care rights in a resource-constrained environment?

Non-deliberation may diminish the chances of disclosure to family members and even sexual partners. This in turn may lead to:

- a loss of emotional support;
- a lost opportunity to speak about the risk in the family;
- a lost opportunity to decrease stigma by more sharing; and
- a lost opportunity for the family to plan for illness or loss of income.

The individual may not always benefit from knowing his or her HIV status immediately.

Case 7

The mother of a four-year-old patient who is HIV-positive asks her doctor whether she should inform her friends and the child's crèche of his HIV status.

Response

The possibility of an irrational response to the presence of an HIV-infected child in the crèche should not be discounted. However, it may be seen as a violation of trust not to inform them about potential risks to their own children.

Fear is often based on misinformation, and the process of informing others about what may cause contagion needs to be accurate and non-alarmist. The mother is free to decide whether or not to disclose her child's status to her child's playmates' parents. It is worth considering that, should she decide not to disclose, support may not be forthcoming when her child becomes ill, due to a perceived betrayal of trust, among other reasons. This is a good example of the need for more open discussion of HIV/AIDS, so that public understanding of the disease and its transmissibility is improved, and denial and stigma are reduced.

References and further reading:

Jonsen, A. 1982. *Ethics: A practical approach.* New York: Macmillan.

Mash, B. 2000. *Family medicine ethics.* Chapter 11 in: Handbook of family medicine. Cape Town: Oxford University Press.

World Medical Association. 2000. Helsinki Declaration. [Online], Available: http://www.wma.net/e/policy/b3.htm (22 August 2007)

South African Department of Health. 2004. *Ethics in Health Research: Principles, structures and processes.*

South African Medical Association. *Human rights and ethical guidelines on HIV and AIDS, A manual for medical practitioners.* Guidelines approved by the Human Rights, Law and Ethics Committee, and the Board of Directors in 2001, revised 2006.

Healthcare worker burnout

Caring for people in need is both rewarding and uniquely draining work. In particular, it can be highly exhausting in the HIV/AIDS arena. To prevent burnout from the chronic everyday stress of working closely with people in need of continual attention and care, health care providers need to attend to their own well-being. There has to be a balance between giving and taking, between caring for others and caring for oneself.

Stages of burnout

The emotional demands imposed by the interactions between helper and recipient can overwhelm the tolerance of the caregiver, and his or her ability to keep on caring.

Stage 1

The initial warning signs are:
- persistent irritability;
- persistent anxiety;
- periods of high blood pressure;
- bruxism (teeth-grinding at night);
- insomnia;
- forgetfulness;
- heart palpitations;
- inability to concentrate; and
- headaches.

These are clear signs of heightened chronic stress arousal.

Stage 2

If the warning signs in Stage 1 are not recognized, Stage 2 ensues, including the following cognitive behavioural activities to conserve energy:
- lateness for work;
- procrastination;
- taking three-day weekends;

- decreased sexual desire;
- persistent tiredness in the mornings;
- handing in work late;
- social withdrawal (from friends and family);
- cynical attitudes;
- resentfulness;
- increased alcohol consumption;
- increased caffeine consumption; and
- an 'I don't care' attitude.

Stage 3

If the caregiver does not heed the warning signals, exhaustion follows and is characterized by:
- depression;
- chronic stomach or bowel problems;
- chronic mental fatigue;
- chronic physical fatigue;
- persistent headaches;
- the desire to 'drop out' of society;
- the desire to move away from friends, work, and perhaps even family; *and*
- possible suicidal thoughts.

Losing any health caregiver to burnout comes at an unacceptable cost to the individual, the health care system, and society at large.

Causes of burnout

The causes of burnout include:
- overwhelming workload;
- lack of reward – both financial and emotional;
- unfairness and poorly handled evaluations, promotions, or grievances;
- compromised values, owing to high workloads;
- loss of control and inability to finish projects;
- rigid or chaotic health care settings; and
- loss of a sense of community because of tensions with one's employer or colleagues.

Intervention

First, recognize the need for intervention. Too often healthcare providers, especially those dealing with ill, young, HIV-infected patients, persist with the above signs and symptoms without recognizing burnout.

Intervention at an organizational level:

An organization should aim to create a less stressful environment, where burnout is minimized. It may require resourcefulness and tenacity to change the attitudes of colleagues, employers, and institutions.

- *Begin with one person*: Start with one like-minded colleague and be prepared to lead the process of creating awareness and changing attitudes.
- *Make it a group effort*: Awareness will grow if you elicit colleagues' support, by talking and setting priorities. Strength comes in numbers in an organization.
- *Get organizational buy-in*: This will involve all levels of the organization, both above and below. Client/patient gratitude and recognition from management go a long way to making staff feel valued.
- *Tackle one problem at a time*: Identify a problem that has high burnout potential, and make concrete suggestions to alleviate it. Avoid a passive stance.
- *Emphasize process*: The process of problem solving and adapting, on an ongoing basis, is of the essence.

What may be very useful to manage burnout is to set up mentoring and coaching programmes for the healthcare workers. This process would enable them to be contained, supported and have the awareness brought into consciousness, thus sustaining greater effectiveness all round.

Personal intervention:

People who cope well have learned to check their own burnout potential regularly, and restore themselves with practical mental and physical health-enhancing strategies:

- *Control worry:* Prioritize worries into those that can be acted on, and start with the worst. Forget those about which nothing can be done.
- *Eliminate obsessive ruminating:* Don't invest energy in a problem that may never arise, and don't worry about a problem until the appropriate time.

- *Recognize fatigue:* Become aware of energy levels – they have dropped too far when exhaustion prohibits even self-replenishing activities. This requires the development of a mild selfishness, and the need to do personal activities that replenish energy levels.
- *Check perfection:* Check that your standards are not overly high and don't expect perfect performances when energy levels only allow for 75% output. Reduce frustration and irritations while energy levels are low and expect more when feeling better.
- *Delegate:* Call on colleagues for help, and enable fellow health care providers to feel part of the team and to display their own competence – then show appreciation for the shared workload.
- *Play:* As adults, we easily forget the amazingly rejuvenating qualities of play. On occasion, drop adult, result-orientated activity and get lost in the process of play.
- *Humour:* Humour is therapeutic and laughter has an astoundingly liberating effect on the flow of ideas, especially if you can laugh at and about yourself.
- *Exercise:* Inappropriate stress reactions undermine health and immunity. Physical activities such as brisk walking, running, cycling, or swimming alleviate stress and result in feelings of well-being and tranquillity. Avoid overly competitive sports.
- *Eat healthily:* Avoid toxins, pollutants, stimulants, and tranquillizers, and minimize alcohol intake and cigarette smoking. Eat healthy, natural foods, including fish, vegetables, fruit, and cereals and avoid fats, oils, and sweets. Eat regular meals, including breakfast, and reduce caffeine intake.
- *Cultivate friendships:* Friends provide a social network of support.
- *Create a stable home environment:* A stable family or home provides an important refuge to withdraw to.
- *Take time out:* Give yourself time to appreciate nature and beauty and relax regularly.
- *Learn to say 'no' on occasion.*

References and further reading

Cherniss, C. 1995. *Beyond burnout: Helping teachers, nurses, therapists and lawyers recover from stress and disillusionment.* New York: Routledge.

Cheston, R., and Pennell, M. 2000. 'Deconstructing burnout'. *Changes: An International Journal of Psychology and Psychotherapy*; 18 (2):64–68.

Farber, B.A. ed. 1983. *Stress and burnout in the human service professions.* New York: Pergamon Press.

Maslach, C., and M.P. Leiter. 1997. *The truth about burnout.* New York: Jossey-Bass.

Micronutrients and complementary therapies

Complementary and/or alternative (CAM) medicine use is widespread among HIV-infected patients. In South Africa a growing number of herbal and traditional medicines and supplements are promoted for use in HIV disease. These agents may be expensive and are often licensed under the nutriceutical label or sold over-the-counter and thus, do not have the same stringent licensing requirements as other pharmaceuticals. This means that good efficacy and safety data are sparse, and that the quality, and indeed the contents, of the product are not ensured. There is currently no evidence to support prescribing currently available complementary medicines as an alternative treatment to antiretrovirals in patients in whom such treatment is indicated. Studies in the West and in Africa have shown that CAM therapies, however, continue to be popular with patients, and clinicians should therefore be adequately informed of their use and potential safety problems in HIV disease. This chapter discusses dietary supplements and some locally available herbal extracts.

Vitamin and other dietary supplements

There is no evidence supporting routine prescribing of supplements in HIV-infected patients who do not have nutritional deficiencies. However, nutritional deficiencies are common in HIV-infected patients in developing countries, particularly those with advanced disease. It is impractical and expensive to determine individual micronutrient deficiencies in all patients. Wasting, which reflects macronutrient deficiency, may be a useful marker for micronutrient deficiency. In a setting with limited resources, the wasted patient is a good target for supplementation. At all stages of HIV infection, a healthy and well balanced diet should be encouraged. (See Chapter 23: Diet and nutrition.)

In a large Tanzanian randomised placebo controlled trial, daily administration of a multivitamin containing vitamin B complex, vitamin C and vitamin E to pregnant and lactating women was associated with slower HIV disease progression, decreased maternal mortality from AIDS-related causes and improved pregnancy outcomes. Early child mortality was reduced in those women with both nutritional deficiency and advanced disease. Vitamin A supplementation has been shown to be beneficial in HIV-infected children, but not in adults. A Thai placebo controlled study of high dose micronutrient supplementation showed an association between supplementation and decreased mortality among the most immunocompromised group (CD4 counts <100 cells/µl). Zinc in combination with micronutrient supplementation was shown to decrease mortality in HIV and tuberculosis co-infected patients. Selenium supplementation may be of benefit, but further research is needed.

Locally recommended daily doses of micronutrients are outlined in Table 60.1. Excessive doses of vitamin A, zinc and iron may cause harm, and recommended daily doses of these micronutrients should not be exceeded (Table 60.2).

Vitamin D deficiency has been associated with tuberculosis, but the role of vitamin D in HIV-infected patients with tuberculosis is unknown. There is a need for more well-conducted, blinded, randomized controlled studies to explore the value of supplementation in HIV infection.

Table 60.1 Southern African Clinicians society recommendations for daily micronutrient intake for supplementation in adult HIV-infected patients in resource-limited settings

Note: A supplement which provides 100% to 150% of the Recommended Dietary Allowances (RDAs) of the below micronutrients is recommended.

Nutrient	RDA range for female	RDA range for male	Maximum dose for supplementation in HIV/AIDS
Vit E (mg TE)	15 a-TE*	25 a-TE*	1 000 a-TE
Selenium (mg)	55	100	400
Folate (mg)	400	400–800	1 000
Niacin B3 (mg)	14–16	25	35
Thiamine B1 (mg)	1.1–1.2	5.5–6.0	None
Riboflavin B2 (mg)	1.1–1.3	5.5–6.8	None
B6 (mg)**	1.3	6.8	100
B12 (mg)	2.4	5–10	None
C (mg)	75–90	250	2 000
Beta-carotene (mg)		No RDA	15mg
Magnesium (mg)	280	200	350
Chromium (mg)	25–35mg	25mg	
A-Lipoic acid	No RDA	10–15mg	100mg
Glutathion	10mg	50mg	None

* a-TE = a-Tocopherol equivalents or mg of RRR-a-Tocopherol
** Patients receiving isoniazid therapy should receive 25–50mg pyridoxine (Vitamin B6) to prevent peripheral neuropathy.

Table 60.2 Southern African HIV clinician society recommendations for maximum daily doses of zinc, iron and vitamin A in adults

Nutrient	RDA range	Maximum for supplemen-tation in HIV/AIDS	Toxic upper limit
*Zinc (mg)	8–11	11	40
*Iron (mg)	8–18	8 (women); 18 (men)	45
Vitamin A (μg RE)	700–900	800	3 000

Herbal medicines

Echinacea

Echinacea purpurea, *E. angustifolia*, and *E. pallida* are popular health store products. There is no clinical trial evidence demonstrating benefit in HIV infection.

Echinacea is a cytochrome P450 inhibitor, and may therefore interact with hepatically metabolised drugs, including NNRTIs and PIs.

Garlic

Garlic supplementation has not been shown to be of clinical benefit in HIV-infected patients. Garlic supplements can act as both an inducer and an inhibitor of cytochrome P450, and have been shown to significantly decrease saquinavir plasma concentrations.

Phytosterols

A combination of the plant sterols (phytosterols) beta-sitosterol and its glycoside, has been widely promoted as an 'immune booster' in HIV infection. This product has a combination of stimulatory and inhibitory effects on immune function *in vitro*, and *in vivo* effects have not been explored in good quality randomized controlled trials.

Hypoxis hemerocallidea, commonly known as the African potato, has been extensively promoted in South Africa for use in HIV-infected patients. *Hypoxis* can cause bone marrow toxicity, and may lead to worsening of immune suppression, and should therefore be avoided in HIV-infected patients. There is *in vitro* evidence that *Hypoxis* may act as a cytochrome P450 and P glycoprotein inhibitor, or cause increased cytochrome P450 activation, and may therefore interact with non-nucleoside reverse transcriptase inhibitors (NNRTIs) and protease inhibitors (PIs).

Sutherlandia frutescens

The South African medicinal plant *Sutherlandia frutescens* subs. *micro-phylla*, known as Cancerbush, Kankerbos, or Unwele, has a long history of use as a multi-purpose tonic. Animal studies have not shown evidence of toxicity. A randomized placebo controlled clinical trial exploring effects in healthy HIV-infected patients is currently underway in South Africa. *In vitro* evidence suggests that *Sutherlandia* may act as a cytochrome P450 and P glycoprotein inhibitor, or cause increased cytochrome P450 activation, and may therefore interact with NNRTIs and PIs.

St John's Wort

St John's wort has been shown to be effective for treatment of mild to moderate severity depression. It is an inducer of cytochrome P450 and may result in sub-therapeutic concentrations of NNRTIs or PIs.

Doctors and patients should be aware that many complementary therapies have side-effects and may cause clinically significant drug interactions. All patients should be asked about concurrent use of herbal and traditional remedies before initiating antiretrovirals, and all should be asked to report initiation of new medications, including those obtained over-the-counter or from a traditional healer.

There is a need for further research in the fields of efficacy, mechanism, and interactions of complementary/alternative agents. A guiding principle for any practitioner in the field is that proven therapies should never be undermined by experimental ones. Until evidence for benefit exists, HIV patients should use CAMs with circumspection.

References and further reading

Irlam, J.H., Visser, M.E., Rollins, N., Siegfried, N. 2005. 'Micronutrient supplementation in children and adults with HIV infection.' *Cochrane Database of Systematic Reviews* Issue 4. Art. No.: CD003650. DOI: 10.1002/14651858.CD003650.pub2.

Fawzi, W., Msamanga, G.I., Spiegelman, D., Wei, R., Kapiga, S., Villamor, E., Mwakagile, D., Mugusi, F., Hertzmark, E., Essex, M., Hunter, D.J. 2004. 'A randomized trial of multivitamin supplements and HIV disease progression and mortality.' *New England Journal of Medicine*; 35(1), 23-32.

Southern African HIV clinicians society nutrition guidelines, 2004. Available: http://www.sahivsoc.org/index.php/guideline/index/1/21.

Index

Please note: Page references to tables and figures are in *italics*.

A

abnormal cytology 278–279
acute HIV infection following sexual exposure 54–56
acute interstitial nephritis 315
acute respiratory disease 322
acute severe malnutrition 150
acute (renal) tubular necrosis 314–315
adherence to antiretroviral therapy
  defined 512
  factors influencing *517*
  interventions to improve 516–518
  measuring 513–515
  and resistance, relationship 512–513
  risk factors for poor adherence 515–516
  sufficiency? 512
adult antiretroviral therapy
  efficacy, monitoring 470–471
  goals 465
  safety monitoring 471
  salvage therapy 471–472
  when to start 465–470
adults with HIV infection
  clinical assessment 189–197
  contraception 280–284
  diet and nutrition 224–230
  emergencies, common 198–212
  evaluation of fever 213–217
  primary prophylaxis and immunization 219–222
  sexual assault 285–289
  tuberculosis 232–261
adverse drug reactions, managing
  dysglycaemia 540–541
  dyslipidaemia 537–538
  gynaecomastia 541
  haematological toxicity 531–532
  hepatitis in patients on ART and TB therapy 534–535
  hepatoxicity 532–534
  hyperlactataemia 536–537
  hypersensitivity 539–540
  lipodystrophy 538
  nephrotoxicity 540
  neurophychiatric toxicity 540
  pancreatitis 541
altered mental states, aggressive or agitated behaviour 208–211
anaemia
  aetiology, tests for 304
  of chronic disease 304
  infections 305
  leucopenia 308
  lymphopenia 308
  management 307–308
  myelosyppression 306
  neutropenia 308
  nutritional deficiency 227, 304–305
  red cell destruction 306–307
analgesics and local anaesthetics 212
anorexia 226
antenatal HIV seroprevalence, trends 4–6
antibody responses during HIV-1 infection 28
antigens 24–26
antimicrobial resistance of STD pathogens 262
antiretroviral and immune restorative therapy 34–35
antiretroviral drug classes
  combination antiretroviral regimen, constructing 463–464
  HIV replication cycle *459*
  integrase inhibitors 462–463
  non-nucleoside reverse transcriptase inhibitors 460, *461*
  nucleoside reverse transcriptase inhibitors 460, *461*
  protease inhibitors 462
antiretroviral drug management
  adherence to antiretroviral therapy 512–519
  adult antiretroviral therapy 465–473
  antiretroviral drug classes 459–464
  antiretroviral drug resistance 508–511
  drug-drug interactions 520–525
  mother-to-child transmission, prevention of 498–507
  paediatric antiretroviral therapy 474–496
antiretroviral drug resistance
  assays to detect 511
  induced resistance 508–509
  integrase inhibitors 510
  mechanisms 508
  non-nucleoside reverse transcriptase inhibitors (NNRTIs) 510
  nucleoside reverse transcriptase inhibitors (NRTIs) 509–510
  primary resistance 509
  protease inhibitors (PIs) 510
  specific drug classes, resistance 509–510
antiretroviral drug therapy
  adverse drug reactions, managing 531–541
  immune reconstitution inflammatory syndrome 526–529
  impact 10–11

nutritional effects on children with HIV infection 147
occupational post-exposure prophylaxis 543–549
antiretroviral treatment, and tuberculosis 38–39
antituberculosis therapy, in patients with hepatitis or jaundice 243–244
antituberculous drugs
    adults infected with HIV 239–241
    and antiretroviral therapy 241–242
    breastfeeding mothers 243
    liver failure 243
    pregnant mothers 243
    side-effects 241–242
    specific categories of patients 243–244
ascites, response to 239
assembly, budding and maturation of HIV virus 22
autoimmune responses during HIV infection 33

B
babies, tests for HIV 47
bacterial vaginosis 273–274
Bartholin's gland abscess 277
B-cell abnormalities during HIV infection 32
BCG adverse events in children, suggested diagnostic workup and management 119–120
binding, fusion and virus entry of HIV virus 20
biological factors affecting transmission of HIV 53–54
biomedical interventions for prevention of HIV infection
    barrier methods 88
    cervical barrier methods 88–89
    female condoms 88
    male circumcision 85–89
    microbicides 87–88
    vaccines 86–87
bone marrow examination 309
breastfeeding 121–122, 124–125, 243
    see also expressed breastmilk feeding in hospital
bronchiestasis 328
burnout in healthcare workers
    causes 625
    intervention 626–627
    stages 624–625

C
cardiac failure 203–204
cardiology
    adult cardiology 295
    cardiovascular and ischaemic heart disease 301
    cardiovascular therapy 295
    dilated cardiomyopathy 298–299
    drug interactions with HIV-cardiology 302
    infective endocarditis 300
    myocarditis 300–301
    myocarditis and cardiomyopathy 293
    pericardial disease 296–297

pericardial effusions 294
pulmonary hypertension 294–295, 299
cardiovascular and ischaemic heart disease 301
cardiovascular therapy 295
CD4 cells
    counts 49–50, *61, 62*
    counts, and common HIV-associated disorders of the eye *389*
    loss and viral load , relationship 60
CD4+ T-cells
    abnormalities during HIV infection 31
    depletion and dysfunction during HIV infection, proposed mechanisms 32
CD8+ T-cell abnormalities during HIV infection 31–32
cell types infected by HIV 26–27
cervical cancer 278–279
cervical infection 267
chancroid 270
chest radiography 162, 235–239
childhood vaccination
    BCG adverse events, suggested diagnostic workup and management 119–120
    BCG vaccine in HIV-infected children 110
    conclusions 117
    diphtheria-tetanus-pertussis vaccines 112–113
    Haemophilus influenzae type b (Hib) conjugate vaccine (HicCV) 115
    hepatitis B vaccine 114
    immune responses 109
    immunization schedule 118
    influenza vaccine 116
    measles vaccine 113
    mumps and rubella vaccines 114
    normal reaction vs BCG adverse event 111
    other vaccines 116–117
    polio vaccine 112
    rotavirus vaccine 114
    Streptococcus pneumoniae vaccination 115–116
    systemic or disseminated disease 111–112
    vaccine safety 110
    vaccine schedule 109
    varicella vaccine 114
children with HIV infection
    clinical assessment (paediatric) 95–107
    clinics, setting up 178–185
    nutrition 145–151
    paediatric tuberculosis 160–168
    pharmacological preparations for nutrition 150
    sexual abuse 174–177
chronic HIV infection in adults 57–58
chronic lung disease 327–328
chronic non-infectious (respiratory) diseases 328–329
classification of HIV infections, in children 98–101
clinical assessment of adults with HIV infection
    assessment 194

examination 192–194
follow-up visits 194–195
history taking 189–191
initial investigations 195–196
Karnofsky score 197
clinical assessment of children
classification 98–101
diagnosis 102–103
epidemiology 95
hidden effects, of HIV 101–102
HIV exposed uninfected infants and children 103–104
natural history and prognosis 95–96
pathogenesis, difference between children and adults 96
transmission modes 96–98
clinical features of TB infection in HIV 36–37
clinics for children with HIV/AIDS, setting up 178–179
apparatus 184
data capturing 184–185
drug supply 184
laboratory support 184
nature of HIV clinic 178–181
paediatric services, practical issues 181–183
public-private partnerships, value of 184–185
quality of care, supporting 181
space 183
staff requirements 183
colitis, in children with HIV infection 155
commercial pasteurization of expressed breastmilk 135
community-acquired pneumonia 199–200
condom use, and SDI management 264
contraception
contraceptive choices in the era of HIV *283*
counselling 281
drug interactions with hormonal contraceptives 282–284
emergency 281–282
introduction 280
non-nucleoside reverse transcriptase inhibitors (NNRTIs) 282
nucleoside reverse transcriptase inhibitors (NRTIs) 282
Protease inhibitors (PIs) 284
Rifampicin, interactions 282
counselling
aims 69–70
contraception 281
ethical issues, post-test counselling 611–612
further options 76–77
gay patients 604
for the healthcare worker 77
HIV testing 70
issues that may arise 71, 75–76
mother-to-child transmission, risk reduction 500–501
necessity of 69
negative result 72, 78
positive result 73–74, 78

post-test 71–76, 78, 611–612
pre-test 70–71, 78
sexually transmitted infections 263–264
counselling lines for sexual assault 289
couple counselling 76
crisis situations 75
crystalluria 315
culturing, as HIV test 45

D

data capturing, in clinics for children with HIV/AIDS 184–185
dehydration 203
denial 76
dermatology
bacillary angiomatosis 431–432
bacterial infections 435–436
blisters, erosions, or crusts 435–439
blue nails 440
crusted ('Norwegian') scabies 429
cutaneous drug reactions, common 442
drug hypersensitivity syndrome 429–430
drug reaction erosions and blisters 438–439
drug reaction lesions 435
dry skin or ichthyosis 429
ecthyma 439
folliculitis 433–434
fungal infection (tinea) 427–428
hair changes 441
herpes simplex 437–438, 439–440
itchy bump disease 432
itchy papules 432–434
Kaposi's sarcoma 434–435
moluscum contagiousum 430–431
moluscum-like papules due to other organisms 431
nail abnormalities 440–441
nodulo-ulcerative syphilis 440
non-itchy papules and nodules 430–432
photosensitive dermatosis 428–429
pigmentation, changes in 440
pre-existing dermatosis, worsening 428
puritic papular eruption of HIV 432
purple-brown skin lesions 434–435
scabies 433
scaly rashes 426–430
seborrhoeic eczema/dermatitis 426–427
skin and mucosal ulcers 439–440
skin nodules 432
varicella-zoster virus 436–437
warts 431
white discolouration of the nails 440–441
yeast infections 438
destructive pneumonia 328
developmental milestones from six months to six years of life 378–379
diagnosis of HIV infection, in children 102–103
diagnostic tests for HIV 42–45
diarrhoea
antiretroviral-induced 405
chronic 582–583

and dehydration 206–207
emergencies of adults with HIV infection 206–207
HIV-infected patients 402–406
and malnutrition 226
palliative care in adults 590
diarrhoea in children with HIV infection
colitis 155
diagnostic approach 153
drugs & dosages for organisms causing *156–157*
examination 153
fermented milk, preparation *156*
general remarks 153–154
history 152
hydration status, evaluation 158–159
invasive investigations 155–156
milk ladder *154*
nutritional support 157
opportunistic infections 154–155
stool 154
treatment 156–158
dietary management 149–150
diet & nutrition of adults with HIV infection
energy requirements 227
fat requirements 228
food and medication interactions 227–228
key nutritional messages 228–229
macronutrient requirements 228–229
malnutrition 224–227
micronutrient requirements 227–228
protein requirements 228
symptoms of HIV, practical guidelines for coping *229–230*
dilated cardiomyopathy 298–299
disclosure, to HIV-exposed and infected children 107
disease progression profiles 58–60
dislipidaemias 150
doctors and sexually abused children 174–175
drug-drug interactions
anticonvulsants 522–523
complementary medicines 522
drug absorption 521
frequency of 522–524
mechanism 520–522
metabolic interactions 521–522
other interactions between antiretrovirals 524
P-glycoprotein 522
protease inhibitor boosting 524
rimafpicin 523–524
therapeutic drug monitoring 524–525
traditional medicines 522
drug interactions with HIV-cardiology 302
drug resistance tests for HIV 50–52
drug supply to clinics for children with HIV/AIDS 184

E

emergencies of adults with HIV infection
abdominal pain 211
altered mental states, aggressive or agitated behaviour 208–211
analgesics and local anaesthetics, use of 212
diarrhoea and dehydration 206–207
fluids, feeds and medications, providing 211–212
headache, severe 207–208
respiratory distress 198
emergency contraception 281–282
endocrinology & metabolic abnormalities
adrenal insufficiency 351–352
in adults 347–352
in children 346–347
hypothyroidism 351
immune reconstitution Grave's disease 350–351
lipodystrophy, metabolic syndrome & artherogenesis 347–350
metabolic bone disease 352
poor growth and pubertal delay 346–347
sick euthyroid syndrome 351
energy requirements 227
enzyme-linked immunosorbent assay (ELISA) 42
epiglottitis 323
ethical issues
access to treatment 621
children, HIV testing 612
confidentiality 560–561, 612–613
death certificates 620
employment issues 618–620
family members, notifying 614–615
healthcare workers 615–616
insurance issues 617–618
medical certificates 617
notification to authorities 621
occupational injury 620–621
other ethical considerations 622–623
post-test counselling 611–612
pre-test 610
research and HIV 621–622
rights and responsibilities 608–609
sexual partners 613–614
testing for HIV 609
unaccompanied children, testing 612
evaluation of fever in adults with HIV infection
acute presentation 213–214
sub-acute or chronic presentation 214–217
expressed breastmilk feeding in hospital
administering expressed breastmilk 134
containers and labelling 131
contamination, handling to prevent 132
to HIV-exposed VLBW infants 141–143
HIV-positive mothers 132–133
infant exposed to another mother's breastmilk 138–141
mothers who refuse to be tested 133
pasteurization techniques 135–138
pasteurized donor expressed breastmilk (PDEBM) 141–143
storage of expressed breastmilk 133–134

thawing of expressed breastmilk 134
see also breastfeeding
expressed breastmilk, heat-treated 126
extrapulmonary tuberculosis 238, 244–245

F
family counselling 76
fat requirements 228
feeds, providing 211–212
fermented milk, preparation *156*
fever, and malnutrition 226
Flash Heating method for pasteurizing
expressed breastmilk 135–138
fluids, providing 211
food and medication interactions 227–228
food preparation 148
food security and nutrition of children with HIV
infection 146
forensic specimens, in cases of sexual assault 288
formula feeding, safe conditions for 125–126
frequent vomiting 226
fungal infections 221

G
gastroenterology and herpetology
abdominal pain 408
acalculous cholecystitis 411
AIDS cholangiopathy 411–412
antiretroviral-induced diarrhoea 405
aphthous ulcers 401
atypical mycobacteria – *Mycobacterium
avium* complex 406
billiary tree, diseases 411
cytomegalovirus oesophageal ulceration 401
diarrhoea 402–406
drug-induced hepatotoxicity 409–410
endoscopic procedures 405
hepatobiliary disease 408–412
herpes simplex ulcers 401
HIV enteropathy 405
imaging for biliary dilation or gallstones
408–409
liver function tests 408
oesophageal disorders 400–401
opportunistic diseases and the liver 411
perianal disease 412
rehydration 406
Salmonella septicaemia 406
viral hepatitis 410–411
weight loss and the HIV wasting syndrome
407–408
gay sex and sexuality
ability to cope, assessing 605
counselling gay patients for testing 604
education 606
HIV and the gay community 602
issues 602
lesbian sex and safer sexual practices 604
male rape survivors, care of 606
men, risk of HIV infection 603
positive HIV test result, discussing 605

risk assessment 604–605
support systems, assessing 605
general immune responses to HIV 27
genital ulceration 267–268
genital ulcer syndrome *268*
genital warts 276–277
genotype assays 50–51
glomerulonephritidies, other 318
granuloma inguinale (Donovanosis) 271–272
gynaecological problems
abnormal cytology 278–279
abnormal vaginal discharge 273
bacterial vaginosis 273–274
Bartholin's gland abscess 277
cervical cancer 278–279
genital warts 276–277
pelvic inflammatory disease 274–276
vulval conditions, other 277
vulvovaginal candidiasis 274

H
haematology
anaemia 303–308
blood cell production, effects of HIV infection
303
haemophilia 310
haemostasis disorders 310
thrombocytopenia 308–309
haemophilia 310
haemostasis disorders 310
headache, severe 207–208
healthcare workers, counselling 77
hepatitis B 222
hepatitis or jaundice, management of
antituberculosis therapy 243–244
herpes simplex virus (HSV) 268–269
herpetic genital ulcer disease control,
prevention of HIV infection 89
hidden effects of HIV, in children 101–102
hilar and mediastinal adenopathy, radiological
signs 257–261
HIV-associated nephropathy (HIVAN) 316–317
HIV-cardiology, and drug interactions 302
HIV epidemic in South Africa
aetiology 12
antenatal HIV seroprevalence, trends 4–6
antiretroviral therapy, impact 10–11
factors influencing 11–14
future 8–10
local studies of HIV prevalence and incidence
7–8
national HIV prevalence surveys 6–7
sources of data 3–4
transmission 12–14
HIV epidemiology in Africa, lessons for
prevention of HIV infection 84–85
HIV genes, proteins and their function 18
HIV immune complex kidney disease 317–318
HIV-positive mothers, expressed breastmilk
feeding in hospital 132–133
HIV seroconversion syndrome 56–57

HIV testing
counselling 70
referral after testing 74
of sexually abused children 176
HIV transmission
sexual assault, prevention 288–289
and sexually transmitted infections 262
HIV virus
binding, fusion and virus entry 20
cellular receptors and viral tropism 19
life cycle 20–22
structure and function 17–18
tuberculosis, interactions with 36–39
Holder Method for pasteurizing expressed
breastmilk 135
holistic management of renal disease 319–320
holistic patient care
burnout in healthcare workers 624–627
ethical issues 608–623
gay sex and sexuality 602–606
micronutrient and complementary therapies
629–632
palliative care in adults 585–595
palliative care in children 576–585
primary care approach 553–568
tuberculosis and HIV services, integrating
569–575
women's health 596–601
hormonal contraceptives, drug interactions
282–284
human leukocyte antigen (HLA), role in immune
recognition 25
hydration status of children with HIV infection,
evaluation 158–159
hyperlactaemia and lactic acidosis 201–206

I
immune competence, immunotherapies
designed to restore 33–34
immune priming by antigens within lymphoid
tissue 25–26
immune recognition
antigen processing 25
human leukocyte antigen (HLA), role in 25
immune reconstitution inflammatory syndrome
(IRIS)
categories 527
children 528
diagnosis and management 529
other manifestations 529
paediatric antiretroviral therapy 486
paediatric tuberculosis 165
paradoxical cryptococcal IRIS 528–529
proposed IRIS case definition 526
immune restorative and antiretroviral therapy
34–35
immune system
antigen processing and immune recognition
25
antigens and receptors 24
described 23–24

and HIV infection 26–33
human leukocyte antigen (HLA), role in
immune recognition 25
immune priming by antigens within
lymphoid tissue 25–26
treatment options 33–35
immunization 221
immunopathological mechanisms in TB/HIV
coinfection 37–38
immunopathology of HIV 30–33
immunotherapies designed to restore immune
competence 33–34
infant exposed to another mother's breastmilk
138–141
infant feeding
alternatives to breastfeeding 125
avoidance of breastfeeding 127
breastfeeding 121–122, 124–125
contraindications to breastfeeding 127
expressed breastmilk, heat-treated 126
formula feeding, safe conditions for 125–126
mother on lifelong ART treatment 124
nevirapine prophylaxis and exclusive
breastfeeding 124–125
South African guidelines 123–124
stopping breastfeeding 125, 127
WHO guidelines 122
infections, HIV and opportunistic, treatment 147
infective endocarditis 300
influenza vaccine 222
inguinal bubo 271
integration, of HIV virus 20–21
intensive care management
adults 343
antiretroviral therapy in the ICU 344
children 342–343
respiratory failure 343–344
sepsis, severe 344
ventilation in newborn and older children
342–343
interferon-gamma Release Assays (IGRAs)
161–162
intermediate progressors 58–59
ischaemic and cardiovascular heart disease 301
isoniazid preventive treatment [IPT] 163

J
jaundice, and treatment of tuberculosis in adults
infected with HIV 243–244

K
Karnofsky score 197

L
laboratory diagnosis
of MDR-TB 246
of tuberculosis in adults 233–234
lactic acidosis and hyperlactaemia 201–206
laryngotracheobronchitis 323
leucopenia 308
lipodistrophy syndrome 150

liver failure and antituberculous drugs 243
local anaesthetics and analgesics, use of 212
local studies of HIV prevalence and incidence 7–8
long-term non-progressors 58–60
lower respiratory tract infections 323–325
lymphocytic interstitial pneumonias (LIP) 329
lymphogranuloma venereum (LGV) 271
lymphoid tissue, role during HIV-1 infection 29
lymphopenia 308
lymphoid tissue destruction during HIV infection 30–31

M
malaria prophylaxis 221
malignancy, pulmonary 329
mediastinal & hilar adenopathy, radiological signs 257–261
medication for HIV-exposed and infected children 106–107
medications, providing to adults with HIV infection, in emergencies 211–212
micronutrient and complementary therapies
    echinacea 631
    garlic 631
    herbal medicines 631–632
    phytosterols 631
    St John's Wort 632
    Sutherlandia frutescens 632
    vitamin and other dietary supplements 629–631
molecular biology of HIV
    cellular receptors and viral tropism 19
    classification 16–17
    virus life cycle 20–22
    virus structure and function 17–18
monitoring tests for HIV 47–50
monocytes/macrophanges, role during HIV-1 infection 30
mothers who refuse to be tested, expressed breastmilk feeding in hospital 133
mother-to-child transmission, prevention
    antiretroviral prophylaxis 505
    antiretroviral treatment in pregnancy 502–504
    child mortality rates 498
    contraception 506
    family planning 506
    HIV infected women, management in pregnancy 499–500
    intrapartum care 501
    laboratory tests 500
    opportunistic infections (OIs), prophylaxis 502
    paediatric antiretroviral therapy 498–507
    postpartum care 501
    postpartum care of HIV-exposed neonates 506
    risk reduction counselling 500–501
    statistics 498
    WHO four-pronged approach 498
    see also prevention of HIV infection

multi-drug resistant tuberculosis 245–248
myelosyppression 306

N
national HIV prevalence surveys 6–7
nausea and frequent vomiting 226
negative result, counselling 72, 78
nephrology (kidney disease)
    assessment 311–313
    direct renal involvement 316–318
    holistic management 319–320
    indirect renal involvement 314–315
neurodevelopmental disorders in children and infants 374–375
neurodevelopmental screen for first six months 376–377
neurological diseases in adults
    acute disseminated encephalomyelitis (ADEM) 370
    Bell's palsy 372
    cryptococcal meningitis 360–362
    dementia, HIV-associated 364–366
    encephalitis and viral meningitis 364
    HIV-associated dementia 364–366
    HIV-related neuropathy 371–372
    inflammatory demyelinating polyneuropathy 371
    intercranial mass lesions on CTR or MRI scan 367, 380
    meningitis 359–360
    meningovacsular syphilis 363–364
    myopathy 372–373
    pheumococcal meningitis 364
    polyradiculopathy 372
    primary CNS lymphoma 369
    progressive multifocal leukoencephalopathy (PMLE) 369–370
    radiculopathy and neuropathy 371–372
    seizures 366
    single lesion on CT scan 368–369
    spinal cord involvement 370–371
    stroke 366–367
    toxoplasma encephalitis 368
    tuberculour meningitis 362–363
    vacuolar myelopathies 371
    viral meningitis and encephalitis 364
neurological diseases in children
    cryptococcal meningitis 356–357
    HIV encepalopathy 354–355
    HIV myelopathy 358–359
    immune reconstitution inflammatory syndrome (IRIS) 355
    seizures 359
    stroke 358
    tuberculous meningitis 356
neutropenia 308
nevirapine prophylaxis and exclusive breastfeeding 124–125
non-nucleoside reverse transcriptase inhibitors (NNRTIs) 282
non-specific interstitial pneumonitis 328–329

normal chest radiograph, response to 238–239
nutritional deficiency anaemia 304–305
nutritional support 148–149
    diarrhoea in children with HIV infection 157
nutrition of children with HIV infection
    acute severe malnutrition 150
    antiretroviral therapy, nutritional effects 147
    dietary management 149–150
    dislipidaemias 150
    food preparation 148
    and food security 146
    growth, disturbed or failed 145–146
    infections, HIV and opportunistic, treatment
      147
    lipodistrophy syndrome 150
    megesterol acetate 150
    nutritional support 148–149
    nutritional value of meals, improving 148–149
    pharmacological preparations 150
    wasting syndrome 146

O

oncology
    common malignancies 443
    Kaposi's sarcoma 443–446
    lymphoid neoplasms 446–447
    secondary neoplasms 446–447
ongoing counselling after an HIV-positive
    result 74
ophthalmology
    abnormal appearance on inspection 390–392
    abnormal appearance on ophthalmoscopy
      393
    abnormal eye movements 399
    CD4 counts and common HIV-associated
      disorders of the eye *389*
    conjunctival neoplasia 391–392
    cytomegalovirus retinitis (CMV) 394–396
    herpes zoster ophthalmicus (HZO) 390–391
    herpes zoster retinitis 396–398
    Kaposi's sarcoma of the eyelid and
      conjunctiva 391–392
    microangiopathy 393
    molluscum contagiosum 392
    ophtalmic manifestations in developed and
      developing world, compared *389*
    optic disc swelling 393
    painful red eye 394, *395*
    painless visual loss 394–398
    proptosis 392
    syphilis 398
    toxoplasmosis 398
opportunistic infections, diarrhoea in children
    with HIV infection 154–155
oral medicine
    adult 417–420
    children 413–417
    gingival and periodontal lesions 416, 423–424
    herpes simplex virus infections 414–415
    Kaposi's sarcoma 422
    molluscum contagiosum 417

    Non-Hodgkin's lymphoma 422–423
    oral candidiasis 413–414, 418–420
    oral hairy leukoplakia 421–422
    oral ulceration 420–423
    paediatric 413–417
    parotid enlargement 417
    recurrent aphthous ulcers 415–416
    salivary gland diseases 424–425
oral rehydration solution 230
oral thrush 226
otological diseases 322
outpatient care for HIV-exposed and infected
    children
    disclosure 107
    first visits 104–105
    medication 106–107
    regular outpatient visits 104–105
    second visits 104–105

P

p24 antigen 45
paediatric antiretroviral therapy
    abacavir hypersensitivity 488–489
    adherence to therapy, how to promote
      483–484
    adolescents 492–496
    and adult, compared 474
    adverse drug reactions 485–486
    antiretroviral therapy registered in South
      Africa 477–480
    changing 490–491
    class-specific adverse events, particularly
      harmful or life threatening 487–489
    complications 485–486
    dosages 482–483
    dosing 496
    guidelines for starting 475–476
    hepatoxity 487–488
    immune reconstitution inflammatory
      syndrome (IRIS) 486
    lactic acidosis 487
    lipodystrophy/lipoatrophy syndrome 488
    mother-to-child transmission, prevention
      of 498–507
    pubertal staging 494–495
    resistance testing 484
    safe monitoring of therapy 489–490
    treatment, choice of 476–482
    and tuberculosis therapy 491
    when to start 474–475
paediatric tuberculosis *see* tuberculosis in
    children infected with HIV
palliative care in adults
    adjuvant analgesics 589
    anorexia 590
    anxiety 593–594
    carers, caring for 595
    constipation 590
    cough and dyspnoea 589
    defined 585
    delirium and dementia 593

denture care 592
diarrhoea 590
fatigue 594
home-based care 586
hospices 586
incontinence 593
insomnia 593–594
morphine, use of 588
mouth care 592
nausea 590
pain 587–588
physical care 586
pressure care 592–593
pruritus and other skin conditions 590–591
psychological support 594
social support 594
symptom control 587–589
vomiting 590
weakness 594
xerostomia 591–592
palliative care in children
    anorexia 583
    anxiety 583–584
    chronic diarrhoea 582–583
    cough 579
    depression 583–584
    drooling 581
    dyspnoea 580–581
    end of life and palliative care 584–585
    excessive secretions 581
    nausea 582
    pain 577–579
    painful swallowing 582
    predominant symptoms 576
    pruritis and painful skin conditions 584
    QUESTT 577
    symptom control 577
    vomiting 582
    wasting 583
    weakness 583
    WHO pain ladder 578–579
pasteurization techniques for expressed
    breastmilk 135–138
pasteurized donor expressed breastmilk
    (PDEBM) 141–143
pathogenesis of HIV infection, difference
    between children and adults 96
pelvic inflammatory disease 274–276
pericardial disease 296–297
pericardial effusions 294
persistent pneumonia 327
pharmacological preparations for nutrition of
    children with HIV infection 150
pleural effusion, response to 237
pneumococcal vaccine 222
Pneumocytis jirovecii pneumonia (PCP) 323–325
Pneumocytis pneumonia 201
polymerase chain reaction 45
positive result, counselling 73–74, 78
post-exposure prophylaxis (PEP) of recipient
    baby of donated breastmilk 139–141

post-test counselling 71–76, 78
post-traumatic stress disorder 75
pregnancy , safety of antituberculous drugs 243
pre-test counselling 70–71, 78
Pretoria Pasteurization of expressed breastmilk
    135–138
preventative and therapeutic vaccines 34
prevention of HIV infection
    biomedical interventions 85–89
    conclusions 90–91
    herpetic genital ulcer disease control 89
    lessons from HIV epidemiology in Africa
        84–85
    sexual assault 288–289
    sociobehavioral interventions 89–90
    vaccines 34
    women 599
    see also mother-to-child transmission,
        prevention
primary care approach
    antiretroviral waiting lists 557
    burnout, of staff 561
    clinics 555–556, 559–560, 568
    community services 564–567
    confidentiality issues 560–561
    decanting antiretroviral patients to nurse-
        based primary care 562–563
    disclosure 561
    donor organizations 564–567
    equipment for clinics, essential 568
    goals 553–555
    infection control 557
    interpreters 561
    nurse-based primary care 562–563
    patient booking 556–557
    patient referral 557–559
    systematic improvements 563
primary prophylaxis and immunization
    co-trimoxazole 219–220, 223
    fungal infections 221
    hepatitis B 222
    immunization 221
    influenza vaccine 222
    malaria prophylaxis 221
    pneumococcal vaccine 222
    tuberculosis, preventing 220–221
    vaccination for travellers 222
profiles of disease progression 58–60
proposed mechanisms for CD4+ T-cell depletion
    and dysfunction during HIV infection 32
Protease inhibitors (PIs) 284
psychological problems
    anxiety disorders 386
    children's mental health and AIDS 387
    context 381–382
    delirium 384–385
    dememtia, HIV-related 385–386
    depression 382–383
    mania 383
    other psychiatric problems 386
    pregnancy and mental health 386–387

psychoses, HIV-related 383–384
psychosocial treatment and rehabilitation 387–388
suicide 383
public-private partnerships, value of 184–185
pulmonary diseases occurring in HIV infected adults
bronchial carcinoma 337
bronchiolitis obliterans organizing pneumonia 338
chest radiographic patterns & common diagnosis in HIV 340
chronic bronchitis and bronchiectasis 337–338
community-acquired pneumonia 332–335, 341
cytomegalovirus (CMV) 336
fungal infections 335–336
infectious complications 331–335
Kaposi's sarcoma 336–337
neoplastic diseases of the lung 336–337
non-Hodgkin's lymphoma 337
non-specific interstitial pneumonitis 338
Pneumocytis jirovecii pneumonia 333–335
primary pulmonary hypertension 339
smoking 337
spontaneous pneumothorax 338
upper respiratory tract infections 331
pulmonary diseases occurring in HIV infected children
acute respiratory disease 322
bacterial infections 325–326
chronic lung disease 327–328
chronic non-infectious diseases 328–329
fungal infections 327
lower respiratory tract infections 323–325
malignancy 329
table of diseases 330
upper respiratory tract infections 322–323
viral infections 326
pulmonary hypertension 294–295, 299

Q

quality of care, supporting 181

R

radiological signs of mediastinal & hilar adenopathy 257–261
rage reaction 75
rapid progressors 58–59
rapid test devices 44
recurrent pneumonia 327–328
red cell destruction 306–307
regular outpatient visits for HIV-exposed and infected children 104–105
rehydration solution 230
renal failure and antituberculous drugs for adults infected with HIV 243
restoration of immune competence, immunotherapies 33–34
reverse transcription 20

rheumatology
acute HIV 455
arthritis and HIV infection 449–451
athralgia, HIV-associated 448
autoimmune diseases, other 453–454
benign conditions, common 448–449
children 455
diffuse infiltrative lymphocytosis syndrome 452–453
extraglandular features of DILS 453
HIV-associated arthritis 450–451
HIV-associated polymyositis 452
immune reconstitutory inflammatory syndromes (IRIS) 455
muscle disease, HIV-associated 451–452
musculoskeletal complications, other 454
musculoskeletal infections in HIV-positive patients 454
myalgia and fibromyalgia 449
osteoarticular tuberculosis (TB) 454
painful articular syndrome 448–449
psoriatic arthritis 450
pyomyositis 452
reactive arthritis 449
septic arthritis and acute osteomyelitis 454
zidovudine-associated myopathy 452
rhinitis 323
Rifampicin, interactions 282

S

scrotal swelling 266
sedation of aggressive & agitated patients in accordance with Mental Health Care Act 209–211
sepsis, severe 200–201
sex and sexuality
history taking, orientation, terminology and culture 79–80
risk taking 81
special issues 82–83
sexual abuse of children, and HIV infection 174–177
sexual assault
counselling lines 289
critical factors 286–287
evidence collection kit (SAECK) 289
examination of victim 287
forensic specimens 288
history taking 286
HIV transmission, prevention 288–289
investigations 287
medical objectives 286
in South Africa 289
special issues 285–286
treatment of victims 288
sexual assault evidence collection kit (SAECK) 289
sexually transmitted infections
antimicrobial resistance of pathogens 262
chancroid 270
counselling 263–264

genital ulceration 267–268
granuloma inguinale (Donovanosis) 271–272
herpes simplex virus (HSV) 268–269
history taking 263
and HIV transmission 262
inguinal bubo 271
lymphogranuloma venereum (LGV) 271
management 262
scrotal swelling 266
syndromic approach to treatment 262–263
syphilis 269–270
treatment 264–272
urethral discharge syndrome 264–266
vaginal discharge syndrome 266–267
sinusitis 323
slow progressors 58–60
smear-negative and extrapulmonary TB,
   antituberculous drugs in adults infected with
   HIV 244–245
smear-negative pulmonary tuberculosis 235
smear-negative tuberculosis, treatment
   monitoring 244–245
smear-positive pulmonary tuberculosis,
   diagnosis 234
sociobehavioral interventions in the prevention
   of HIV infection 89–90
staff requirements of clinics for children with
   HIV/AIDS 183
steady state viral dynamics 58
support groups 76–77
syphilis 269–270
systemic approach to HIV infection
   cardiology 293–302
   dermatology 426–442
   endocrinology and metabolic abnormalities
      346–352
   gastroenterology and hepatology 400–412
   haematology 303–310
   intensive care management 342–345
   nephrology 311–321
   neurology 354–380
   oncology 443–447
   ophthalmology 389–399
   oral medicine 413–425
   psychiatry 381–388
   pulmonology 322–341
   rheumatology 448–455

T
TB control in HIV prevalence communities 39
T-cell responses during HIV-1 infection 28–29
tests for HIV
   babies 47
   diagnostic 42–45
   drug resistance 50–52
   monitoring 47–50
   window period 45–46
therapeutic and preventative vaccines 34
therapeutic drug monitoring (TDM) 51–52
thrombocytopenia
   bone marrow examination 309

management 309
mechanism of 308–309
thymic dysfunction in HIV infection 32–33
transcription and translation of HIV virus 21
transmission and natural history of HIV
   acute HIV infection following sexual exposure
      54–56
   biological factors affecting transmission
      53–54
   chronic HIV infection in adults 57–58
   clinical progression of HIV disease 63–65
   HIV seroconversion syndrome 56–57
   profiles of disease progression 58–60
   relationship between viral load and CD4 cell
      loss 60
   steady state viral dynamics 58
   virological and immunological evolution
      60–62
   WHO clinical staging 67–68
transmission modes in children 96–98
travellers' vaccination 222
treatment of MDR-TB 245–246
treatment options 33–35
tuberculin skin test 161
tuberculosis
   and antiretroviral treatment 38–39
   clinical features of TB infection in HIV 36–37
   epidemiology 36
   high HIV prevalence communities, control
      in 39
   HIV virus, interactions with 36–39
   immunopathological mechanisms in TB/HIV
      coinfection 37–38
   infection control 249
   izoniazid preventative therapy 249–251
   prevention 220–221
   urological tract 315
tuberculosis and HIV services, integrating
   core services list 569
   infection control procedures 571
   monitoring of patients antituberculosis
      therapy 573–574
   sputum smears 574–575
   TB/HIV healthcare workers, care of 571–572
   TB patients, diagnosis and treatment for HIV
      569–570
   treatment outcomes, recording 574–575
   WHO's DOTS strategy 573
tuberculosis & HIV services, integrating,
   diagnosis, treatment & prevention of TB in
   HIV-infected patients 570–571
tuberculosis in adults infected with HIV,
   diagnosis
   algorithm for TB suspects 254–256
   chest radiography 235–239
   extrapulmonary tuberculosis 238
   laboratory diagnosis of MDR-TB 245–246
   laboratory diagnosis of TB 233–234
   multidrug resistant tuberculosis 245–248
   pleural effusion, response to 237
   pregnancy 243

radiological signs of mediastinal & hilar
adenopathy 257–261
renal failure 243
smear-negative and extrapulmonary TB
244–245
smear-negative pulmonary tuberculosis 235
smear-negative or GXP-negative tuberculosis
235
smear-positive pulmonary tuberculosis 234
symptoms 232–233
tuberculosis in adults infected with HIV,
treatment
antituberculous drugs 239–241
antituberculous drugs in specific categories
of patients 243
antituberculous therapy & antiretroviral
therapy 241–242
ascites, response to 239
breastfeeding mothers 243
hepatitis or jaundice 243–244
holistic care 251
monitoring and adherence 244
multidrug resistant tuberculosis 246–248
tuberculosis in children infected with HIV
chest radiography 162
clinical features 160–161
expectorated sputum 169–170
gastric sputum 170–172
immune reconstitution inflammatory
syndrome (IRIS) 165
interferon-gamma Release Assays (IGRAs)
161–162
microscopy and culture 162
non-tuberculous mycobacteria infection 166
overlapping drug side-effects 165
patient history 160–161
physical examination 161
prognosis 165–166
prophylaxis (isoniazid preventive treatment
[IPT]) 163
special investigations 161–163
sputum samples, procedure for obtaining
169–173
supportive investigations 162
therapeutic trial of antituberculosis treatment
162

treatment 163–165
tuberculin skin test 161
WHO strategy to control tuberculosis 166–168
two-glass urine test 265

U

uninfected infants and children exposed to HIV
103–104
upper airway obstruction 323
upper respiratory tract infections 322–323
urethral discharge syndrome, treatment 264–266
urological tract tuberculosis 315

V

vaccination for travellers 222
vaccines 34, 86–87, 222
    see also childhood vaccination
vaginal discharge, abnormal 273
vaginal discharge syndrome 266–267
viral load 48–49
viral load and CD4 cell loss, relationship 60
virology *see* molecular biology of HIV
visits for HIV-exposed and infected children
104–106
vomiting, frequent 226
vulvovaginal candidiasis 274

W

wasting syndrome 146
weight loss and malnutrition 224–227
Western blot 44
window period 45–46
women's health
    antiretroviral therapy in women 597
    domestic violence 600–601
    epidemiology and transmission of HIV in
        women 596
    gynaecological disease in HIV-infected
        women 597–598
    HIV, impact on women's health care 598–599
    laboratory testing and monitoring 597
    natural history of HIV in women 597
    pregnancy 598
    prevention of HIV infection in women 599
    testing for HIV in women 599–600